FOOD AND NUTRITION BOARD, NATIONAL ACADEMY OF SCIENCES—NATIONAL RESEARCH COUNCIL, RECOMMENDED DAILY DIETARY ALLOWANCES,[a] REVISED 1980

	Age (years)	Weight (kg)	Weight (lb)	Height (cm)	Height (in)	Protein (g)	Fat-Soluble Vitamins			
							Vitamin A (μgRE)[b]	Vitamin D (μg)[c]	Vitamin E (mgα-TE)[d]	Vitamin C (mg)
Infants	0.0–0.5	6	13	60	24	kg × 2.2	420	10	3	35
	0.5–1.0	9	20	71	28	kg × 2.0	400	10	4	35
Children	1–3	13	29	90	35	23	400	10	5	45
	4–6	20	44	112	44	30	500	10	6	45
	7–10	28	62	132	52	34	700	10	7	45
Males	11–14	45	99	157	62	45	1,000	10	8	50
	15–18	66	145	176	69	56	1,000	10	10	60
	19–22	70	154	177	70	56	1,000	7.5	10	60
	23–50	70	154	178	70	56	1,000	5	10	60
	51+	70	154	178	70	56	1,000	5	10	60
Females	11–14	46	101	157	62	46	800	10	8	50
	15–18	55	120	163	64	46	800	10	8	60
	19–22	55	120	163	64	44	800	7.5	8	60
	23–50	55	120	163	64	44	800	5	8	60
	51+	55	120	163	64	44	800	5	8	60
Pregnant						+30	+200	+5	+2	+20
Lactating						+20	+400	+5	+3	+40

[a] The allowances are intended to provide for individual variations among most normal persons as they live in the United States under usual environmental stresses. Diets should be based on a variety of common foods to provide other nutrients for which human requirements have been less well defined. See text for detailed discussions of allowances and of nutrients not tabulated.

[b] Retinol equivalents. 1 retinol equivalent = 1 microgram of retinol or 6 micrograms of β-carotene. See text for calculation of vitamin A activity of diets as retinol equivalents.

[c] As cholecalciferol; 10 micrograms of cholecalciferol = 400 International Units of vitamin D.

[d] αTocopherol equivalents; 1 milligram of d-α-tocopherol = 1 α-TE. See text for variation in allowances and calculation of vitamin E activity of the diet as α-tocopherol equivalents.

[e] 1 NE (niacin equivalent) is equal to 1 milligram of niacin, or 60 milligrams of dietary tryptophan.

[f] Folacin allowances refer to dietary sources as determined by *Lactobacillus casei* assay after treatment with enzymes (conjugases) to make polyglutamyl forms of the vitamin available to the test organism.

Water-Soluble Vitamins						Minerals					
Thia-mine (mg)	Ribo-flavin (mg)	Niacin (mg NE)[e]	Vita-min B$_6$ (mg)	Fola-cin[f] (µg)	Vita-min B$_{12}$ (µg)	Cal-cium (mg)	Phos-phorous (mg)	Mag-nesium (mg)	Iron (mg)	Zinc (mg)	Iodine (µg)
0.3	0.4	6	0.3	30	0.5[g]	360	240	50	10	3	40
0.5	0.6	8	0.6	45	1.5	540	360	70	15	5	50
0.7	0.8	9	0.9	100	2.0	800	800	150	15	10	70
0.9	1.0	11	1.3	200	2.5	800	800	200	10	10	90
1.2	1.4	16	1.6	300	3.0	800	800	250	10	10	120
1.4	1.6	18	1.8	400	3.0	1,200	1,200	350	18	15	150
1.4	1.7	18	2.0	400	3.0	1,200	1,200	400	18	15	150
1.5	1.7	19	2.2	400	3.0	800	800	350	10	15	150
1.4	1.6	18	2.2	400	3.0	800	800	350	10	15	150
1.2	1.4	16	2.2	400	3.0	800	800	350	10	15	150
1.1	1.3	15	1.8	400	3.0	1,200	1,200	300	18	15	150
1.1	1.3	14	2.0	400	3.0	1,200	1,200	300	18	15	150
1.1	1.3	14	2.0	400	3.0	800	800	300	18	15	150
1.0	1.2	13	2.0	400	3.0	800	800	300	18	15	150
1.0	1.2	13	2.0	400	3.0	800	800	300	10	15	150
+0.4	+0.3	+2	+0.6	+400	+1.0	+400	+400	+150	[h]	+5	+25
+0.5	+0.5	+5	+0.5	+100	+1.0	+400	+400	+150	[h]	+10	+50

[g] The recommended dietary allowances for vitamin B$_{12}$ in infants are based on the average concentration of the vitamin in human milk. The allowances after weaning are based on energy intake (as recommended by the American Academy of Pediatrics) and consideration of other factors, such as intestinal absorption; see text.

[h] The increased requirement during pregnancy cannot be met by the iron content of habitual American diets or by the existing iron stores of many women; therefore the use of 30 to 60 milligrams of supplemental iron is recommended. Iron needs during lactation are not substantially different from those of nonpregnant women, but continued supplementation of the mother for 2 to 3 months after parturition is advisable to replenish stores depleted by pregnancy.

Source: From Recommended dietary allowances (9th ed). Washington, D.C.: National Academy of Sciences, 1980, by permission of the Academy.

THE NURSE'S
GUIDE TO
DIET THERAPY

THE NURSE'S GUIDE TO DIET THERAPY

Lois H. Bodinski, R.N., M.Ed.
Professor and Department Chairman
Associate Degree Nursing Program
Dr. William F. Flanagan Campus
Community College of Rhode Island
Lincoln, Rhode Island

In consultation with

Roba Ritt, R.D., M.S.
Consulting Nutritionist
Wilmington, Delaware

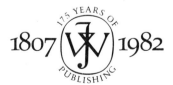

1807 1982

A Wiley Medical Publication
JOHN WILEY & SONS
New York • Chichester • Brisbane • Toronto • Singapore

Cover design: Wanda Lubelska
Production Editor: Rosalind Straley

Library of Congress Cataloging in Publication Data
Bodinski, Lois H.
  The nurse's guide to diet therapy.

  (A Wiley medical publication)
  Includes index.
  1. Diet therapy. 2. Nursing. I. Title. II. Series. [DNLM: 1. Diet therapy—
Nursing. WY 150 B667n]
RM216.B658   615.8′54   82-6954
ISBN 0-471-08167-1   AACR2

Printed in the United States of America

10 9 8 7 6 5 4 3 2 1

TO MY HUSBAND
CHESTER BODINSKI
AND TO THE MEMORY OF MY PARENTS
AMANDA AND RALPH HARDEN

Preface

Dietary aspects are an essential component of total patient care. These aspects must be considered in assessing, planning, implementing, and evaluating nursing care. A wealth of dietary information exists that would be valuable to nurses if it were readily available. Many excellent nutrition and diet therapy books tend to contain more depth and detail than nurses need. Much of the content related to diet therapy is concerned with the disease process, information that nurses usually do not need. Finding practical, concise dietary information is difficult.

This book compiles and organizes dietary information for nurses and presents it in a concise manner. Some background nutritional principles are included; however, the primary purpose of the book is to discuss therapeutic diets for specific disorders. Data were obtained from many reliable sources, and the entire manuscript was reviewed by a qualified nutritionist for nutritional accuracy.

A body system approach to disorders is used. The pathophysiology and treatment of each condition are described to enable nurses to recognize the rationale for diet therapy and its contribution to the total treatment regimen. Other aspects of the disease process are not included because they are considered irrelevant to the purpose of this book.

This book is intended for practicing nurses in hospitals, clinics, nursing homes, and communities. It is designed to be used as a dietary reference when planning nursing care. The nursing implications that follow the discussion of each diet are intended to help nurses care for or teach patients who are receiving therapeutic diets. Nursing students in any type of program can use the book to help them integrate dietary aspects into their nursing care. Community health nurses and nurse practitioners can use the book effectively in counseling their clients. The influences of culture and age on diet are included to help individualize dietary care to specific patient needs. A generic listing of drugs and their relationship to food intake and diet comprises the final chapter. Nurses will be able to find specific diet therapy for a patient's condition, implications for his or her age and culture, and factors to consider if the patient is receiving one of the listed drugs.

Diet therapy is a neglected area in overall health care. This book is intended to increase the nurse's understanding, interest, and support of the dietary regimen.

L.H.B.

Acknowledgments

I express my appreciation to the following people who helped make this book a reality:

To my editors at John Wiley & Sons, Cathy Somer, Linda Turner, and Rosalind Straley, who provided guidance, encouragement, and support.

To Roba Ritt, who served as my nutritional consultant and reviewed the entire manuscript. Her many helpful suggestions and comments were gratefully received.

To Betty McCool and Frank St. Pierre of the Learning Resource Center, Flanagan Campus, Community College of Rhode Island, whose unfailing pleasantness and help aided in locating resource materials.

To Dr. and Mrs. John Harrison, who assisted in researching material for Chapter 10.

To Dr. and Mrs. Peter Schwartz, who provided reference material for Chapters 23 and 24.

To Colette Durand, who painstakingly typed the manuscript. Her skill, interest, and support were greatly appreciated.

To my family, coworkers, and friends, who graciously accepted my altered priorities during the preparation of the manuscript.

L.H.B.

Contents

THE NURSE'S
GUIDE TO
DIET THERAPY

1
The Nurse's Role in Diet Therapy

Diet therapy is only one of the many treatment modalities available to the health team in preventing disease and in maintaining and restoring health. The modification of food intake in the treatment of disease is one of the oldest forms of therapy even though the science of nutrition is relatively young.

The earliest people who cared for the sick had little to offer their patients; they could only try to keep them clean, comfortable, and provided with food to maintain their body's strength to fight disease. From successes in patient care evolved recognition of foods that appealed to sick people and that were likely to be retained by a diseased body. Lacking knowledge about other methods to help their patients, these earliest nurses concentrated on food preparation and administration. This information about diets for invalids was shared and incorporated into medical writings.

Florence Nightingale, the founder of modern nursing, said that "Nursing . . . ought to signify the proper use of fresh air, light, warmth, cleanliness, quiet and the proper selection and administration of diet—all at the least expense of vital power to the patient" (Nightingale, 1859). She included two chapters related to food in her *Notes on Nursing*. Early nursing schools provided instruction in foods for invalids and their preparation. The trained nurses from these schools worked primarily in the homes of the sick and were responsible for the preparation and serving of the patient's diet regardless of the number of servants employed. Before World War II, most nursing schools included in their curriculums courses in nutrition, laboratories in food preparation, classes in diet therapy, and clinical practice in the preparation and serving of special diets.

World War II saw a tremendous change in health care and the public's attitude toward hospitalization. There was a massive increase in knowledge about disease and injury. The public no longer thought of hospitals as places to go to die but, rather, as sources of health restoration. These changes were reflected in an increase in the responsibilities of nurses coupled with a shortage of nurses to meet the demands for hospital staffing. Numerous ancillary services sprang up to meet the increased demand for nursing care, and nurses delegated some of their functions to these new workers. Dietitians had been providing services to patients before the war, but their responsibilities also increased. The hospital dietitians became responsible for all the food served in the hospital and all special diet plans and preparation. They shared with the nurses responsibility for teaching patients about diets.

Concurrently, an explosion occurred in the number of drugs used in the treatment of disease. This explosion started with the discovery of the chemotherapeutic agents, the sulfonamides, before the war, and continued with the discovery of penicillin and the antibiotics. Surgeons who had perfected radical lifesaving operations during the war became more daring in their surgical approaches and offered hope to many previously doomed patients.

Nurses who willingly accepted the administration of the many new miracle drugs and the numerous complex treatments associated with the new surgical procedures turned over even more of their other tasks to the growing number of technicians and aides.

Some of the tasks most willingly relinquished were related to diet therapy. Teaching patients about diets was viewed as a responsibility of the dietitians, whose number in the hospital setting had increased. Preparing patients for meals was delegated to nurse's aides, and serving meals became the responsibility of dietary aides. Recording the patient's dietary intake deteriorated into writing meaningless generalizations in the nurse's notes.

Compared to diet therapy, drug therapy was a direct, dramatic, and definitive attack on disease. Patients tended to favor drugs over diet therapy. It was far less disturbing to their life-style to add a pill or two or even an injection than to alter their food intake. Nurses, impressed with the responses of patients to drug therapy, jealously guarded their right to be completely responsible for the administration of medications. Dietitians continued to prepare special diet plans and to teach patients about them, but rarely were they given more than token support by the rest of the medical team. In clinics, ambulatory care centers, and physicians' offices, mimeographed diets became the chief form of dietary instruction. Patients already disenchanted by the idea of food deprivation quickly sensed the attitude of the health team and felt less bound by the dietitian's recommendations.

Meanwhile, schools of nursing, faced with the massive increase in medical knowledge, began to integrate such courses as nutrition and diet therapy. In many instances, this integration consisted only of reading assignments and vague references to diet included in the discussion of nursing needs. In schools that retained nutrition and diet therapy courses, these courses were taught by nonnursing faculty and lacked reinforcement in the clinical component of the curriculum. Nursing students, like patients, sensed the indifferent attitude of their faculty and coworkers toward diet therapy and concentrated their attention on other aspects of patient care.

Today the medical team has many forms of therapy to offer to patients. In some instances, patients are able to choose the therapeutic regimen that they prefer. The rapid proliferation of new drugs has slowed. Drugs are being studied more carefully, particularly their long-term effects and safety. Awareness of drug interactions with other drugs and with food is increasing. Patients are finding that, although taking medications may not alter their life-style, the side effects of certain drugs very well may.

The public has developed an interest in foods and their role in health. Natural food stores and organically grown vegetables have found an enthusiastic following. Reliable authors in the nutrition field, with few exceptions, did not write for the lay audience. But self-proclaimed nutrition experts have flooded the market with books about food and health. Suggestions in many such books are nutritionally unsound and expensive. What these writers lack in scientific knowledge, they have made up for in missionary zeal.

Research is beginning to uncover some of the relationships between our dietary practices and the causes of disease. Nursing students are seeking more nutritional information as it pertains to themselves and to their patients. Nutritionists are setting up private practices to provide consultation services to the public. The future will provide definitive answers from sound research related to diet and health.

Economic pressures are forcing a reexamination of our food intake in terms of availability and the highest nutrient return for food dollars spent. Federal law requires that labels must provide the following information:

- Serving size
- Number of servings per container
- Calories per serving
- Grams of protein, carbohydrate, and fat per serving
- Percentages of U.S. recommended daily allowances (RDA) for protein, vitamins A and C, thiamine, riboflavin, niacin, calcium, and iron per serving

Competition has forced many manufacturers to provide certain information in addition to what is required by law. This additional information usually pertains to vitamin and mineral contents expressed as percentages of the RDA. Cholesterol, polyunsaturated fat content, and sodium content are included on some labels, whereas others state the procedure for obtaining this information. Consumer advocates have sparked interest in more informative labeling and dating to ensure good quality. Concern for the shopper on a special diet has prompted some food chains to flag dietary products. Color-coded tags identify foods that are Calorie controlled, cholesterol controlled, free of added sodium, and combinations of these categories.

In the future, people will be expected to assume more responsibility for their own health. The prevention of disease and the maintenance of health may finally be given the emphasis that they deserve. Primary nursing, in which one nurse assumes responsibility for a small group of patients throughout their hospital stay, may permit nurses to observe how all aspects of treatment relate to a patient's progress. Continuity of care and observation over an extended period should improve patient teaching in all areas, including diet therapy. Nurse practitioners will assume more responsibility for health maintenance and could easily incorporate nutritional assessment and counseling for clients on normal and therapeutic diets.

The nurse's role in diet therapy has come full circle from complete responsibility through complete neglect to recognition of its role in the total care of the individual. Nutritionists and dietitians are the experts in the field, but they cannot do the job alone. Nurses are in a unique position to assess nutritional status, observe nutritional intake, evaluate response to diet therapy, and support the dietary teaching and regimen ordered for the patient.

Diet therapy is only one of the many forms of treatment available in the prevention and treatment of disease. Diet therapy is not the only answer or, in many situations, the best answer. But in conjunction with other treatment modalities, it may lessen the severity of symptoms, decrease the need for medication, delay the progression of disease, or increase stamina and improve outlook. At the very least, it gives the patients some control over their care.

Our bodies require food for fuel to function, and so food is consumed. Research has identified many nutritional components essential to our survival and health. It is possible that soon we will be able to select foods that will make us feel better and stay healthier.

References

McDaniel, J. M. Diet therapy in nursing school curriculum. *Journal of the American Dietetic Association*, March 1977, *70*, 3.

Nightingale, F. *Notes on nursing*. London: Harrison and Sons, 1859.

2
Principles Underlying Diet Therapy

This chapter presents a simplified and summarized discussion of the principles underlying diet therapy. The reader is referred to the excellent textbooks listed in the references for more complete and in-depth coverage of the subject.

Our bodies require food for the following purposes:

- To provide energy for organ function
- To provide energy for body movement and work
- To maintain body temperature
- To provide materials for enzyme production
- To provide materials for growth, replacement, and repair

The body needs six categories of nutrients to carry out these functions. Nutrients are foods that contain the necessary elements for body function. The six nutrients are:

Water
Carbohydrates
Proteins
Lipids
Vitamins
Minerals

Energy Requirements

Food is ingested, digested, and absorbed for the major purpose of producing energy. The unit used to measure energy is the Calorie, which is also referred to as the kilocalorie and is abbreviated kcal. A Calorie is the amount of heat energy required to raise the temperature of one kilogram of water one degree Celsius. A calorie (lower case *c*) is 1/1000th of a Calorie, also called a gram-calorie.

In metric measure, the energy unit is a joule (J). One kilocalorie equals 4.184 joules, which is usually rounded off to 4.2 joules. Most tables of nutrient composition in the United States continue to use Calorie; however, this value is easily converted to joules by multiplying the caloric value by 4.2.

Energy requirements of people differ and are influenced by many factors. The energy needs of the awake person at rest are expressed as the basal metabolic rate (BMR). The BMR is, in turn, influenced by the person's:

Age
Body size
Body temperature
Physical activity
Environmental temperature
Growth rate
Sex
Nutritional state
Emotional state
Food intake

The total energy needs of any person are the sum total of the factors just listed, reflecting body size and composition; basal needs for cellular activity augmented or reduced by environment, activity, physical and emotional state, and what food is available; and the nutritional status of the body at any given time. If energy requirements are met, people maintain their activity levels without weight change. If more food is ingested than is needed for energy, the person gains weight; if less, the person loses weight. The body meets its energy requirements through the intake of proteins, lipids, carbohydrates, and alcohol. Vitamins and minerals are involved in the release of energy.

Water

Water is the most important nutrient. Our bodies are composed of 60 to 70% water. Our cells function in a fluid medium. Depending on environmental circumstances, we can survive for only a few hours to a few days without fluid.

The water needs of the body are met by the fluids that we drink, by the large fluid component of most solid foods and, to a smaller degree, by the water produced by the body when food is oxidized.

In health, fluid intake from all sources equals fluid output from all sources. An elevated body temperature increases fluid needs, as do many specific disease conditions. Diseases that impair kidney function and reduce urinary output reduce the body's ability to handle the usual fluid intake.

The body's need for fluid is usually signaled by thirst. Thirst is a protective symptom that alerts the conscious person to the need for fluids, and if fluids are available, the person will drink. Thirst is a less reliable guide to the need for fluids in the older, confused person.

Even though water does not provide Calories, it is essential for energy production since no cells can function without it. Most of the activity in digestion and absorption requires that nutrients be in solution.

Carbohydrates

Carbohydrates are nutrients composed of the elements carbon, hydrogen, and oxygen. Carbohydrates account for about 50% of the caloric intake in the usual American diet. The caloric contribution of carbohydrates to the diet tends to increase in poorer families and to decrease in wealthier families. In other parts of the world, carbohydrates may account for as much as 90% of the caloric intake. For the most part, plants are our source of carbohydrates; the only important animal source of carbohydrates is the lactose in milk. Metabolism of carbohydrates provides 4 Calories (17 joules) for every gram digested and absorbed.

Carbohydrates are classified according to their sugar units, or saccharides. A monosaccharide is a simple sugar. It cannot be broken down into any simpler sugar unit. Glucose, galactose, fructose, and mannose are monosaccharides. They have the same chemical formula, $C_6H_{12}O_6$, but the arrangement of the molecules differs.

A disaccharide has two sugar units. It is the result of the combination of two monosaccharides and the loss of one molecule of water:

Monosaccharide	Monosaccharide	Disaccharide	Water

$$C_6H_{12}O_6 \;+\; C_6H_{12}O_6 \;=\; C_{12}H_{22}O_{11} \;+\; H_2O$$

During the digestive process, disaccharides are split into simple sugars for absorption. Sucrose, lactose, and maltose are disaccharides.

Polysaccharides are complex compounds made up of many simple sugar units. Polysaccharides are insoluble in water and are digested with varying degrees of completeness. Glycogen is a polysaccharide and is the body's storage form of carbohydrate. Glycogen is synthesized from glucose in the liver and muscles.

Starch is the plant storage form of carbohydrate and consists of granules surrounded by cellulose walls. Cooking causes these granules to swell and burst the cellulose wall; this action increases the granules' contact with digestive enzymes and increases the degree of digestion.

When starch is digested, it is first broken down into dextrins, then into maltose, and finally into glucose. Dextrin, the intermediate product of starch digestion, is produced in small amounts when bread is toasted or flour browned. Dextrin is also produced commercially and used in baby foods and cereals to make them easier to digest.

There are some polysaccharides that are classified as nondigestible. These polysaccharides include cellulose, hemicellulose, pectin, agar, carrageenan, and lignin. The body does not have enzymes capable of digesting these substances; however, they are useful sources of fiber in the diet. Agar and pectin have the ability to form gels and are used as thickeners. Carrageenan (Irish moss) imparts a smoothness to products and is a useful additive to sauces and ice cream. Lignin is a woody substance that has been used to increase the fiber content of bread.

Carbohydrates are stored to a limited degree in the body as glycogen. Approximately 300 to 350 grams of carbohydrate are stored in the healthy adult body. About 100 grams are stored in the liver; 200 to 250 grams in the muscles of the heart, the skeletal muscles, and the smooth muscles of the body; and 15 grams in the extracellular fluid.

Specific RDAs for carbohydrate are not given; they are part of the energy requirement. At least 50 to 100 grams of carbohydrate are needed daily to prevent ketosis. Carbohydrates are the body's preferred source of energy and are needed for the oxidation of fats. The United States Dietary Goals recommend that 55 to 60% of the caloric intake come from the carbohydrate group (U.S. Senate, 1977).

Carbohydrates digested by the body meet one of three fates: They may be metabolized to meet the body's energy needs; they may be converted to glycogen and stored in the liver or muscles; or they may be converted to fat and stored for future energy needs. The end products of carbohydrate digestion are monosaccharides. The end products of carbohydrate metabolism are carbon dioxide, water, and energy.

Proteins

Proteins are nutrients composed of carbon, hydrogen, oxygen, and nitrogen. In addition, almost all proteins contain some sulfur and phosphorus. Proteins are large-molecular-weight compounds that contain nitrogen; they form colloidal solutions that do not pass through body membranes readily. The most important components of proteins are amino acids. Amino acids are essential for the synthesis of body tissues in growth, maintenance, and repair. Proteins can also be used as energy sources.

Proteins account for approximately 15% of the caloric content of the American diet. As income increases, protein intake tends to increase. Limited income in the United States is reflected in reduced protein intake.

Proteins are classified as simple, conjugated, or derived. A simple protein is one that when hydrolyzed will yield only amino acids or their derivatives. Albumin and globulin are examples of simple proteins.

Conjugated proteins are composed of a simple protein and a nonprotein substance. Mucoproteins and lipoproteins are examples of conjugated proteins.

Derived proteins are formed in the various stages of breakdown of the protein molecule. Proteoses and peptides are derived proteins.

Proteins are also classified according to their nutritional value. A complete protein contains all the essential amino acids in sufficient quantity to maintain nitrogen balance and support growth. A complete protein is also said to have high biologic value. Meat, poultry, fish, milk, and eggs are proteins with high biologic value, or complete proteins.

Incomplete proteins do not have sufficient amounts of the essential amino acids necessary for nitrogen balance and growth. Cereals, legumes, and vegetables are examples of incomplete proteins.

Amino acids are classified as essential or nonessential. An essential amino acid is one that the body is unable to synthesize and therefore must be present in the diet. The essential amino acids are:

Histidine
Isoleucine
Leucine
Lysine
Methionine
Phenylalanine
Threonine
Tryptophan
Valine

The nonessential amino acids can be synthesized in the body in amounts needed for normal function. The nonessential amino acids are needed by the body; however, since they can be manufactured by the body from other amino acids, they are not considered essential to the diet. When the body needs these amino acids, it can synthesize them from components of protein foods. The nonessential amino acids are:

Alanine

Arginine

Aspartic acid

Citrulline

Cysteine

Cystine

Glutamic acid

Glycine

Hydroxyglutamic acid

Hydroxyproline

Norleucine

Proline

Serine

Tyrosine

Protein is the body's only source of dietary nitrogen; protein is 16% nitrogen. Every 6.23 grams of protein ingested provides the body with 1 gram of nitrogen. Nitrogen balance is an important concept in health and disease. When nitrogen intake in the diet equals nitrogen output in the urine, feces, and perspiration, the body is in nitrogen equilibrium, or balance. When the nitrogen intake exceeds the nitrogen output, the body is in positive nitrogen balance. The nitrogen retained in the body is used for body protein synthesis. Examples of positive nitrogen balance are growth, pregnancy, tissue repair, and muscle development. When the nitrogen output exceeds the nitrogen intake, the body is in negative nitrogen balance. More nitrogen is leaving the body than is being taken into the body. Negative nitrogen balance occurs in starvation, infection, kwashiorkor, fever, injury, and prolonged immobilization.

In addition to including essential amino acids, it is important that the diet contain enough carbohydrate for energy so that the protein is spared for growth and repair. Protein in excess of the body's need for growth and repair can be converted to carbohydrate and used as fuel or stored as fat.

Meats, fish, poultry, and dairy products provide the bulk of essential amino acids. Vegetable sources of protein are apt to lack some of the essential amino acids or contain insufficient amounts for the body's needs. Well-planned vegetarian diets provide for combination dishes of cereals and legumes that correct amino acid deficiencies in one another. Amino acid supplementation can also be used to increase the biologic value of foods. The addition of synthetic lysine to wheat is an example of amino acid supplementation.

The end result of protein metabolism is amino acids that can be anabolized into tissues, enzymes, hormones, or fat or catabolized into energy, carbon dioxide, and water.

Proteins yield 4 Calories per gram (17 joules) in addition to the nitrogen and amino acids that they supply in the diet. Recommended daily allowances for protein intake are found in Table 2-1.

Lipids

Lipids are composed of a heterogeneous group of substances that share the common property of insolubility in water but solubility in organic solvents, such as ethanol, ether, benzene, and acetone. Lipids are composed of carbon, hydrogen, and oxygen but in proportions differing from carbohydrates. Lipids account for 35 to 45% of the American diet. Fat intake tends to increase with affluence. *Lipids* is the preferred term for fats because it refers to oils as well as fats. Oils are fluid at room temperature, whereas fats are solid at room temperature.

Lipids are classified as simple, compound, or derived. Simple lipids are esters of glycerol and fatty acids. (An ester is a compound formed from alcohol and fatty acids by the removal of water. Glycerol is a three-carbon alcohol with three hydroxyl groups [OH], each of which can combine with a fatty acid.) Examples of simple lipids are monoglycerides, diglycerides, and triglycerides. A monoglyceride contains one fatty acid, a diglyceride contains two fatty acids, and a triglyceride contains three fatty acids.

Compound lipids are composed of esters of glycerol, fatty acids, and other substances, such as carbohydrate, phosphate, or nitrogen compounds. Examples of compound lipids include phospholipids, lipopro-

TABLE 2-1
RECOMMENDED DAILY ALLOWANCES FOR PROTEIN

Age	Grams per Day
Birth to 6 months	2.2/kg of body weight
6 months to 1 year	2.0/kg of body weight
1–3 years	23
4–6 years	30
7–10 years	34
11–18 years (girls)	46
19–51 + years (women)	44
11–14 years (boys)	45
15–51 + years (boys and men)	56
Pregnant women age requirement	+ 30
Lactating women age requirement	+ 20

Source: Adapted from *Recommended dietary allowances* (9th ed.), 1980, with permission of the National Academy of Sciences, Washington, D.C.

teins, and glycolipids. Derived lipids (fat substances produced from simple and compound lipids by hydrolysis or enzymatic breakdown) include fatty acids, glycerol, sterols, carotenoids, and the fat-soluble vitamins: A, D, E, and K. Examples of derived lipids are cholesterol, steroid hormones, and ergosterol.

Triglycerides account for approximately 98% of the fat in foods and 90% of the fat in the human body. Triglycerides are classified as simple or mixed. A simple triglyceride contains three fatty acids, all of which are the same. A mixed triglyceride contains at least two different fatty acids.

Of increasing interest in the field of medicine is the saturation level of fatty acids in relation to blood levels of cholesterol. A saturated fatty acid contains the maximal number of hydrogen atoms that it can hold. An unsaturated fatty acid can form a bond with another hydrogen atom. A polyunsaturated fatty acid can take up more than one additional hydrogen atom. Unsaturated and polyunsaturated fatty acids have lower melting points and are liquid at room temperature.

Hydrogenation is a process in which hydrogen atoms are added to unsaturated fatty acids to make them more solid and saturated. Saturated fatty acids appear to raise blood levels of cholesterol. Unsaturated fatty acids do not appear to affect blood levels of cholesterol appreciably. Polyunsaturated fatty acids appear to lower blood levels of cholesterol.

Most animal fats are saturated, whereas most vegetable oils and fish contain higher amounts of unsaturated and polyunsaturated fatty acids. Coconut oil, palm oil, and chocolate, although vegetable products, contain larger amounts of saturated than of unsaturated and polyunsaturated fatty acids.

There is one fatty acid that the body is unable to synthesize, so it becomes an essential component in the diet. Linoleic acid is the essential fatty acid. It is a polyunsaturated fatty acid found in safflower, soybean, corn, cottonseed, and peanut oils.

Since fat is insoluble in water, it circulates in the blood in the form of lipoproteins. Of more recent interest to the medical community is the relationship between high-density lipoproteins and heart disease. Two types of lipoproteins have been identified. High-density lipoproteins contain a large proportion of protein, phospholipids, and cholesterol and do not appear to be affected to any great degree by diet or age. Low-density lipoproteins are composed of triglycerides, cholesterol, phospholipids, and protein and appear to be related to diet and age. An inverse relationship has been identified between high levels of high-density lipoproteins in the blood and heart disease.

Fat is the body's form of stored energy. The glycerol portion of fat can be converted to glucose by the process of gluconeogenesis. All the cells of the body, except those of the central nervous system and the red blood cells, can oxidize fatty acids to yield energy. Although the central nervous system cells require glucose for energy, after a period of starvation they can adapt by using amino acids and ketone bodies obtained from fats for their energy needs.

The final products of fat metabolism are fatty acids and glycerol. These products can be anabolized into adipose tissue or catabolized into carbon dioxide, water, and energy.

One gram of fat provides 9 Calories (38 joules). Fats are also sources of the fat-soluble vitamins: A, D, E, and K.

Recommended daily allowances are not listed for fats except in the sense that they contribute to the energy requirement and the requirements for fat-soluble vitamins. Linoleic acid, the essential fatty acid, must be provided by dietary intake.

Vitamins

Vitamins are organic compounds that act as catalysts in the biochemical reactions of the body. Since the body is unable to synthesize these compounds in the required amounts, it must rely on ingested sources. There is probably much more to be learned about the role of vitamins in human physiology.

Vitamins occur naturally in our foods and are affected by processing, storage, and preparation (see Chapter 4). Vitamins are classified according to their solubility as water soluble or fat soluble.

Water-Soluble Vitamins	*Fat-Soluble Vitamins*
Vitamin B complex	Vitamin A
Vitamin B_1 (thiamine)	Vitamin D
Vitamin B_2 (riboflavin)	Vitamin E
Niacin	Vitamin K
Vitamin B_6	
Pantothenic acid	
Biotin	
Folic acid	
Vitamin B_{12}	
Vitamin C (ascorbic acid)	

Water-Soluble Vitamins

VITAMIN B COMPLEX

The B vitamins are usually considered as a group because they tend to be present in the same foods and because a deficiency of one rarely occurs without concurrent deficiencies of some of the others.

Vitamin B$_1$, thiamine, is needed by the body as a component of enzymes; it is important in the breakdown and oxidation of carbohydrates. Deficiency of thiamine results in beriberi (see Table 2-2 for the RDAs for thiamine).

Sources of Thiamine

Pork
Fish
Eggs
Poultry
Dried beans
Whole grains

Vitamin B$_2$, riboflavin, is essential to the metabolism of food and is needed for growth. Sources of riboflavin tend to be low in the usual American diet. Deficiency of riboflavin causes ariboflavinosis (see Table 2-3 for the RDAs for riboflavin).

Sources of Riboflavin

Milk
Whole grains
Green vegetables
Liver

TABLE 2-2
RECOMMENDED DAILY ALLOWANCES FOR THIAMINE

Age	Milligrams per Day
Birth to 6 months	0.3
6 months to 1 year	0.5
1–3 years	0.7
4–6 years	0.9
7–10 years	1.2
11–22 years (girls and women)	1.1
23–51+ years (women)	1.0
11–8 years (boys)	1.4
19–22 years (men)	1.5
23–50 years (men)	1.4
51+ years (men)	1.2
Pregnant women age requirement	+ 0.4
Lactating women age requirement	+ 0.5

Source: Adapted from *Recommended dietary allowances* (9th ed.), 1980, with permission of the National Academy of Sciences, Washington, D.C.

Niacin, nicotinic acid, is essential to protein utilization. The body is able to synthesize niacin from the essential amino acid tryptophan. A deficiency of niacin results in pellagra (see Table 2-4 for the RDAs for niacin).

Sources of Niacin

Meats

Dairy products

Whole-grain cereals

Vitamin B_6, a complex of pyridoxine, pyridoxal, and pyridoxamine, is utilized by the body to metabolize nutrients, to synthesize nonessential amino acids, to convert tryptophan to niacin, and to ensure proper functioning of the blood and central nervous system cells. Deficiencies of vitamin B_6 do not appear to occur when a variety of foodstuffs is ingested, but such deficiencies have been produced in the laboratory. Vitamin B_6 reverses the antiparkinson effect of levodopa (L-dopa; see Table 2-5 for the RDAs for vitamin B_6).

Pantothenic acid is so named because it is found in all living things. It functions in the metabolism of nutrients, the synthesis of cholesterol and steroid hormones, and the functioning of the adrenal cortex. Due to its wide distribution in foods, deficiencies have not been identified nor are they likely to occur. RDAs have not been established.

Biotin also occurs in almost all living things. It is important in the synthesis of fatty acids, the utilization of glucose, the metabolism of protein,

TABLE 2-3
RECOMMENDED DAILY ALLOWANCES FOR RIBOFLAVIN

Age	Milligrams per Day
Birth to 6 months	0.4
6 months to 1 year	0.6
1–3 years	0.8
4–6 years	1.0
7–10 years	1.4
11–22 years (girls and women)	1.3
23–51 + years (women)	1.2
11–14 years (boys)	1.6
15–22 years (boys and men)	1.7
23–50 years (men)	1.6
51 + years (men)	1.4
Pregnant women age requirement	+ 0.3
Lactating women age requirement	+ 0.5

Source: Adapted from *Recommended dietary allowances* (9th ed.), 1980, with permission of the National Academy of Sciences, Washington, D.C.

TABLE 2-4

RECOMMENDED DAILY ALLOWANCES FOR NIACIN

Age	Milligrams[a] per Day
Birth to 6 months	6
6 months to 1 year	8
1–3 years	9
4–6 years	11
7–10 years	16
11–14 years (girls)	15
15–22 years (girls and women)	14
23–51 + years (women)	13
11–18 years (boys)	18
19–22 years (men)	19
23–50 years (men)	18
51 + years (men)	16
Pregnant women age requirement	+ 2
Lactating women age requirement	+ 5

Source: Adapted from Recommended dietary allowances (9th ed.), 1980, with permission of the National Academy of Sciences, Washington, D.C.

[a]Milligrams of niacin equivalents; 1 niacin equivalent is equal to 1 milligram of niacin or 60 milligrams of dietary tryptophan.

and the body's use of vitamin B_{12} and folic acid. A protein substance in raw egg white, avidin, binds biotin to itself and prevents its absorption. Deficiency of biotin has been produced by the ingestion of large quantities of raw egg whites. RDAs have not been established.

Folic acid, folacin, is essential for the metabolism of certain amino acids and the maturation of red blood cells. Deficiency of folic acid causes anemia (see Chapter 7). Recommended daily allowances for folacin are given in Table 2-6.

TABLE 2-5

RECOMMENDED DAILY ALLOWANCES FOR VITAMIN B_6

Age	Milligrams per Day
Birth to 6 months	0.3
6 months to 1 year	0.6
1–3 years	0.9
4–6 years	1.3
7–10 years	1.6
11–14 years	1.8
15–51 + years (girls and women)	2.0
15–18 years (boys)	2.0
19–51 + years (men)	2.2
Pregnant women age requirement	+ 0.6
Lactating women age requirement	+ 0.5

Source: Adapted from Recommended dietary allowances (9th ed.), 1980, with permission of the National Academy of Sciences, Washington, D.C.

TABLE 2-6

RECOMMENDED DAILY ALLOWANCES FOR FOLACIN[a]

Age	Micrograms per Day
Birth to 6 months	30
6 months to 1 year	45
1–3 years	100
4–6 years	200
7–10 years	300
11–51+ years	400
Pregnant women age requirement	+ 400
Lactating women age requirement	+ 100

Source: Adapted from *Recommended dietary allowances* (9th ed.), 1980, with permission of the National Academy of Sciences, Washington, D.C.

[a]The folacin allowance refers to dietary sources.

Sources of Folic Acid

Leafy green vegetables

Liver

Yeast

Vitamin B_{12}, cobalamin, is required in the manufacture of enzymes needed to metabolize foods, nucleic acid, and folic acid. It is also needed for the proper functioning of all cells, particularly those of the bone marrow, gastrointestinal tract, and nervous system. Absence of the intrinsic factor in the gastric secretion prevents the absorption of vitamin B_{12} and results in pernicious anemia. Vitamin B_{12} is referred to as the extrinsic factor (see Chapter 7). Vitamin B_{12} is plentiful in foods of animal origin. Recommended daily allowances for vitamin B_{12} are listed in Table 2-7.

VITAMIN C

Vitamin C, ascorbic acid, is needed for the production of collagen, the integrity of capillary walls, the formation of red blood cells, the metabolism of amino acids, and the reduction of iron salts. A deficiency of vitamin C causes poor wound healing and scurvy. Recommended daily allowances for vitamin C appear in Table 2-8.

Sources of Vitamin C

Citrus fruits

Potatoes

Cabbage

Tomatoes

Broccoli

Strawberries

Cantaloupe

TABLE 2-7
RECOMMENDED DAILY ALLOWANCES FOR VITAMIN B$_{12}$

Age	Micrograms per Day
Birth to 6 months	0.5[a]
6 months to 1 year	1.5
1–3 years	2.0
4–6 years	2.5
7–51 + years	3.0
Pregnant women age requirement	+ 1.0
Lactating women age requirement	+ 1.0

Source: Adapted from *Recommended dietary allowances* (9th ed.), 1980, with permission of the National Academy of Sciences, Washington, D.C.

[a]Based on the average concentration of this vitamin in human milk.

The water solubility of vitamin B complex and vitamin C is a protection against overdosage because any excess is excreted in the urine. However, this property also affects the body's ability to store water-soluble vitamins and results in losses in food preparation (see Chapter 4).

Fat-Soluble Vitamins

VITAMIN A

Vitamin A is needed for growth and maintenance of epithelial tissue, for bone development, and for the maintenance of visual acuity in dim light. A precursor of vitamin A, carotene, is found in yellow and green vegetables. The body can convert carotene into vitamin A. Deficiency of vitamin A causes night blindness, rough, scaly skin, dry mucous membrane with resulting decreased resistance to infection, and faulty bone and tooth development. Excessive amounts of vitamin A cause toxic symptoms (see Chapter 17).

TABLE 2-8
RECOMMENDED DAILY ALLOWANCES FOR VITAMIN C

Age	Milligrams per Day
Birth to 1 year	35
1–10 years	45
11–14 years	50
15–51 + years	60
Pregnant women age requirement	+ 20
Lactating women age requirement	+ 40

Source: Adapted from *Recommended dietary allowances* (9th ed.), 1980, with permission of the National Academy of Sciences, Washington, D.C.

Sources of Vitamin A

Liver
Butter
Cream
Whole milk
Egg yolk
Green and yellow vegetables
Fortified margarine
Fortified skim milk

Recommended daily allowances for vitamin A are found in Table 2-9.

VITAMIN D

Vitamin D is involved in the absorption and utilization of calcium in bone and tooth development. A deficiency of vitamin D causes rickets in children and osteomalacia in adults. Excessive vitamin D results in toxicity (see Chapter 17).

Sources of Vitamin D

Exposure to sunlight (vitamin D synthesized in the skin)
Fortified milk
Fish liver oils
Butter, egg yolk, and liver (contain small amounts of vitamin D)

Recommended daily allowances for vitamin D appear in Table 2-10.

TABLE 2-9
RECOMMENDED DAILY ALLOWANCES FOR VITAMIN A

Age	Micrograms[a] per Day
Birth to 6 months	420
6 months to 3 years	400
4–6 years	500
7–10 years	700
11–51+ (girls and women)	800
11–51+ (boys and men)	1,000
Pregnant women age requirement	+ 200
Lactating women age requirement	+ 400

Source: Adapted from *Recommended dietary allowances* (9th ed.), 1980, with permission of the National Academy of Sciences, Washington, D.C.

[a]Micrograms of retinol equivalents; 1 retinol equivalent is equal to 1 microgram of retinol or 6 micrograms of beta-carotene.

TABLE 2-10
RECOMMENDED DAILY ALLOWANCES FOR VITAMIN D

Age	Micrograms[a] per Day
Birth to 18 years	10
19–22 years	7.5
23–51+ years	5
Pregnant women age requirement	+ 5
Lactating women age requirement	+ 5

Source: Adapted from Recommended dietary allowances (9th ed.), 1980, with permission of the National Academy of Sciences, Washington, D.C.

[a]As cholecalciferol; 10 micrograms is equal to 400 International Units.

VITAMIN E

The specific role of vitamin E in human nutrition is that of a cellular antioxidant. Vitamin E is found in many food sources, so that deficiency is unlikely on a varied diet. In premature infants, however, vitamin E deficiency may result in oxidation of red blood cells in an environment of increased oxygen tension.

Sources of Vitamin E

Vegetable oils
Leafy green vegetables
Milk
Eggs
Meat
Cereal

Recommended daily allowances for vitamin E are given in Table 2-11.

VITAMIN K

Vitamin K is essential for prothrombin formation and therefore for proper blood clotting. It is synthesized by *Escherichia coli* in the large intestine; it also occurs widely in foods. Deficiency of vitamin K, which occurs only in newborn infants, results from the sterility of their intestines or from diseases in which vitamin K absorption is compromised. Excessive intake of vitamin K causes toxicity (see Chapter 17). Recommended daily allowances for vitamin K have not been established.

The fat-soluble vitamins are more stable than the water-soluble vitamins. The body is able to store them. Toxicity can occur, usually a result of excessive vitamin supplementation than of dietary intake. Deficiencies of fat-soluble vitamins occur when fat intake is drastically limited or when fat absorption is reduced or altered. The use of water-miscible forms of fat-soluble vitamins is important in these instances.

TABLE 2-11
RECOMMENDED DAILY ALLOWANCES FOR VITAMIN E

Age	Milligrams[a] per Day
Birth to 6 months	3
6 months to 1 year	4
1–3 years	5
4–6 years	6
7–10 years	7
11–51 + years (girls and women)	8
11–14 years (boys)	8
15–51 + years (boys and men)	10
Pregnant women age requirement	+ 2
Lactating women age requirement	+ 3

Source: Adapted from Recommended dietary allowances (9th ed.), 1980, with permission of the National Academy of Sciences, Washington, D.C.

[a]Alpha-tocopherol equivalents; 1 milligram of d-alpha-tocopherol is equal to 1 alpha-tocopherol equivalent.

Minerals

Minerals are inorganic elements that are needed by the body to act as catalysts in biochemical reactions. Minerals are classified as macrominerals or microminerals, depending on the daily amount needed by the body. Macrominerals are those needed in amounts at or above 100 milligrams per day. Only a few milligrams or a trace of the microminerals is needed daily. Microminerals are also referred to as trace elements.

Macrominerals	*Microminerals*
Calcium	Arsenic
Chloride	Cadmium (possibly)
Magnesium	Chromium
Phosphorus	Cobalt
Potassium	Copper
Sodium	Fluoride
Sulfur	Iodine
	Iron
	Manganese
	Molybdenum
	Nickel
	Selenium
	Silicon
	Tin
	Vanadium
	Zinc

CALCIUM

Calcium is needed by the body for the following functions.

- Formation of bones and teeth
- Contraction of muscle fibers
- Transmission of nerve impulses
- Activation of enzymes
- Permeability of cell membranes
- Coagulation of blood
- Cardiac function

Calcium and phosphorus have a reciprocal relationship in that an increase in the blood level of one causes a decrease in the blood level of the other. A deficiency of calcium in the extracellular fluid can result from:

- Metabolic abnormalities of the parathyroid gland
- Inadequate dietary intake
- Excessive losses, as in diarrhea and wound drainage

Calcium deficiency is often associated with the following conditions:

- Tropical sprue
- Acute pancreatitis
- Hypoparathyroidism
- Massive cellulitis
- Burns
- Peritonitis

The major dietary sources of calcium are milk and milk products. Recommended daily allowances for calcium are given in Table 2-12.

CHLORIDE

Chloride, although a mineral, is more important for its role as an electrolyte in the human body. Most of the body's chloride exists as chloride ions (atoms carrying electrical charges). Chloride is the chief anion (negatively charged ion) in the extracellular fluid. The functions of chloride include:

- Regulation of osmotic pressure
- Component of gastric juice
- Activation of the enzyme amylase in saliva
- Regulation of acid-base balance

TABLE 2-12
RECOMMENDED DAILY ALLOWANCES FOR CALCIUM

Age	Milligrams per Day
Birth to 6 months	360
6 months to 1 year	540
1–10 years	800
11–18 years	1,200
19–51 + years	800
Pregnant women age requirement	+ 400
Lactating women age requirement	+ 400

Source: Adapted from *Recommended dietary allowances* (9th ed.), 1980, with permission of the National Academy of Sciences, Washington, D.C.

Chloride deficiency is associated with severe vomiting, drainage losses, and diarrhea. Recommended daily allowances have not been determined. The major dietary source of chloride is salt that is added to food in preparation, preservation, and processing and as seasoning.

MAGNESIUM

Magnesium is another mineral whose role as an electrolyte has been emphasized. It ranks second to potassium as the most important cation (positively charged ion) within the cells. Functions of magnesium include its role in activating enzyme systems related to the:

- Functioning of B vitamins
- Utilization of potassium, calcium, and protein
- Maintenance of electrical activity in nerves and muscles

Magnesium and calcium appear to share a control system in which renal reabsorption of magnesium varies inversely with renal reabsorption of calcium.

Magnesium deficiency is seen in the following disease states:

- Chronic alcoholism
- Severe renal disease
- Toxemia of pregnancy
- Cirrhosis of the liver

Magnesium deficiency can also occur with the use of some diuretics, the loss of gastrointestinal secretions, and the sustained use of magnesium-free intravenous solutions.

Sources of Magnesium

Whole grains
Fish
Nuts
Legumes

Recommended daily allowances for magnesium appear in Table 2-13.

PHOSPHORUS

Phosphorus, along with calcium, is a major component of bones and teeth. As an electrolyte, it is the chief intracellular anion. Phosphorus functions in:

- Activation of B vitamins
- Transferral of energy within cells
- Promotion of normal nerve and muscle action
- Carbohydrate metabolism
- Regulation of acid-base balance
- Cell division
- Transmission of hereditary traits

Phosphorus deficiency rarely occurs because this mineral is widely distributed in foods. Phosphorus excess may occur in renal failure.

TABLE 2-13
RECOMMENDED DAILY ALLOWANCE FOR MAGNESIUM

Age	Milligrams per Day
Birth to 6 months	50
6 months to 1 year	70
1–3 years	150
4–6 years	200
7–10 years	250
11–14 years (boys)	350
15–18 years (boys)	400
19–51+ (men)	350
11–51+ (girls and women)	300
Pregnant and lactating women age requirement	+ 150

Source: Adapted from *Recommended dietary allowances* (9th ed.), 1980, with permission of the National Academy of Sciences, Washington, D.C.

Sources of Phosphorus

Pork
Beef
Dried peas and beans

Recommended daily allowances for phosphorus are listed in Table 2-14.

POTASSIUM

Potassium is the chief intracellular cation. Its functions include:

• Maintenance of intracellular osmotic pressure
• Participation in intracellular enzyme reactions
• Participation in the conversion of glucose to glycogen
• Transmission of nerve impulses
• Contraction of muscle fibers
• Transmission of electrical impulses within the heart

Potassium deficiency is associated with the loss of gastrointestinal secretions, therapy with some diuretics and corticosteroid drugs, surgery, trauma, gastrointestinal drainage and suction, vomiting and diarrhea. Potassium excess can occur soon after burns and crushing injuries. However, potassium excess is most often the result of oral or intravenous overdosage of potassium in the correction of electrolyte imbalances.

Sources of Potassium

Apricots
Oranges and orange juice
Bananas
Tomatoes and tomato juice
Potatoes

Although no RDAs have been established, 1 to 3 milliequivalents per kilogram of body weight is thought to be adequate as a daily intake.

SODIUM

Sodium is the chief cation in the extracellular fluid and has important functions within the cell as well. The functions of sodium include:

• Maintenance of osmotic balance within the body compartments
• Maintenance of blood volume

TABLE 2-14

RECOMMENDED DAILY ALLOWANCES FOR PHOSPHORUS

Age	Milligrams per Day
Birth to 6 months	240
6 months to 1 year	360
1–10 years	800
11–18 years	1,200
19–51+ years	800
Pregnant women age requirement	+ 400
Lactating women age requirement	+ 400

Source: Adapted from *Recommended dietary allowances* (9th ed.), 1980, with permission of the National Academy of Sciences, Washington, D.C.

- Participation in intracellular chemical reactions
- Participation in acid-base balance

Sodium deficiency is related to decreased intake or increased loss of sodium or to increased intake or decreased output of water. These situations alter the ratio of sodium to body fluid and upset the osmotic balance. Clinical situations in which sodium deficiency may occur are related to the replacement of body fluid losses by water alone. Sodium excess is associated with excessive intake of sodium or excessive loss of fluid without comparable loss of sodium.

Sources of Sodium

Salt
Salted foods
Ham
Preserved meats
Milk
Meats
Eggs
Carrots
Beets
Celery

Although RDAs have not been established, it is believed that sodium intake in most American diets is more than adequate and probably excessive.

SULFUR

Sulfur is a mineral found chiefly in the amino acids methionine, cysteine, and cystine. It is also a component of the B vitamins thiamine and biotin. Sulfur's functions in the human body include:

- Activation of many oxidation-reduction reactions
- Participation in detoxification of harmful compounds

There is much more to be learned about sulfur's role in human physiology. There are no specific descriptions of deficiency or excess; RDAs have not been established. Dietary sources of sulfur are protein foods that contain the amino acids methionine, cysteine, and cystine. Cheeses, eggs, poultry, and fish contain these amino acids.

COBALT

Cobalt is a component of vitamin B_{12}. This vitamin is the only known nutritional source of this micromineral. Recommended daily allowances have not been established, although 15 micrograms per day has been suggested as an adequate amount. Organ meats are the best dietary sources of cobalt.

COPPER

Copper is found in various proteins and is essential to hemoglobin formation (see Chapter 7). Copper participates in the formation and activity of some enzymes, its most important function being a cofactor in the synthesis of phospholipids. Copper deficiency is associated with protein-Calorie malnutrition, sprue, cystic fibrosis, and kidney disease. Wilson's disease is characterized by low serum levels of copper and deposition of copper in the tissues.

Sources of Copper

Liver
Kidney
Shellfish
Nuts
Raisins

Recommended daily allowances for copper have not been established, although 0.08 milligram per kilogram per day for children and 1.3 to 2 milligrams per kilogram per day for adults appear to be adequate.

IODINE

Iodine is a basic component of the thyroid hormones thyroxine and triio-dothyronine, which are necessary for normal growth and development and for metabolic regulation. Iodine deficiency in the fetal or newborn period can cause cretinism (see Chapter 10). Iodine deficiency in children and adults results in goiter (thyroid enlargement in an attempt to compensate for the lack of iodine). Iodine excess can result in toxic goiter (enlargement of the thyroid gland due to hyperthyroidism).

Sources of Iodine

Iodized salt
Seafood
Food additives
   Dough oxidizers
   Dairy disinfectants
   Coloring agents

Table 2-15 lists the RDAs for iodine.

IRON

Iron is perhaps the best known of the microminerals because of its essential role in hemoglobin formation. Iron is also found in myoglobin (the iron-protein complex in muscles responsible for oxygen transport). Iron deficiency anemia is the result of inadequate iron intake (see Chapter 7). Excessive iron intake results in hemosiderosis, a condition in which iron is deposited in the liver and other body tissues.

TABLE 2-15
RECOMMENDED DAILY ALLOWANCES FOR IODINE

Age	Micrograms per Day
Birth to 6 months	40
6 months to 1 year	50
1–3 years	70
4–6 years	90
7–10 years	120
11–51 + years	150
Pregnant women age requirement	+ 25
Lactating women age requirement	+ 50

Source: Adapted from *Recommended dietary allowances* (9th ed.), 1980, with permission of the National Academy of Sciences, Washington, D.C.

Sources of Iron

Liver
Lean meats
Whole grains
Enriched breads and cereals
(see Chapter 7 for additional sources)

The RDAs for iron appear in Table 2-16.

MANGANESE

Manganese is involved in bone formation, reproduction, and central nervous system function. It is a component of enzyme systems. No instances of deficiency in humans have been reported.

Sources of Manganese

Whole grains
Nuts
Fruits
Vegetables

Although no RDAs have been established, a daily intake of 2.5 to 7 milligrams appears to be adequate.

MOLYBDENUM

Molybdenum is a mineral involved in bone formation, growth, and metabolism. Deficiencies of molybdenum have not been identified in human

TABLE 2-16
RECOMMENDED DAILY ALLOWANCES FOR IRON

Age	Milligrams per Day
Birth to 6 months	10
6 months to 3 years	15
4–10 years	10
11–50 years (girls and women[a])	18
51+ years (women)	10
11–18 years (boys)	18
19–51+ years (men)	10

Source: Adapted from *Recommended dietary allowances* (9th ed.), 1980, with permission of the National Academy of Sciences, Washington, D.C.

[a]Pregnant and lactating women need 30 to 60 milligrams of supplemental iron because the increased requirements of pregnancy and lactation cannot be met by the habitual American diet or by existing iron stores.

beings. Excessive amounts of molybdenum appear to interfere with copper metabolism.

Sources of Molybdenum

Beef liver
Whole-grain cereals
Legumes

Recommended daily allowances for molybdenum have not been established; 150 micrograms has been suggested as the result of research studies.

ZINC

Zinc is a micromineral vital to the formation of enzymes needed in the major aspects of metabolism. Zinc deficiency is associated with extreme undernutrition and impairs wound healing. Zinc deficiency also decreases taste and smell sensations. Zinc excess can result from ingestion of acid foods stored in zinc-lined (galvanized) containers.

Sources of Zinc

Oysters
Liver
Meats
Poultry
Legumes
Nuts

The bioavailability of zinc is greater in animal sources than in vegetable sources. Recommended daily allowances for zinc are listed in Table 2-17.

TABLE 2-17
RECOMMENDED DAILY ALLOWANCES FOR ZINC

Age	Milligrams per Day
Birth to 6 months	3
6 months to 1 year	5
1–10 years	10
11–51+ years	15
Pregnant women age requirement	+ 5
Lactating women age requirement	+ 10

Source: Adapted from *Recommended dietary allowances* (9th ed.), 1980, with permission of the National Academy of Sciences, Washington, D.C.

CHROMIUM

Chromium is needed for proper glucose metabolism and the efficient use of insulin by the body. It is also responsible for the activation of several enzymes. Body stores of chromium decline with age.

Sources of Chromium

Whole grains
Animal proteins (except fish and cheeses)

Refinement of sugar and wheat results in loss of chromium. Enrichment does not replace chromium at the present time. The estimated daily requirement for chromium is 50 to 200 micrograms.

FLUORIDE

Fluoride is the mineral associated with tooth formation and prevention of dental caries. Fluoride has been suggested in conjunction with vitamin D and calcium in the treatment of bone disease. The addition of fluoride to drinking water supplies continues to be controversial in some areas. Fluoride deficiency results in poor dental health. Fluoride excess causes tooth enamel to become mottled, pitted, and discolored. Sources of fluoride include fluoridated drinking water and seafoods. Fluoride is also available in toothpastes, mouthwashes, and tooth gels. Recommended daily allowances have not been established.

SELENIUM

Selenium is an important mineral because it is a component of the enzyme that protects red blood cells against destruction. Selenium can also replace some of the vitamin E needed for antioxidation. Neither deficiency nor excess has been described. Food sources include meats and seafood. Grains vary in their selenium content, depending on the selenium level of the soil in which they are grown.

OTHER MICROMINERALS

Silicon, vanadium, nickel, arsenic, tin and, possibly, cadmium have been found to be necessary in animal studies, and it is believed that they are probably essential for human beings as well.

The expansion of knowledge in the field of minerals is one of the major areas of nutritional research at present.

Digestion

The only nutrients in the diet that the body can use in the form in which they are ingested are simple sugars, water, vitamins, some minerals, and alcohol. All other foods must be altered by digestion into a form suitable for absorption.

Digestion includes the mechanical breakdown of food by chewing, churning, and mixing of the food with fluid and the chemical processes by which nutrients are reduced into their simplest form for absorption. The stimulation of the flow of digestive juices is under hormonal control. An essential component of the chemical breakdown is the enzyme system. Enzymes are proteinlike substances that function as catalysts to increase the speed of a reaction. As catalysts, enzymes do not become part of the products of the reaction. Most enzymes participate in only one type of chemical reaction; some enzymes are able to enter into several reactions on related substances. Enzyme activity is regulated by intestinal pH. Each enzyme functions best at a specific pH and will be inactivated by major variation from this pH. Movement along the gastrointestinal tract results in progressive changes in the pH of gastrointestinal fluids, from the relatively neutral saliva to the highly acid gastric juices to the alkaline pancreatic juice and bile.

The mechanical, chemical, and hormonal activities of digestion are interdependent. Enzyme activity depends on mechanical breakdown of food to increase the surface area exposed for chemical reaction. Interference with the secretion of juices under hormonal control slows the digestive process. The secretions of digestive juices, as well as the motility of the intestinal tract, are regulated by physical, chemical, and hormonal factors and intricately tied into psychologic, emotional, and nervous system changes.

The following review of the digestive process is provided to refresh the nurse's understanding of physiology and to promote the recognition of the connection between pathologic states and the digestive activity in the area of the gastrointestinal tract affected.

Food is taken into the mouth, where it is chewed and mixed with saliva. The chewing process increases the surface area of the food for enzyme activity and also reduces the pieces of food into particles suitable for swallowing. Saliva lubricates the food for ease in swallowing. Ptyalin, an enzyme in saliva, acts on cooked starch and starts its breakdown into maltose. The longer food is chewed, the more starch digestion occurs in the mouth. Action on proteins and fats in the mouth is solely mechanical because there are no enzymes in the mouth to act on these food groups.

From the mouth, the swallowed food is moved along the esophagus by peristalsis. When the food reaches the cardiac sphincter at the entrance to the stomach, its presence causes relaxation of the muscle, permitting food to enter the stomach.

The stomach acts as a reservoir for food. The length of time that food stays in the stomach depends on the type of food, gastric motility, and psychologic factors. Carbohydrate foods leave the stomach quickly, protein foods are held longer, and lipid foods stay in the stomach the longest period. Large amounts of food delay gastric emptying by decreasing motility. The average length of stay for food in the stomach is three hours, with a range of one to seven hours.

In the stomach, the action of ptyalin continues until the falling pH, due to the presence of hydrochloric acid, inactivates the ptyalin. Food is mixed with gastric juice, and the churning action of the stomach promotes further breakdown and mixing of the food. The enzymes pepsin and lipase are present in the gastric juice; for optimal function, they require the acid environment provided by hydrochloric acid. Pepsin begins to act on proteins, breaking them into proteoses and peptones. Lipase splits emulsified fats, such as butter, egg yolk, milk, and cream, into fatty acids and glycerol. Lipase functions best in the alkaline medium but is able to act on emulsified fats when the pH is near neutral.

When the food mass leaves the stomach, it is in the form of the acid, liquefied mass called chyme. Chyme passes through the pyloric sphincter into the duodenum. About four inches below the pylorus, pancreatic juice, bile, and intestinal juice flow into the duodenum to mix with the chyme. Pancreatic juice contains five enzymes: trypsin, chymotrypsin, and carboxypolypepidase, which enter into reactions with proteins; amylase, which acts on starch; and lipase, which acts on emulsified fats.

Intestinal juice contains seven enzymes: two, aminopolypeptidase and dipeptidase, act on proteins; one, lipase, acts on fats; and four, amylase, sucrase, lactase, and maltase, act on carbohydrates.

Bile emulsifies fats to permit their digestion and holds fatty acids in solution to aid in their absorption.

The mechanical action in the small intestine is called peristalsis; reverse peristalsis mixes the juices and chyme. The pH of the partially digested food mass becomes progressively alkaline. The small intestine is the site of most digestion, and the end products of carbohydrate, protein, and lipid digestion are glucose, fructose, galactose, amino acids, fatty acids, and glycerol.

Absorption

Absorption occurs in the small intestine, which is physically structured for that purpose, containing numerous villi that greatly increase the absorptive surface area. Table 2-18 illustrates the site of absorption of the various nutrients. No further absorption occurs after the intestinal contents move into the large intestine, except for the absorption of water.

TABLE 2-18
SITES OF ABSORPTION OF NUTRIENTS

Upper Duodenum	Lower Duodenum	Upper Jejenum	Lower Jejenum	Ileum
	← Glucose →	→		
	← Amino Acids →	→		
	← Fats →	→		
			← Sucrose →	→
			← Lactose →	→
			← Maltose →	→
	← Lumen of the small intestine →			
Cholesterol				
	← Iron			
	← Calcium →	→		
	Vitamin A			
		Vitamin D^a ←	→	→
			Vitamin B$_6$ ←	
Vitamin E				
Vitamin K				
Folic Acid		Minerals		
Riboflavin			Absorbic acid	
Thiamine				Vitamin D^a
				Vitamin B$_{12}$

^{a}Site of absorption controversial.

Elimination

The materials in the large intestine are propelled by peristalsis to the rectum. The longer materials remain in the colon, the more water is absorbed from them. The end products of the digestive process include cellulose and similar substances for which the body has no digestive mechanism, sloughed cells from the intestinal tract, mucus, digestive secretions, water, and microorganisms.

References

Fleck, H. *Introduction to nutrition* (3rd ed.). New York: Macmillan Publishing Company, 1976.

Goodhart, R., & Shils, M. (Eds.). *Modern nutrition in health and disease* (6th ed.). Philadelphia: Lea & Febiger, 1980.

Howard, R., & Herbold, N. *Nutrition in Clinical Care*. New York: McGraw-Hill Book Company, 1978.

Howe, P. *Basic nutrition in health and disease* (6th ed.). Philadelphia: W. B. Saunders Company, 1976.

Krause, M., & Mahan, L. K. *Food, nutrition and diet therapy*. Philadelphia: W. B. Saunders Company, 1979.

Mayer, J. *Health*. New York: D. Van Nostrand Company, 1974.

Mertz, W. Trace elements. *Contemporary Nutrition*, February 1978, *3*, 2.

Mitchell, H., Rynbergen, H., Anderson, L., et al. *Nutrition in health and disease* (16th ed.). Philadelphia: J. B. Lippincott Company, 1976.

Robinson, C., & Lawler, M. *Normal and therapeutic nutrition* (15th ed.). New York: Macmillan Publishing Company, 1977.

United States Senate Select Committee on Nutrition and Human Needs. *Dietary goals for the United States*. Washington, D.C., 1977.

3
Nutritional Assessment

Importance of Individualizing Diet Prescriptions

The cells of the body need food as a source of energy, for metabolic support, for the production of enzymes, and for growth, maintenance, and repair. However, food serves many other functions. Food intake is related both to physiologic processes and to other totally unrelated variables, such as family ties, security, comfort, status, tradition, religion, and culture. A given food preference has its basis in a person's past; the reason may no longer be remembered, although the food remains a favorite. Food aversions may also be linked to the forgotten past but are more apt to remind the person of the unpleasant circumstances associated with the disliked food. Troubled times are apt to prompt a desire for milk or another food of early infancy, when the person felt secure and protected. Foods commonly served to the childhood family unit may be favorites of the adult who remembers childhood as pleasant or may be rejected by the adult who had a traumatic childhood. Adoption of the likes and dislikes of parents by the child may persist into adult life. Ethnic foods may be served proudly or rejected in favor of foods that are identified with a new life-style or environment. People's food preferences and aversions are intricate parts of their total being, and no two patterns of food selection are likely to be the same.

Diet modification that does not take into consideration feelings about food as well as physiologic needs is likely to fail. Diet modification does more than change food intake; it may threaten security, stir memories, symbolize rejection or denial, compete with religious values, jeopardize status, or disrupt social and family equilibrium. It is essential to determine a person's food intake, complete with food likes and dislikes, before attempting any modification of his or her diet. Information about the social and physical environment of meals is also of prime importance.

The old diet should form the basis for the new diet, with food aversions respected and favorites retained when possible. The inclusion of a favorite food, although less than ideal dietarily, often improves compliance. Ruthless elimination of preferred foods in the structuring of an ideal diet may result in total rejection of the dietary plan.

Nutritional Assessment

If nurses are truly committed to health maintenance and promotion, nutritional assessment must be a part of every nurse-patient relationship. Assessment is the first step in the nursing process. The nursing process is a framework that provides a systematic approach to identifying and meeting a patient's needs. The goal of the nursing process is to provide comprehensive care based on a plan that identifies unmet needs, initiates strategies to meet these needs, evaluates the effectiveness of the plan, and revises it accordingly. The nursing process is ongoing, constantly changing to adapt to the dynamic state of the patient's condition. Assessment is the collection and analysis of data. Data may be collected through observation, interviewing, and monitoring by patients.

Food and fluid are basic biologic needs of all human beings. Disease and trauma frequently interfere with people's ability to meet their needs for food and fluids. Nutritional assessment is essential as part of the overall nursing assessment. If the treatment regimen calls for dietary modification, a deeper analysis of a patient's food habits and former meal patterns becomes critical as a basis for the diet prescription.

OBSERVATION

Nurses have been observing patients throughout the history of the profession. Recently, physical assessment has become an activity of some levels of nurses. Physical assessment skills are being included in basic nursing programs and in continuing education courses. Physical assessment includes careful observation of the patient, usually following a body system approach. The examiner is assisted by guidelines that direct attention to common deviations from normal findings.

Improper nutrition affects all body systems, and clues to malnutrition may be overlooked. It is possible to combine the observations that are particularly pertinent to nutritional status into guidelines for physical assessment. Table 3-1 is an example of such a guideline.

Patients in clinical facilities are often exposed to numerous examinations and interviews by various professionals. The nurse should review the recorded data about a patient to determine whether any information being sought is available in the physician's record of the physical examination. Nurses may wish to make their own observations despite similar

TABLE 3-1
PHYSICAL SIGNS INDICATIVE OF NUTRITIONAL STATUS

Body Area	Signs of Good Nutrition	Signs of Poor Nutrition
Hair	Shiny, lustrous; firm, healthy scalp	Dull, dry, brittle, depigmented, easily plucked
Face	Skin color uniform; healthy appearance	Skin dark over cheeks and under eyes, skin flaky, face swollen
Eyes	Bright, clear, moist	Eye membranes pale, dry (xerophthalmia); Bitot's spots; increased vascularity, cornea soft (keratomalacia)
Lips	Good pink color, smooth	Swollen and puffy (cheilosis), angular lesion at corners of mouth (angular fissures)
Tongue	Deep red; surface papillae present	Smooth appearance; swollen, beefy red, sores; atrophic papillae
Teeth	Straight, no crowding, no cavities, bright	Cavities, mottled appearance (fluorosis), malpositioned
Gums	Firm, good pink color	Spongy, bleed easily, marginal redness, recession
Glands	No enlargement of the thyroid	Thyroid enlargement (simple goiter)
Skin	Smooth, good color, moist	Rough, dry, flaky, swollen, pale, pigmented; lack of fat under skin
Nails	Firm, pink	Spoon shaped, ridged
Skeleton	Good posture, no malformation	Poor posture, beading of ribs, bowed legs or knock knees
Muscles	Well developed, firm	Flaccid, poor tone, wasted, underdeveloped
Limbs	No tenderness	Weak and tender; presence of edema
Abdomen	Flat	Swollen
Nervous system	Normal reflexes	Decrease in or loss of ankle and knee reflexes

Source: Brunner, L., & Suddarth, D. *Textbook of medical-surgical nursing* (4th ed.). Philadelphia: J. B. Lippincott Company, 1980, p. 142, by permission of the publisher.

notations by others. When this is the case, it may be wise for the nurse to mention to the patient that she realizes that the physician has already checked the area and to ask if she may also. Patients often feel that professionals do not communicate with one another and resent reexamination unless the repetition is introduced as an extension or reevaluation of the previous examination.

Anthropometric measurements that help identify nutritional problems include height, weight, mid-upper arm circumference, and triceps skin fold measurements. In most clinical facilities, admission weights are recorded routinely only for patients from the medical service. Heights are rarely recorded for adults. It is important in nutritional care in the hospital setting that all ambulatory patients be weighed and measured on admission. Bed scales should be used for nonambulatory patients if this activity does not jeopardize their condition or plan of care. For patients who cannot be weighed and measured, information about height and weight should be obtained from them or their families. General observations about body weight can also be made on the basis of overall appearance. Loose skin folds, temporal hollowing, sunken eyes, and wasted muscles are common clues.

Information about the state of skeletal muscle mass is obtained by measuring the mid-upper arm circumference and comparing the results to normal values. The triceps skin fold measured by special calipers and compared to a table of normal values provides information about the amount of subcutaneous fat.

Laboratory tests useful in nutritional assessment include a complete blood count, serum levels of albumin and transferrin, and urinary levels of sodium, potassium, urea nitrogen, and creatinine. The blood count may reveal leukopenia or anemia reflected in depressed white and red blood cell counts. Hemoglobin and hematocrit values give information about hydration and anemia. The serum levels of albumin and transferrin are helpful in diagnosing protein-Calorie malnutrition (PCM). Reduced serum levels of albumin and transferrin reflect a visceral protein deficit in adults. In catabolic states, protein is rapidly depleted. Transferrin, an iron-carrying protein in the blood, is rapidly lost in acute illnesses.

Urinary values are also helpful in assessing nutritional problems. Twenty-four or 48-hour urine specimens are usually collected. Urinary levels of sodium and potassium give information about renal function and the body's response to intravenous electrolyte therapy. The urea nitrogen level is related to the utilization of exogenous protein and to the rate of anabolism or catabolism as it affects nitrogen balance. Creatinine is another by-product of protein metabolism that is used in conjunction with height as an indicator of the gain or loss of lean tissue mass.

Laboratory test results provide early clues to nutritional deficiencies. Nurses who suspect nutritional problems in their patients can find relevant information to confirm or disprove their suspicions in the results of laboratory tests and in the results of other diagnostic procedures. They should also take into account the patient's diagnosis and other influences on the laboratory test results.

In addition to noting physical examination and laboratory results, nurses should be alert to high-risk patients. Some people, because of their nutritional status at the time of the disease or injury, are particularly jeopardized by nutritional problems that may affect the outcome of the disease process.

Both overweight and underweight patients are at risk. Usually a 20% deviation from ideal body weight is required for a patient to be considered at high risk. Both gross increases and gross decreases in weight may be associated with lack of protein reserve.

Any patient with a disease that interferes with the ability to ingest, digest, or absorb adequate nutrients should be considered at risk from a nutritional standpoint. Celiac disease, pancreatic insufficiency, and Crohn's disease are examples of such diseases. Congenital anomalies of the gastrointestinal tract and surgical revisions of the gastrointestinal tract also place patients at risk as a result of interference with ingestion, digestion, or absorption. Another group of patients at risk nutritionally are those maintained more than 10 days on intravenous glucose solutions, saline solutions, or both.

Increased demand for nutrients to meet higher metabolic requirements heightens the risk for infants, pregnant women, and patients with burns, fevers, and infections. Increased losses of body fluids also place patients in a nutritional high-risk category. Patients with draining wounds, abscesses, blood loss, vomiting, or diarrhea are in this category.

The nurse can use the physical examination, the patient's history, the laboratory data, and the diagnosis to identify the potential for problems in meeting the nutritional needs of the patient. Once the nutritional needs of the patient are established, the next step is to formulate a plan to meet those needs.

INTERVIEWING

If the nurse is to provide nutrients that will meet the needs of a patient, she must know which foods are acceptable to the patient. The best diet plan is of no use if the patient is unwilling to follow it.

Some form of food intake survey should be performed for every patient before or soon after admission. If a patient is unable to be interviewed, information should be obtained from family members or others familiar with the patient's eating habits. This information can be part of the nursing history or, when diet modification will be part of long-term nursing goals, a separate and more detailed survey may be used.

The survey should include information relative to the pattern of food intake, the number of meals and snacks eaten during the day, and a typical daily intake. Food allergies, preferences, and aversions should be specifically sought and recorded.

Ideally, a three-day food intake should be obtained. At least one day should reflect weekend intake; the other day or days should reflect weekday intake. It is possible to evaluate three-day intakes against RDAs to screen for possible inadequacies. Recommended daily allowances are intended as a standard of nutritional adequacy for groups of healthy people. These allowances provide generous safety margins to cover individual differences. Recommended daily allowances for protein, carbohydrate, fat, vitamins, and six minerals have been determined.

It is also possible to evaluate intake using the basic four food groups as a criterion. If the intake contains the recommended number of servings from each group, it can be assumed that the diet is adequate in protein, vitamins A and C, thiamine, riboflavin, niacin, and calcium. If the intake is inadequate in any of the four groups, it should be examined for compensatory foods that contribute the same nutrients.

At some point in a patient's hospitalization, it may become crucial to have the patient eat or drink. The patient is much more likely to comply if the nurse offers a favorite food or beverage. It is far better to know what the patient likes to drink and bring it to the bedside than to try to find out from the patient what might be sipped when the patient is really not interested in drinking or even talking. The realization that the nurse cared enough to check for preferences in previously given information might be sufficiently comforting to encourage the patient to drink.

Background information on usual food intake becomes more important when the nurse is dealing with infants and children and with adults who have communication problems. A confused and frightened child may respond to familiar foods or meal patterns based on information from a diet history. An adult who cannot communicate any of his or her needs and concerns will become further frustrated by being served foods that he or she will not or cannot eat due to preference, custom, culture, or religion. Anorexia might often be alleviated if there were a diet history and if it were used to meet the patient's nutritional needs on an individual basis.

Table 3-2 is an example of a diet history. The person conducting the dietary interview should get as much information as possible from the chart before questioning the patient and should refer to previous patient interviews when asking for clarification and amplification.

The diet history can be used as a basis for planning a therapeutic diet based on the patient's present food intake. It can also be used as the starting point in planning a prudent diet and for teaching sound nutritional principles.

TABLE 3-2
DIET HISTORY

Name _____ Date _____

Age _____ Hospital number _____

Family composition _____

Present weight _____ Usual weight _____

Height _____ Recent changes in weight _____

Number of meals per day _____ Number of snacks per day _____

Meals prepared by _____

TABLE 3-2 (Continued)

Appetite _____ Recent changes in appetite _____

Breakfast at _____ AM With _____

Usual breakfast   Serving size

_____   _____
_____   _____
_____   _____
_____   _____
_____   _____

Occasional breakfasts _____

Weekends _____ Holidays _____ Special _____

Eats lunch/dinner at _____ PM With _____

At home _____ At work _____

Usual lunch/dinner   Serving size

_____   _____
_____   _____
_____   _____
_____   _____
_____   _____

Occasional lunches/dinners _____

Weekend _____ Holiday _____ Special _____

Eats supper/dinner at _____ PM With _____

Usual supper/dinner   Serving size

_____   _____
_____   _____
_____   _____
_____   _____
_____   _____

Occasional supper/dinner _____

Weekends _____ Holidays _____ Special _____

Snacks   Time   Serving size

_____   _____   _____
_____   _____   _____
_____   _____   _____
_____   _____   _____

TABLE 3-2 (Continued)

Food preferences	Food allergies	Food aversions	Nonfavored but acceptable foods

List any foods that cause indigestion.

List any foods that cause diarrhea.

List any foods that cause flatulence (gas).

Any difficulty chewing or swallowing?

Dentures?

Usual bowel habits.

History of dietary problems.

History of diseases, surgical procedures, or weight problems.

Physcial activity.

TABLE 3-2 (Continued)

Weekdays ————————————— Weekends —————————————

Vitamin or mineral supplements taken?

Usual method of meat preparation. Bake ——————— Broil ——————— Boil ———————

Fry ———————

Usual method of vegetable preparation ——————————————————————————————

References

Brunner, L., & Suddarth, D. *Textbook of medical-surgical nursing* (4th ed.). Philadelphia: J. B. Lippincott Company, 1980.

Buergel, N. Monitoring nutritional status in the clinical setting. *Nursing Clinics of North America*, 1979, *14*, 2.

Butterworth, C. L., & Blackburn, G. L. Hospital malnutrition and how to assess the nutritional status of the patient. *Nursing Digest*, November/December 1976, *4*, 6.

Caly, J. Assessing adult's nutrition. *American Journal of Nursing*, October 1979, *77*, 10.

Greenburg, J. Why your hospitalized patient won't eat. *Consultant*, September 1979, *19*, 9.

Keithley, J. Proper nutritional assessment can prevent hospital malnutrition. *Nursing '79*, February 1979, *9*, 2.

Krause, M., & Mahan, L. K. *Food, nutrition and diet therapy* (6th ed.). Philadelphia: W. B. Saunders Company, 1979.

Modrow, C. L., & Modrow, R. E. Nutritional concerns in long term care. *Journal of Long Term Care Administration*, Fall 1978, *6*.

Saperstein, A., & Frazier, M. *Introduction to nursing practice*. Philadelphia: F. A. Davis, 1980.

Suitor, C., & Hunter, M. *Nutrition: Principles and application in health promotion*. Philadelphia: J. B. Lippincott Company, 1980.

Watson, J. *Medical-surgical nursing and related physiology* (2nd ed.). Philadelphia: W. B. Saunders Company, 1979.

Wellman, N. The evaluation of nutritional status. In R. Howard & N. Herbold *Nutrition and clinical care*. New York: McGraw-Hill Book Company, 1979.

4

Diet Therapy for High-Level Wellness

High-level wellness is a concept developed by Dr. Halbert Dunn (1959), who thought that there should be a distinction between health and wellness. He defined health as a passive state, an absence of illness, and a state of homeostasis. He perceived wellness as a dynamic state with forward movement toward a higher level of bodily function. Dr. Dunn envisioned high-level wellness and death at opposite ends of a continuum.

Between these poles lay varying degrees of wellness or illness affected by a hostile or supportive environment. Functioning at the highest level of wellness means being in peak physical condition in an optimal, highly supportive environment.

High-level wellness is more than the absence of disease, and the goal of high-level wellness means a great deal more than preventing illness; it means providing the optimal internal and external environments for the achievement of the highest potential of which the person is capable.

Diet therapy contributes to high-level wellness. As our understanding of the essential nutrients and the dietary genesis of some diseases continues to increase, diet therapy will have an even greater role in the future.

Search for the Optimal Diet

With the identification of essential nutrients and the establishment of the approximate amounts of these nutrients required by the body, interest began to focus on formulating a diet that would promote healthful living. One of the earliest dietary recommendations was a well-balanced diet. Since almost every living thing depends on similar amounts of the same chemicals to maintain health, it was reasoned that selecting foods from a wide variety of animal, vegetable, and fish products would ensure the intake of the necessary nutrients in the required amounts.

The well-balanced diet was an excellent idea but was too general to provide direction for meal planning. The concept of the basic seven food groups was introduced to give specific instructions on daily food intake. Every day, foods from each of seven categories were to be included in the diet to provide all the known essential nutrients. The seven food groups were:

Leafy green and yellow vegetables
Citrus fruits, tomatoes, cabbage, and salad greens
Potatoes, vegetables, and fruits
Milk and milk products
Meat, poultry, fish, eggs, and dried beans and peas
Bread, flour, and cereals
Butter or fortified margarine

The basic seven food groups were replaced by the basic four food groups. This system divides food into groups with similar nutrient content and lists amounts for each group based on age and condition. The basic four food groups are:

Meat, fish, poultry, eggs, and dried beans and peas
Milk and milk products
Fruits and vegetables
Grains, bread, and cereals

The recommended selections from these groups include:

Meat group: 2 or more servings daily
Milk group   3 or more glasses for children
             4 or more glasses for adolescents
             2 or more glasses for adults
             4 or more glasses for pregnant and lactating women
Fruits and vegetables: 4 or more services, 1 citrus fruit daily
                       1 green or yellow vegetable every other day
Grains: 4 or more servings

Serving sizes for the basic four food groups include:

Meat group
  2 ounces of lean, cooked meat, fish, or poultry
  2 eggs

    2 ounces of hard cheese

    ½ cup of cottage cheese

    1 cup of cooked dried beans, peas, or lentils

    ½ cup of nuts

    4 tablespoons of peanut butter

Milk group

    1 cup of milk or yogurt

    1 ounce of hard cheese

    ½ cup of ice cream or ice milk

    1 serving of milk-based pudding, soup, or beverage

Fruit and vegetable group

    1 apple, banana, tomato, or potato

    ½ grapefruit or cantaloupe

    ½ cup of cooked fruit or vegetable

    1 cup of raw fruit or vegetable

Grain group

    1 slice of bread

    1 ounce of cereal

    1 roll or muffin

    ½ cup of cooked rice, pasta, or cereal

The basic four food groups in the recommended amounts provide approximately 1,200 kcal. Additional Calories to meet the energy demands may be provided by additional servings of the listed foods and by the foods not included in the basic four food groups. These nonlisted foods, such as butter or margarine, shortening, condiments, sugars, candies, jams, and syrups, provide neglible nutrients in proportion to the Calorie content.

The basic four food group approach to meal planning takes into consideration the RDAs set up by the Food and Nutrition Board of the United States government. Recommended daily allowances are not intended as guidelines for individual food intake but may be used to evaluate food intake in assessing the nutritional value of diets. These allowances were formulated to be estimated amounts of the essential nutrients needed to meet the physiologic needs of healthy people. Recommended daily allowances are set high enough to cover people with the greatest needs and exceed the requirements of most people.

Modern technology has greatly improved the availability of food. Perishable foods can be shipped throughout the world to make most foods available in any season. Modern processing techniques have made available foods that require a minimum of preparation and few cooking skills. Scientific advances have increased the shelf life of foods and have provided protection from food spoilage.

Nonetheless, modern technology, instead of improving our ability to select nutritious foods, has focused its attention on convenience. Convenience foods, while reducing preparation time, rely heavily on additives to improve appearance, taste, texture, and shelf life.

As our standard of living has risen, our food choices have changed. North Americans prefer soft, white, rich foods, and industry caters to these desires. Grains have been bleached and refined to remove the bran and the germ for a finer, whiter product. This process also removes essential nutrients. To compensate for the loss of nutrients in food processing, "enrichment" is used. Enriched foods have some nutrients lost in processing returned to them, but enriched foods are not nutritionally equivalent to their preprocessed, preenriched forms because not all removed nutrients are returned and because the amount of nutrient added may be greater or less than the original product contained.

In response to studies that have demonstrated widespread nutritional deficiencies, the food industry introduced the concept of fortification. Fortified foods have nutrients added to them that were not originally present or, if present, were at considerably lower levels.

Enrichment increases the cost of food—the consumer pays for the refining process and then pays for the enrichment process. The enriched product is more expensive and less nutritional than the unrefined food. Fortification may have advantages in providing essential nutrients in commonly eaten foods to prevent deficiencies, but widespread fortification could result in excessive intake of certain nutrients. A new cereal advertises that 1 ounce of the fortified cereal has 100% of the RDAs for 10 essential vitamins and minerals.

Recent studies have suggested that excessive processing and food additives may be dangerous to health. In addition, specific food intake patterns have been linked to disease processes. Although definitive proof is still lacking, there is increasing support for the prudent diet. Proponents of the prudent diet argue that it can do no harm and probably will improve health.

The prudent diet suggests:

- Increased consumption of fruits, vegetables, and grains
- Reduced consumption of fat and partial replacement of saturated fats with polyunsaturated fats
- Reduced consumption of animal fats
- Reduced intake of cholesterol
- Reduced intake of salt
- Reduced intake of alcohol

Meals can still be planned using the basic four food groups with the following adaptations: In the meat group, increase consumption of fish, chicken, turkey, and veal, and reduce consumption of beef, lamb, and pork. Increase the use of legumes, nuts, and seeds as sources of protein, and limit egg yolks to two to three weekly, including those used in cooking. In the milk group, substitute low-fat and nonfat milk for whole milk, and use low-fat dairy products, such as skim milk cheeses and low-fat yogurt. Increase the total intake of both fruits and vegetables. Select whole-grain products and starches as sources of carbohydrate. The rationale behind some of these suggestions is worth considering more fully.

Fats

Fats now represent a larger portion of our caloric intake than they did in the past. Increased fat intake is related to an increased standard of living. Affluence is generally coupled with a desire to increase the intake of status foods, such as well-marbled beef, buttery sauces, and rich desserts. Along with an increase in fat intake in present-day America, there has been a decrease in the level of activity. High intake of fat in the absence of exercise leads to obesity, which is an important factor in coronary heart disease and hypertension. Hyperlipidemia, an elevation of the serum level of cholesterol and/or triglycerides, has been linked to atherosclerosis and ischemic heart disease. Although definitive proof is lacking, it seems prudent to reduce fat intake because this dietary change can cause no harm and may well be helpful.

Fats can be safely reduced from the approximately 40% of caloric intake that they now comprise to 30%. Not only should total intake of fat be reduced, but the intake of saturated fats should be reduced to about 10% of the caloric intake and replaced in part by polyunsaturated fats to account for at least 10%. The remaining 10% comes from unsaturated fat intake. Polyunsaturated fats have the ability to reduce the serum level of cholesterol. The physiologic implications of limiting intake of cholesterol in an attempt to reduce the serum level of cholesterol are still being debated. Because the body manufactures cholesterol on a feedback basis, some authorities believe that there is no point in limiting cholesterol intake (if dietary cholesterol is reduced the body will produce more). Other authorities recommend limiting intake of cholesterol to 300 milligrams per day as a prudent step that can do no harm because the body will be able to manufacture sufficient cholesterol for its needs.

Meats are a major source of fat. Choice cuts from grain-fed animals tend to contain the largest amount of saturated fat. Substitution of chicken, turkey, fish, and veal for some of the beef, pork, ham, and lamb in the diet is recommended. Removal of the skin from chicken and turkey before eating further reduces fat intake. Turkeys, formerly a holiday meal, are now available year-round. Turkey meat is being processed into cold cuts, and turkey parts are available for small families.

Nonmeat sources of protein can also be used. Macaroni, low-fat cheeses, and meals containing dried beans, peas, and lentils are good sources of protein and are lower in fat and less expensive than most meats. Sesame seed, soybean, cottonseed, corn, safflower, and sunflower oils are good sources of polyunsaturated fats. The liquid forms of these oils, tub margarines, contain more polyunsaturated fats. Hydrogenation, the process that hardens these fats into stick margarines, saturates some of the fatty acids.

In general, vegetable oils contain higher percentages of polyunsaturated fatty acids than of animal fats; however, there are important exceptions. The consumer must read beyond "all vegetable oil" on the label to be sure that the product is high in polyunsaturated oils. Palm oil and coconut oil, although of vegetable origin, are highly saturated fats. Palm oil and coconut oil are used in nondairy creamers and whipped toppings as well as in bakery products and other products that claim to use only vegetable oil. Peanut oil and olive oil are unsaturated oils that are believed to reduce serum levels of cholesterol minimally.

Food preparation methods can be an important influence on fat intake. Meats should be well trimmed, with all visible fat removed before cooking. Broiling, roasting, or baking permits more fat to cook out of meat. The use of a rack to allow the fat to drip away from the meat during cooking promotes the removal of all the cooked-out fat. Gravies made from pan drippings should be avoided. Soups and stews can be prepared in advance and refrigerated. The hardened fat can then be easily skimmed from the top before reheating and serving. Vegetables should be seasoned with herbs in preference to rich sauces or butter. Water-packed tuna in place of tuna packed in oil would further reduce intake of fat. Deep-fat frying should be avoided, and frying of any kind should be limited in an attempt to avoid adding fat to the diet.

Low-fat milk and skim milk should replace whole milk for everyone except very young children. Nonfat dry milk can be used in cooking. Ice cream can be replaced by ice milk or sherbet or, better yet, fresh fruit. Cheeses should be selected from those made wholly or in part from skim milk.

Limiting saturated fats tends to limit cholesterol intake, but there are important exceptions. Shellfish are low in fat, but shrimp is high in cholesterol. Kidney, brain, liver, and sweetbreads are rich sources of cholesterol. A diet high in fiber and low in refined sugar also aids the body in eliminating cholesterol from the blood. Egg yolks are a source of both fat and cholesterol; eggs also contain choline and lecithin, which are believed by some authorities to help the body control levels of serum cholesterol.

Sugar

The prudent diet calls for a reduction of the intake of refined sugar. Sugar is a source of Calories but provides few other nutrients. Sugar increases the body's need for thiamine and chromium. It is recommended that intake of refined sugar be reduced from 45% of the total Calories to 10%. This reduction applies to corn syrup, honey, and fructose as well as to granulated, confectioner's, and brown sugar. There is no appreciable difference in nutritional value among these sugars; however, fructose and honey are sweeter, so smaller amounts of these sugars can be used to achieve the desired sweetness, thereby reducing total intake of sugar.

Sugar is an important ingredient in processed foods and snack foods. The addition of sugar to baby foods has been discontinued, except for some dessert items, but older children and adults ingest large amounts of sugar hidden in processed foods. Refined sugar is an important factor in tooth decay and has been linked to coronary heart disease, cancer of the colon, and diabetes mellitus.

Soft drinks are rapidly replacing coffee and milk as the most popular beverages in North America and are an important dietary source of sugar. Replacing refined sugars in the diet is difficult because most people find the sweet taste satisfying as a comfort food, a snack, or at the end of a meal. Home-prepared products contain known amounts of sugar; adding sugar to beverages, fruits, and cereals should be discouraged but is still preferable to eating presweetened varieties. It is possible that if our taste buds were stimulated by less sugar, smaller amounts might be sufficient to satisfy our desire for sweetness.

Fresh fruits are perhaps the best substitutes for desserts that contain large amounts of sugar. Some canned fruits are available packed in water or in natural juices. Some fruits are flash-frozen without sugar. Replacing sugary snacks with fruit, raw vegetables, nuts, popcorn, or seeds would provide additional fiber as well as reduce intake of refined sugar. The use of artificial sweeteners is not recommended because of controversy over their possible carcinogenicity.

Alcohol

Consumption of alcohol is of concern nutritionally as well as because of the increasing incidence of alcoholism. Alcohol is a source of Calories but contains little else of nutritional value. Some wines contain iron, and some liquors appear to stimulate appetite. However, excessive intake of alcohol destroys appetite and the utilization of essential nutrients. Alcohol results from the fermentation of sugar. Throughout history, people have found ways of producing alcoholic beverages by the fermentation of various fruits, vegetables, and grains. Alcohol yields 7 kcal for every gram ingested and can account for a considerable portion of the caloric intake of people who routinely drink large quantities of alcohol. Moderation in the use of alcohol is advised to permit caloric intake from more nutritious foods.

Salt

Salt is a compound of sodium and chloride, both of which are essential minerals in the human diet. The exact requirements for sodium and chloride have not been determined. The average intake of salt in North America is thought to be vastly greater than the body's need. Excess intake of salt has blunted our taste buds and increased our consumption of salt. People who are accustomed to a limited intake of salt are quick to react negatively to a salty taste.

Salting food has become such a habit that many people automatically reach for the saltshaker before tasting their food. Salting is a method of preserving food. Salt is an important ingredient in processed foods, snacks, and condiments. It is difficult to find processed foods that have been prepared without salt.

Excessive intake of salt has been linked to hypertension and cardiac disease. About 1 teaspoon of salt per day is considered adequate for most people but represents a severe limitation to a society that presently uses three times that amount.

Fresh or flash-frozen vegetables contain less salt than do canned vegetables. Salt should be omitted from food preparation when possible, and smaller amounts should be used when it must be used. Cured meats and cold cuts contain large amounts of salt and should be used sparingly in the diets of people who seek to reduce their intake of salt. Revival of the old-fashioned salt dish and spoon might make people who overuse the saltshaker more aware of their salt intake. Light salts are available that contain one-half of the sodium chloride content of regular salt.

Fiber

The content of fiber in the present-day North American diet has decreased as a result of modern technology and food preference. Fiber consists of substances in plant foods that the body is unable to digest. Although fiber does not provide nutrients to the body, it does affect health. Fiber has the ability to absorb fluid, to form a gel, and to bind substances to itself. By absorbing fluid and increasing the bulk of fecal matter, fiber helps prevent constipation and disorders related to constipation, such as hemorrhoids. By decreasing the amount of time that fecal material is in contact with the intestinal mucosa, fiber decreases the incidence of cancer of the colon. It is believed that carcinogens in the fecal material are removed from the body before they can damage cells. Low-fiber diets have been implicated in the development of diverticulosis. Fiber can bind cholesterol to itself and assists in its removal from the body. Dietary deficiency of fiber is associated with appendicitis, diverticular disease, varicose veins, hemorrhoids, irritable bowel syndrome, hiatal hernia, dental caries, obesity, diabetes mellitus, coronary heart disease, and ischemic heart disease.

The dietary content of fiber can be increased by substituting whole-grain breads for white bread and whole-grain cereals for highly processed cereals and by increasing intake of fruits and vegetables. Snacks of popcorn, nuts, and seeds would also increase fiber intake.

Our modern way of life has created a market for fast-foods and convenience products. It appears that time is saved at the expense of health. To gain more control over food intake, people must either prepare more meals from raw materials or pressure food manufacturers into providing foods that satisfy the recommendations of the Dietary Goals for the United States prepared by the United States Senate Committee on Nutrition and Human Needs.

It is interesting to note the interrelationships among the recommendations, the role of both refined sugars and lack of fiber in colon cancer, the ability of fiber to promote cholesterol excretion, and the part that fats and refined sugars play in obesity, which is the forerunner in many cases of heart disease, diabetes mellitus, and hypertension.

Obesity

Obesity is a major health problem in North America. It cuts across all socioeconomic levels. It is an added risk factor for many of the leading causes of death. Excessive weight is unattractive; it causes psychologic problems, inconvenience, and unhappiness.

There are countless diets for weight loss. The most popular ones promise rapid weight loss with a minimum of deprivation. The sheer number of these diets indicates their lack of effectiveness in helping most people attain and maintain ideal body weight. Most people talk about "going on a diet" to lose a specified number of pounds. In other words, when that poundage is lost, they will go off their diets and back to their former eating habits.

To lose weight, a person must take in fewer Calories than the body burns for daily energy requirements, forcing the body to burn fat stores for energy. This goal can be accomplished either by reducing food intake or by increasing energy output, with a combination of the two being the most desirable plan. Increasing exercise at the same time as reducing food intake provides a distraction from the thoughts of food, firms tissues as weight is lost, and may even decrease appetite (Mayer, 1979). Once the ideal body weight is attained, the diet is adjusted to maintain this weight. The successful dieter does not go off the diet. This plan requires adopting for life a new style of food intake and exercise.

The best treatment for obesity is modification of food intake. The use of drugs or surgical procedures to bypass food digestion or absorption is an extreme measure that carries attendant dangers and often lacks the commitment of the individual.

A low-Calorie diet that contains the essential amounts of nutrients in the proper proportions is prescribed. The basic four recommendations provide approximately 1,200 kcal and should form the basis for any diet plan. The proportions of the prudent diet also supply guidelines: 50% of the total daily calories from carbohydrates, mainly complex carbohydrates instead of concentrated sweets, 20% from proteins, and 30% from fats, with 10% saturated and 10% polyunsaturated. Weight loss should average 1 to 2 pounds (1 kilogram) per week (see Table 4-1 for a 1,200-Calorie prudent diet).

It is advisable to measure body weight every week during the weight loss phase. Daily measurements may help maintain the desired weight after the excess pounds have been lost.

It is important to encourage clients to think in terms of adopting a more healthful diet than in terms of giving up certain foods. It is also important that the diet retain some foods that the patient associates with rewards. One of the most difficult periods of weight reduction is the plateau period, when body weight remains stationary even though the dieter has adhered faithfully to the diet plan. Nurses and other health workers should be particularly supportive during these periods.

TABLE 4-1
1,200-CALORIE PRUDENT DIET

Breakfast
½ cup of orange juice
1 shredded wheat biscuit
1 cup of skim milk
1 banana
Black coffee

Lunch
3 ounces of water-packed tuna
½ cup of tomato
Lettuce as desired
2 tablespoons of low-Calorie dressing
2 slices of whole-wheat bread
1 cup of skim milk

Dinner
3 ounces of chicken with skin removed
½ cup of brown rice with herbs
½ cup of broccoli
½ cup of carrots
2 teaspoons of sunflower oil margarine
1 medium peach
Tea with lemon

Keeping graphs of weight or records of intake are positive ways to reinforce the weight loss plan. Breads, cereals, and potatoes are frequently omitted foods in many diets, but these foods provide satiety and have a positive place in the menu of the dieter; in fact, increased intake of bread has been associated with weight loss in one study (Mayer, 1979).

Vegetarian Diets

Some people have adopted a diet free of meats, and others elect not to ingest dairy products and eggs as well. Vegetarian diets incorporate some components of the prudent diet; however, such diets must be carefully planned to ensure adequate intake of complete proteins. If milk is included, it provides complete protein when served in the same meal with grains. Other combinations that provide the essential amino acids include grains plus legumes and legumes plus seeds. Other limitations of vegetarian diets include inadequate intake of vitamin B_{12}, which is present only in foods containing animal proteins, and, possibly, inadequate intake of iron.

Food Preparation

Even preparation of food from basic ingredients may destroy nutrients. Vitamins B and C are water soluble and are easily destroyed by certain preparation methods. Fruits and vegetables are most nutritious if they are served raw or after a brief cooking time. Copper-lined pots destroy vitamin C. Fruits and vegetables should be prepared as close to serving time as possible. Cutting, crushing, soaking, and exposure to air reduce vitamin content. The use of unpeeled fruits and vegetables is recommended as a means of preserving vitamin content and also of providing fiber. Nutrient content is preserved if fruits and vegetables are not cut into small pieces. Steaming vegetables is preferable to boiling, and the water in which vegetables are cooked should be saved for stews and soups. Serving vegetables as soon as they are ready prevents the loss of vitamins that occurs when they are held over heat before serving. Reheating vegetables as leftovers increases vitamin loss. The addition of baking soda may improve the color of green vegetables, but it causes vitamin loss and should be avoided. Milk should be stored in opaque containers and should not be exposed to direct sunlight, to prevent riboflavin loss.

Dental Health

Sound teeth and healthy gums are dependent, as are all body tissues, on an adequate supply of blood to carry essential nutrients to the oral cavity. Adequate sources of calcium, phosphorus, and vitamin D are essential for tooth development and calcification of teeth. Once tooth formation and calcification are completed, the prevention of dental caries becomes a major goal in which diet has an influence.

Fluoridation and good hygiene are important in promoting high-level dental health, and diet also has a major role in this regard. Fluoridation of water supplies and the application of fluoride to teeth have reduced the incidence of dental caries. Foods are classified by dental authorities as either detergents or impactants. Detergent foods are those that require thorough chewing. The chewing action cleans by forcing food over the teeth and soft tissues of the mouth. Firm, fresh fruits and raw vegetables are examples of detergent foods. Impacting foods require little chewing and tend to adhere to the teeth and pack into the spaces between teeth. Cookies, crackers, and some candies are impacting foods. A diet that contains adequate amounts of detergent foods and limited amounts of impacting foods is recommended for dental health.

Refined sugar, particularly in sticky forms that adhere to the surfaces of the teeth, has been implicated in dental caries. Reduction of intake of refined sugar, as well as brushing after meals, reduces tooth decay. The substitution of detergent snack foods for sweets is prudent in dental health as well as general health.

Periodontal disease is related to diet as well as dental hygiene. Brushing and flossing combined with a diet low in refined sugars but high in detergent foods and other foods that require chewing aid in the control of plaque (a sticky gelatinous material that has a high bacterial content), which causes periodontal problems.

References

Arlin, M. Controversies in nutrition, a brief review. *The Nursing Clinics of North America,* June 1980, *14,* 2.

Ardell, D. The nature of high level wellness, or why "normal health" is a rather sorry state of existence. *Health Values: Achieving High Level Wellness,* February 1979, *3,* 1.

Bass, L. More fiber—Less constipation. *American Journal of Nursing,* February 1977, *77,* 2.

Bowen, W. Dental caries. *Contemporary Nutrition,* August 1977, *2,* 8.

Collier, D. Fluorine: An essential element for good dental health. *Contemporary Nutrition,* October 1979, *4,* 10.

Dunn, H. What high-level wellness means. *Canadian Journal of Public Health,* November 1959, *50,* 11.

Dwyer, J. Vegetarianism. *Contemporary Nutrition,* June 1979, *4,* 6.

Harland, B., & Hecht, A. Grandma called it roughage. *FDA Consumer,* July/August 1977. Washington, D.C.: U.S. Government Printing Office.

The Institute of Food Technologists' Expert Panel on Food Safety and Nutrition and the Committee on Public Information. Dietary fiber. *Contemporary Nutrition*, September 1979, *4*, 9.

Leslie, J. Commonsense guide to good and healthy eating. *Nursing Mirror*, November 16, 1978.

Lieber, C. Alcohol-nutrition interaction. *Contemporary Nutrition*, September 1978, *3*, 9.

Mayer, J. Food fortification. *Family Health*, February 1979, *11*, 2.

Mayer, J. 10 Nutritional myths. *Family Health*, May 1979, *11*, 5.

Mayer, J. Want to lose some weight? Try bread. *Food For Thought.* Syndicated column. *The Providence Journal*, December 5, 1979.

Stare, F., & Whelan, E. The best diet for you and your health. *Health Values: Achieving High-Level Wellness*, January/February 1977, *1*, 1.

Serrin, W. Let them eat junk—The triumph of food processing. *Saturday Review*, February 2, 1980.

United States Senate Select Committee on Nutrition and Human Needs. *Dietary goals for the United States*. Washington, D.C.: U.S. Government Printing Office, 1977.

Williams, R. *Physician's handbook of nutritional science*. Springfield, Ill.: Charles C Thomas, Publisher, 1975.

The good health food guide menu planner. *Better Homes and Gardens*, January 1979, *57*, 1.

An apple a day. *Nursing Times*, April 12, 1979.

Eating enought high-fiber food? Too much? *Changing Times*, January 1979.

The new nutrition: 101 Ways to feed your family better. *Family Circle*, May 19, 1978.

5
Nutrition for
the Hospitalized
Patient

Hospital Malnutrition

Healthy adults need food for energy production and maintenance of body tissues. Sick adults need food for energy, maintenance, and repair. Children need food for growth in addition to the needs identified for adults. Despite increased need for nutrients, the nutritional needs of many hospitalized persons are ignored or overridden by their other therapies. Dr. Charles Butterworth (1974), among others, has called attention to physician-induced malnutrition, but the situation continues. In some hospitals, concerned physicians have organized nutritional teams to spread the doctrine of the importance of sound nutrition to the hospitalized patient's recovery. Such teams are composed of physicians, dietitians, nurses, and pharmacists whose prime concern is to provide the proper nutrients to patients by the method most appropriate to their needs and illnesses. Hospital practices that contribute to hospital malnutrition include the failure to assess nutritional status on admission by even the simplest measures of height and weight.

Most laboratory tests are thought to have greatest reliability when the specimen is collected from a fasting patient. Many diagnostic procedures require a period of "nothing by mouth" as preparation. Anorexia and loss of regular appetite are accepted without question as part of the disease process. Charting of food intake appears to be a lost art. In rare instances when food intake is evaluated, it is apt to be evaluated in relation to disease rather than to the needs of the body.

Hospitalized patients may not need as many Calories for activity once they are assigned to beds and their ambulation is limited to the length of the unit corridor. However, their needs for nutrients for repair and to offset the changes related to the disease may greatly exceed their normal caloric requirements. Fever increases caloric requirements by 7% for every degree Fahrenheit increase in body temperature. Infection also increases metabolic needs. The popular intravenous feeding of glucose can prevent dehydration and ketosis but not starvation.

Nurses are in a position to protect patients from hospital-induced malnutrition. They can include nutritional assessment in their nursing histories. They can record admission weight and height when a patient's condition permits, rather than limit this procedure to medical admissions. They can remind physicians how long patients have been on inadequate intakes, whether oral or intravenous. Nurses need to become concerned with the nutritional states of their patients to ensure the best outcome of the treatment regimens. They need to become involved in learning why food intake is limited and seek to correct the situation or suggest the need for alternative feeding plans. It is important for nurses to know whether patients are not eating because they are nauseated or because they dislike the food that has been served, or whether the food violates their religious or cultural beliefs.

Withholding food for tests often results in difficulty in obtaining food once the tests have been completed. Trays held on the unit are often cold and unappetizing. Trays held in the main kitchen often take hours to reach the patient. With present-day food packaging and microwave ovens, it should be possible to serve a hot meal promptly when tests are completed.

Some hospitals serve an early continental breakfast, brunch, an early dinner, and a bedtime snack. This meal pattern permits most patients to omit the continental breakfast for test preparation but complete the test in time for brunch. The bedtime snack provides extra nutrition that may allay hunger when fasting is required the next morning.

Nurses need to be aware of the nutritional value of the foods that are served to their patients and to urge nutritional supplementation when inadequate intake lasts more than 1 or 2 days. In the past, nurses were satisfied with the commonly held idea that patients would get their appetites back when they got well. Now, nurses should adopt the attitude that patients must receive an adequate supply of nutrients to get well.

Fluid Intake

The body's need for fluid is critical, and fluids must be provided every day. Withholding food and fluid is permitted for 8 to 10 hours for tests and preoperatively, but even in these instances ample fluid should be provided both before and after the period of abstinence. Unless specific orders urging or limiting fluids are written, the usual fluid intake for the adult patient is 1,500 to 2,000 milliliters. Fever, infection, the withholding of solid food and increased fluid losses through drainage, perspiration, or diarrhea should prompt the nurse to increase the fluid intake to replace the losses and to satisfy the increased need for fluid.

The ease of replacing fluids through the use of the intravenous route has made health care personnel less persistent in urging fluid intake. Intravenous infusions are often lifesaving but should never replace oral intake when the latter is possible. If nurses would consider orders for intravenous feedings as a reflection of nursing care for patients who are capable of oral intake, they would be more insistent, imaginative, persuasive, and probably successful in promoting adequate fluid intake.

Some nursing measures that increase fluid intake include becoming aware of a patient's preferences and offering these beverages when they are permitted in the diet; offering fluids frequently throughout the day, particularly for bedfast patients; and using a variety of textures when the diet permits gelatin or fruit ices or ice cream as alternatives to liquids. Serving fluids in small glasses is often less overwhelming to patients, and they are more apt to drink the entire glassful; large servings of any food are often discouraging to sick people.

Nursing a patient on limited fluid intake is difficult because nurses do not like denying a patient's requests. When fluids must be limited, the total amount permitted should be divided proportionately over the 24-hour period. Nurses on each shift should adhere to the allotted amount to prevent the prescribed amount from being used up, leaving the night nurse with no recourse but to deny the patient fluid throughout the entire shift. Sham drinking is a device that promotes comfort for patients on limited fluids; it consists of allowing patients to hold fluid in their mouths without swallowing to relieve dryness of the mucous membrane of the mouth and its discomfort. If a patient on limited fluids is given ice chips, their intake should be recorded as one-half of the amount of the container. Thus, an 8-ounce glass of ice chips contains 4 ounces of fluid. Adding ice to fluids displaces liquid and should be taken into consideration. Sips of fluid should be taken from a measured amount and recorded in milliliters, not as "sips." Any ice or fluid not taken should be subtracted from the total amount and not simply discarded. Serving liquids separately from meals promotes comfort because the solid foods relieve thirst at mealtime, sparing the liquids to relieve between-meal thirst. Frequent oral hygiene also serves as a comfort measure when fluids are limited. Diverting attention from fluids and the removal of visual reminders of liquids may also be helpful. Hard candy has been found to increase thirst by increasing the osmolarity of saliva and pulling fluid from the cells of the oral mucosa.

Liquid Diets

Intake is restricted to fluids in situations where the person is unable to tolerate solid foods. Patients with febrile illnesses and postoperative patients commonly receive liquid diets. The main nutrients provided are water, sugar, salt, and some vitamins. The content of proteins and Calories is usually low in liquid diets.

CLEAR LIQUID DIET

A clear liquid diet is limited to fluids that are transparent and is usually continued only for 1 to 2 days because of its nutritional inadequacy. A typical clear liquid diet would supply between 400 and 500 Calories, 5 and 10 grams of protein, 100 and 120 grams of carbohydrate, and no fat.

Clear liquids include:
Tea with sugar and lemon
Black coffee
Fat-free broth, bouillon, consomme
Carbonated beverages
Cereal waters
Strained, diluted fruit juice
Fruit ices
Popsicles
Plain gelatin
Ice chips
Water

In an attempt to increase protein and Calorie content in a liquid diet, some protocols permit the addition of egg white and gelatin to clear liquids. Frequent feedings are indicated to increase intake and prevent extreme hunger; however, as soon as the patient's condition permits, expansion of the diet is desirable. Inability to tolerate an increased oral intake would indicate the need for tube feedings or parenteral nutrition.

FULL LIQUID DIET

A full liquid diet includes all liquids and foods that are liquid at body or room temperature. A full liquid diet may contain an adequate amount of Calories, but it tends to be low in iron, and fiber is lacking.

At least six feedings are offered daily. Caloric intake can be increased by the use of 10% cream in place of some of the milk and by the addition of butter or margarine to cereals and soups. If additional fat is not desirable, nonfat dry milk can be added to beverages and soups. The addition of strained baby meats to soups increases protein and iron intake. Sugar can be added to beverages to increase caloric intake.

Foods that are classified as liquids in a full liquid diet include:

Custard
Vanilla pudding
Plain ice cream
Refined cooked cereals
Strained fruit and vegetable juices

Solid Intake

REGULAR DIET

The regular, or house, diet is one that contains from 2,000 to 2,500 kcal. It provides appropriate servings of the basic four food groups. A regular diet is designed to supply approximately 60 to 80 grams of protein, 80 to 100 grams of fat, and 200 to 300 grams of carbohydrate. There are no particular food restrictions in a regular diet; however, foods that commonly cause digestive disturbances are usually limited. Fried foods are also kept to a minimum.

Most hospitals offer patients on a regular diet the opportunity to choose between two or more items. Such patients receive menus the day before and are able to choose between two selections of appetizer, soup, entree, salad, and dessert. Bread and beverage selections may be more numerous. Dietitians presumably review selections and counsel patients whose selections do not constitute an adequate diet. Nonselected items may be served to tempt such patients into a more nutritious intake. Selections that are made the previous day may not reflect a patient's desires the next day, particularly if tests and treatments have been upsetting. Hospital routines require that menus be collected at a specific time, and nurses or visitors may make the selections if a patient is unavailable or uninterested at the time. Dietitians who are responsible for therapeutic diets may not have the time to evaluate the diets selected by patients on regular diets.

Substitutions at mealtime are possible but usually involve delay and are often not worth the persistence required to obtain them while a patient is still interested in eating. A few hospitals are instituting a prudent diet for the regular diet. Table 5-1 is an example of a prudent regular hospital diet.

Patients on regular diets should be receiving adequate nutrition, provided that their nutritional requirements have not been unduly increased by disease and provided that they eat what is served to them on their trays.

TABLE 5-1
A PRUDENT REGULAR HOSPITAL DIET

Breakfast

½ grapefruit

⅔ cup of oatmeal

1 cup of skim milk

2 slices of whole-wheat toast

2 teaspoons of special margarine[a]

Black coffee

10 AM

6 ounces of orange juice

Whole-wheat crackers with peanut butter

Lunch

1 cup of tomato soup

¾ cup of tuna salad (water-packed tuna, special dressing[a])

1 slice of whole-wheat bread with special margarine[a]

1 cup of skim milk

2 PM

Apple with skim milk cheese cubes

Dinner

3 ounces of roast chicken with skin removed

Baked potato with special margarine[a]

½ cup of carrots

½ cup of broccoli

1 whole-wheat roll with special margarine[a]

Fresh fruit in season

Tea with lemon

[a]Made with safflower, sunflower, or corn oil.

SOFT DIET

A soft diet can also be nutritionally adequate. The major modification in the soft diet is texture. A soft diet usually contains sufficient Calories with proportions of protein, carbohydrate, and fat similar to those in a regular diet. A soft diet is designed to be easy to chew, simple to digest, and free from harsh fiber, rich foods, and strongly flavored foods.

The following foods are usually omitted from a soft diet:

Coarse, dark breads

Whole-grain crackers

Hot breads

Pancakes

Waffles

Tough meats

Smoked or salted meats

Fatty or highly seasoned soups

Bran cereals

Unstrained, coarse cereals

Sharp cheeses

Dried fruits and nuts

Rich desserts

Fried foods

Most raw and tough-skinned fruits

Raw vegetables

Chocolate candy

Spices, pepper, and relishes

Table 5-2 gives an example of a soft diet.

Some hospitals include a mechanically soft diet, which differs from the soft diet in that highly flavored foods may be included, as may spices and foods considered difficult to digest. The main consideration in the mechanically soft diet is ease in chewing. This diet is used for dental or edentulous patients.

BLAND DIET

A bland diet is one in which liquids or foods that are chemically, mechanically, or thermally irritating are removed from the diet. A regular soft diet can be made bland by the exclusion of the following:

Tea

Coffee

Colas

Citrus fruits

Meat soups and broths

Highly seasoned foods

Spices

Whole grains

Raw fruits and vegetables

Iced foods and beverages

Very hot foods and beverages

Strong-flavored foods

LOW-RESIDUE DIET

A low-residue diet is frequently ordered preoperatively and before some diagnostic tests when it is desirable to reduce the contents of the intestinal

TABLE 5-2

A SAMPLE SOFT DIET

Breakfast

  1 ripe banana

  ½ cup of strained oatmeal

  2 slices of toasted white bread

  2 teaspoons of butter

  1 tablespoon of jelly

  4 ounces of light cream

  Sugar

  Coffee

10 AM

  Orange juice

  Plain muffin

Lunch

  ½ cup of chicken broth

  ½ cup of mashed potato

  2 ounces of roast chicken

  ½ cup of cooked asparagus tips

  1 slice of white bread

  1 teaspoon of butter

  1 cup of milk

  Tapioca pudding with cream

2 PM

  1 cup of milk

  Plain cookies

Dinner

  ½ cup of tomato juice

  Ground-beef patty

  ½ cup of noodles

  ½ cup of well-cooked carrots

  2 teaspoons of butter

  1 slice of white bread

  ½ cup of vanilla ice cream

  Tea

Bedtime

  1 cup of milk drink

tract. This diet limits not only indigestible fiber but other foods that, although fiber-free, contribute to increased residue. Milk is an example of such a food, and intake of milk and milk products is limited to 8 ounces daily in a low-residue diet. Clear fluids, sugar, salt, meats, fats, and eggs are permitted. Cheeses, fried foods, and highly seasoned foods are avoided. Only refined cereals and white breads are included in a low-residue diet. The only vegetable allowed is peeled white potatoes. Fruit intake is limited to fruit juices. A low-residue diet does not contain suffi-cient calcium, iron, and vitamins, and its use is usually limited to 3 to 4 days.

References

Butterworth, C. The skeleton in the hospital closet. *Nutrition Today,* March/April 1974, *9,* 4.

Howe, P. *Basic nutrition in health and disease* (6th ed.). Philadelphia: W. B. Saunders Company, 1976.

Krause, M., & Mahan, L. K. *Food, nutrition and diet therapy* (6th ed.). Philadelphia: W. B. Saunders Company, 1979.

Massachusetts General Hospital Dietary Department. *Diet manual.* Boston: Little, Brown & Company, 1976.

Mitchel, H., Rynberger, H., Anderson, L., et al. *Nutrition in health and disease* (16th ed.). Philadelphia: J. B. Lippincott Company, 1976.

Robinson, C., & Lawler, M. *Normal and therapeutic nutrition* (15th ed.). New York: Macmillan Publishing Company, 1977.

Thiele, V. *Clinical nutrition.* St. Louis: C. V. Mosby Company, 1976.

Williams, S. *Nutrition and diet therapy* (3rd ed.). St. Louis: C. V. Mosby Company, 1977.

6
Diet Therapy in Gastrointestinal Disorders

The gastrointestinal tract is so intimately related to food intake, digestion, absorption, and elimination that it is no surprise that, historically, gastrointestinal disorders were usually treated by diet modification. More recently, some time-honored diets have been questioned, and research has failed to support some of our commonly accepted beliefs about diet therapy in gastrointestinal disease. A better understanding of the pathophysiology of such diseases as diverticulosis has led to a complete reversal of the diet prescription.

Like the cells in the rest of the body, the cells of the gastrointestinal tract depend on essential nutrients to function and require an extra supply of proteins and vitamins for healing and repair. Patients who have suffered from gastrointestinal complaints for long periods before seeking medical assistance may be malnourished and in need of dietary treatment for nutritional deficiencies as well as for recovery from their disease. Concern about the relationship of saturated fats and cholesterol to atherosclerosis has brought into question the advisability of prescribing diets that consist primarily of milk, cream, and eggs. Patients who have previously thought that what was white, soft, and mild was good in the treatment of gastrointestinal complaints may need extra support in accepting some of the newer dietary modifications.

Achalasia

PATHOPHYSIOLOGY

In achalasia (cardiospasm, esophageal dyssnergia), there is inadequate peristalsis in the upper portion of the esophagus and failure of the lower esophageal sphincter to relax and open during swallowing. As a result, food is unable to enter the stomach and distends the lower portion of the esophagus.

TREATMENT

Achalasia is treated by dilatation of the sphincter or by surgical intervention to split the circular muscle of the cardiac sphincter (cardiomyotomy)

DIET THERAPY

The aim of dietary treatment in achalasia is to provide nutritional support for the patient despite the swallowing difficulty. There are varying degrees of dysphagia, and the dietary regimen may extend from the provision of easy-to-swallow foods through elimination of the foods that increase lower esophageal pressure to nasogastric tube feedings, gastrostomy, or jejunostomy feedings to intravenous nutrition. Liquid or semiliquid diets are frequently used before dilatation or surgical intervention. Fluids are served at a moderate temperature.

Foods that stimulate the gastric hormone gastrin are avoided because gastrin controls the lower esophageal sphincter. Proteins and carbohydrates liberate gastrin and prevent relaxation of the sphincter, whereas, fats lower esophageal pressure and permit relaxation of the sphincter. Coffee and chocolate lower esophageal pressure and would be permitted. Spices, citrus juices, and tomato juice are usually avoided because they may irritate the esophageal mucosa, which may already be traumatized by distention and dilatation.

NURSING IMPLICATIONS

- Avoid temperature extremes. Neither very hot nor very cold foods or fluids should be served.
- Fluids do not require esophageal peristalsis to reach the cardiac sphincter; however, they may be difficult to swallow. Semiliquid foods may be easiest for the patient to swallow.
- Provide plenty of fluids with meals, and encourage the patient to take sips of fluid with the more solid components of the meal.
- Instruct the patient to eat slowly and to chew all food well.
- An alcoholic beverage, such as an aperitif, may be helpful to some patients. Alcohol appears to reduce esophageal pressure and to have a psychologic effect. However, alcohol provides only Calories and should be used only if it permits a substantial increase in nutritional intake.
- Unless contraindicated by other conditions, whole milk should be

used in oral feedings, because its fat content tends to lower esophageal sphincter pressure.

Esophagitis

PATHOPHYSIOLOGY

Esophagitis is inflammation of the esophagus. It is usually the result of reflux of gastric juices into the lower portion of the esophagus due to failure of the cardiac sphincter to close tightly. When the cardiac sphincter fails to close tightly, food that has entered the stomach and been mixed with gastric juice returns to the lower portion of the esophagus. The pressure in the lower portion of the esophagus is reduced, and the sphincter does not close between swallows.

TREATMENT

Antacids are used in the treatment of esophagitis to neutralize the gastric contents and prevent irritation of the esophageal mucosa. Cholinergic blocking agents may be used to reduce the amount of gastric secretions. A mixture of aluminum hydroxide, magnesium trisilicate, sodium bicarbonate, and alginic acid (Gaviscon) has also been tried; this medication prevents acid from entering the esophagus by floating on top of the stomach contents. Surgical treatment can be employed if medical management proves ineffective. A vagotomy (interruption of the impulses carried by the vagus nerve) may be performed to reduce the secretion of the acid gastric juices. The cardiac sphincter can also be tightened surgically.

DIET THERAPY

The aims of diet therapy in esophagitis are to prevent irritation of the esophageal mucosa, to prevent reflux from the stomach, and to reduce the acidity of the gastric contents. A bland, fiber-restricted diet is usually prescribed. A full liquid diet may be ordered initially. Citrus and tomato juices are omitted from the diet because of their irritating effect on the esophageal mucosa.

The effect of classes of food on the gastric hormones and their effect on the pressure in the lower portion of the esophagus are important in selecting foods for this diet. Gastrin increases lower esophageal pressure and protein stimulates gastrin secretions, so that protein feedings would be indicated in esophagitis. Secretin and cholecystokinin reduce lower esophageal pressure. Fatty meals stimulate production of cholecystokinin and should be avoided. Chocolate, coffee, alcohol, peppermint, and spearmint reduce lower esophageal pressure and are limited or excluded from the diet. See Table 6-1 for an example of a bland, fiber-restricted diet.

NURSING IMPLICATIONS

- Feedings should be small, frequent, regular, and of equal size. Patients should be taught how to plan similar meals at home.
- Patients need to be cautioned against lying down, bending over, or straining immediately after eating.
- The final meal of the day should be planned at least 2 to 3 hours before bedtime to reduce reflux related to position change.

TABLE 6-1
BLAND, FIBER-RESTRICTED DIET

Breakfast
  1 ripe banana
  ½ cup of cream of rice cereal
  Skim milk
  Coffee
Midmorning
  1 soft-boiled egg
  1 slice of white toast
  Margarine
  1 cup of skim milk
Lunch
  1 cup of cream of chicken soup
  1 slice of white bread
  ½ cup of carrots with margarine
  ½ cup of canned peaches
Midafternoon
  1 chicken sandwich with mayonnaise
  Baked custard
  1 cup of apricot nectar
Dinner
  1 broiled veal chop
  Baked potato with margarine
  ½ cup of cooked green beans
  1 cup of skim milk
  ½ cup of ice milk
  1 slice of pound cake
Midevening
  3 ounces of Swiss cheese
  Saltines
  1 cup of skim milk
  Applesauce and plain cookies

- Elevation of the head of the bed on blocks 4 to 6 inches high is recommended. The use of the gatch mechanism on hospital beds is not recommended because it tends to jackknife the body rather than provide a gentle slope that uses gravity as an aid to treatment.
- Clothes, dressings, restraints, or anything that is tight around the abdomen should be avoided.
- Obese patients should be supported in their efforts to lose weight since esophagitis improves with weight loss.
- Reflux esophagitis may occur after cardiomyotomy for achalasia.
- Skim milk should be used in preference to whole milk since skim milk increases lower esophageal pressure, whereas whole milk decreases lower esophageal pressure. Skim milk is also preferable when weight loss is indicated.
- When both citrus and tomato juices are omitted from the diet, other sources of Vitamin C should be checked to be sure that an adequate intake is being provided.
- Antacid agents that contain calcium and aluminum tend to be constipating; when such agents are administered along with a low-fiber diet, constipation may become a problem. Consider the inclusion of low-fiber laxative foods and increased fluid intake.
- Antacid agents that contain magnesium tend to cause diarrhea. The alternate use of calcium/aluminum agents and magnesium agents may be considered. Antacids that combine both types of agents may also provide a solution.

Celiac Disease: Gluten-Induced Enteropathy

PATHOPHYSIOLOGY

Celiac disease results from the body's intolerance to gliadin, which is a constituent of the protein gluten. Gliadin has a toxic effect on the mucosa of the small intestine, resulting in destruction of the villi and interference with absorption. Nontropical sprue is adult celiac disease.

TREATMENT

The only known effective treatment of celiac disease is dietary intervention.

DIET THERAPY

The dietary treatment of celiac disease is the removal of the offending protein, gluten, from the diet of the patient, whether adult or child. During celiac crisis, and acute episodes of vomiting and diarrhea, fluids and electrolytes are replaced intravenously. As the diarrhea subsides, the patient progresses to a high-protein, low-fat diet and, eventually, to a regular diet with sources of gluten eliminated.

A gluten-free diet eliminates wheat, rye, barley, and oats but should be rich in other proteins. Because one of the symptoms of celiac disease is steatorrhea (increased fat content of the stools), the initial diet is usually low in fat, particularly saturated fats. The fat in egg yolks and in lean meats is usually well tolerated. Fat restriction may interefere with an adequate intake of fat-soluble vitamins, and supplementation may be needed.

A gluten-free diet makes the selection of breads and cereals critical. The use of flour as a thickening agent in many products, such as puddings and gravies, results in a restricted selection of prepared foods. Rice, corn, and soy flour as well as wheat starch can be used in breads and other baked goods. Corn Flakes, Rice Krispies, Puffed Rice, and precooked rice cereals are acceptable in the diet. Corn meal, hominy, and rice are starches that can be safely used in the diet. Cornstarch is acceptable as a thickening agent to replace flour.

Two to 6 weeks on a gluten-free diet produces dramatic improvement. Absence of symptoms over a long period probably represents a remission of the disease and not a cure. See Table 6-2 for an example of a gluten-restricted diet.

NURSING IMPLICATIONS

- A gluten-free diet is restrictive, and it is important to provide variety. Patients should be directed to sources of recipes for gluten-free breads, cookies, and cakes.
- Special recipes are required when using rice, corn, or soy flour. It is not possible to substitute these flours for wheat flour in regular recipes because other adjustments in ingredients would also have to be made.
- Adequate caloric intake may be a problem, and the diet should be carefully evaluated for adequacy of energy intake.
- The importance of careful reading of product labels cannot be overemphasized. Flour is a hidden ingredient in many prepared foods.
- Small amounts of gluten are often present in the form of fillers, additives, and stabilizers. Check for the possible inclusion in such foods as instant coffee and tea, ice cream, candy, soups, mustard, ground meats, and sausage.
- Patients who rely on convenience foods need additional help in identifying gluten-free selections.

TABLE 6-2
GLUTEN-RESTRICTED DIET

Breakfast

½ grapefruit

½ cup of Rice Krispies with skim milk

2 slices of gluten-free bread (made with potato or soy flour)

Margarine and jelly

Coffee

Lunch

4 ounces of sliced chicken

½ cup of broccoli with margarine

½ cup of boiled rice

Gravy made by thickening chicken broth with cornstarch

Tapioca pudding

Gluten-free cookies

1 cup of skim milk

Dinner

4 ounces of baked fish

1 baked potato

Lettuce and tomato salad with gluten-free dressing

1 cornmeal muffin

½ cantaloupe

1 cup of skim milk

- Unexplained relapses should prompt investigation of the possible source of gluten. Check food intake for the 3 previous days.
- If liberalization of the diet is permitted, it should be accomplished slowly.
- Patients with celiac disease are prone to other food allergies; shellfish are common offenders.
- Assess the need for iron supplements; iron is absorbed in the area of the small intestine affected by celiac disease, and a deficiency may occur despite adequate intake.

Colostomy

PATHOPHYSIOLOGY

A colostomy is an artificial outlet for intestinal wastes that is created by bringing a portion of the colon through the abdominal wall. This surgical procedure diverts fecal material from the distal colon and rectum, where fluid is normally reabsorbed from the intestinal contents. Patients with co-lostomies have stools with a higher than average water content.

DIET THERAPY

A patient with a colostomy needs a well-balanced diet appropriate for the disease that necessitated the colostomy and for other unrelated conditions that the patient may have. In general, the goals for the patient with a co-lostomy are to prevent odor, to prevent constipation, and to prevent diar-rhea. Experience with the diet and the colostomy usually makes it obvious which foods should be limited or avoided. The foods that are most apt to cause gas and odors are beans, cabbage, radishes, onions, cucumbers, fish, broccoli, corn, and nuts. Prune and apple juices may be effective in preventing constipation.

NURSING IMPLICATIONS

- Patients with colostomies have real concerns about flatulence and odors and should be supported in their search for dietary adaptations that can control their occurrence.
- After individual food eliminations have been made, the diet should be reevaluated for the adequacy of essential nutrients.
- The use of a commercial deodorant in the colostomy bag is preferable to eliminating favored foods or foods that contain essential nutrients.
- Check with the physician about the possible oral use of chlorophyll or bismuth subgallate as deodorants. Bismuth subgallate tends to cause constipation.
- Spinach and parsley are foods that have a deodorizing action.
- Encourage patients to eat slowly and to chew their food well to avoid swallowing air or creating food boluses that might obstruct the colostomy.

Constipation

PATHOPHYSIOLOGY

As fecal material moves through the large intestine toward the rectum, water is absorbed, and the stool becomes more solid. The longer fecal material remains in the colon and rectum, the more water is removed and the harder the stool becomes. Constipation is related to transit time of the fecal material, which, in turn, is affected by physical and emotional vari-ables. Normally, waste products from a meal are excreted from the intes-tinal tract 24 to 72 hours after ingestion.

TREATMENT

Treatment of constipation is directed at altering the cause. Many variables have been implicated in the etiology of this symptom, which appears to be related to the stress and strain of modern life. If poor hygienic habits appear to be responsible, the patient is counseled to establish a regular time for bowel evacuation and to adhere to the routine. Regularity of meals, adequate rest, exercise, and relaxation are also advised. Failure to respond to the urge to defecate often contributes to constipation. Medications that contain iron, aluminum, or calcium tend to cause constipation. The consistent use of laxatives can also contribute to the development of constipation.

Suppositories, laxatives, and enemas are used to relieve constipation, but the ideal treatment is the reestablishment of good health habits to restore regularity.

DIET THERAPY

The dietary regimen that aids in preventing constipation is a regular, well-balanced diet with added fiber and fluids. Fiber provides bulk in the stool and draws water into the intestinal contents. It can be provided by whole grains and raw fruits and vegetables. If fiber is undesirable for other conditions that the patient may have, cooked fruits and vegetables provide some laxative effect. Prune and apple juices may also be used. Most people can identify foods that have a laxative effect on them, and they should be encouraged to include these foods in their diets.

Highly refined sugars increase fermentation in the intestinal tract, forming acids that pull fluid and distend the colon, which leads to defecation. The intentional increase of refined sugar in the diet should be discouraged due to the medical problems related to high sugar intake and the availability of better dietary ways to treat constipation.

NURSING IMPLICATIONS

- Adequate fluid intake is a much-neglected aspect in the treatment of constipation. Patients should be advised to plan for fluid intake and to drink at least 8 to 10 glasses of fluid daily.
- Prunes owe their laxative effect to diphenylisatin, which stimulates intestinal motility. Prunes and prune juice are desirable laxative foods because they also contribute calcium, iron, and B vitamins to the diet.
- Increased intake of fiber may be achieved through the addition of bran to foods and the increased use of whole grains in place of refined flour.
- Figs and raisins are helpful in increasing bulk in the diet and can be added to cereals, muffins, and cookies.

- Increasing fiber content in the diet should be approached gradually, or it may cause cramping and discomfort, which might discourage the patient from continuing to include fiber in the diet.
- Patients should be discouraged from regular or excessive use of laxatives. Despite the ease with which they can be obtained, they are drugs and can lead to undesirable dependence and the loss of the normal pattern of defecation.
- Patients should be reassured that a daily bowel movement is not the normal pattern for everyone.

Diarrhea

PATHOPHYSIOLOGY

Diarrhea is a symptom of many disorders in which there is increased peristalsis with a decrease in the transit time of intestinal contents. This situation leads to reduced reabsorption of fluid in the large intestine and to watery stools. Diarrhea is usually classified as functional if it is related to irritation or stress or as organic if it is the result of a lesion in the intestinal tract.

TREATMENT

The treatment of diarrhea is the elimination of the underlying cause. Antidiarrheal drugs may be used to slow peristalsis or to thicken the stool.

DIET THERAPY

In severe diarrhea, all oral feedings are stopped to permit the intestinal tract to rest. During this time, intravenous fluids are used to replace water and electrolytes. Fluid replacement is particularly critical in the infant to avoid dehydration, which can be lethal.

When oral feedings are resumed, they usually consist of clear fluids with a minimum of sugar. Oral electrolyte solutions have been used effectively in pediatric practice. The diet is gradually expanded to include light, easy-to-digest, minimal-residue foods. Boiled skim milk is usually the first milk product permitted. Applesauce and raw apples have been used for the thickening effect of the pectin that they contain. The diet, in general, is low in fiber and low in residue.

An increase in the number of watery stools usually results in a return to "nothing by mouth" and intravenous support. If the need for intravenous feeding persists beyond 72 hours, amino acid preparation may be added to the intravenous intake of glucose and vitamins B and C. Total parenteral nutrition may be used in prolonged, intractable diarrhea.

NURSING IMPLICATIONS

- Meticulous records of intake and output are essential aids in prescribing fluid replacement.
- Daily weights are also indicators of fluid status.
- Carbonated beverages and iced fluids are usually avoided in the management of diarrhea. Flat ginger ale may be used, and coke syrup sometimes relieves nausea.
- The first few bites of food may trigger peristalsis in the recovering patient and may prevent continuation of the meal until after defecation. The tray should be removed and foods kept at appropriate temperatures until the patient has been prepared to resume eating.
- Diversion may be helpful in the management of diarrhea. The bedpan should be readily available but should not be in the direct view of the patient.

Diverticular Disease

PATHOPHYSIOLOGY

Diverticula are herniations of the intestinal mucosa through the muscle fibers of the bowel wall. The presence of diverticula is referred to as diverticulosis. Inflammation of diverticula is called diverticulitis. These conditions can occur in any part of the gastrointestinal tract, but they arise most often in the colon. Herniation of the intestinal wall is due to increased pressure within the lumen of the intestine. Increased segmentation of the bowel, which occurs in diverticular disease, is thought to be related to lack of fecal bulk and to increased intraluminal pressure.

TREATMENT

The treatment of diverticulosis is aimed at preventing inflammation. Severe diverticulitis is treated by temporary colostomy and resection of the involved segment of bowel.

DIET THERAPY

The aim of dietary treatment of diverticular disease is to reduce intraluminal pressure by increasing the size of the stool, thereby distending the bowel wall. A high-fiber diet is usually prescribed. The main dietary sources of fiber are bran, whole grains, fruits, and vegetables. Harsh fiber is apt to be irritating, and such foods as nuts and fibrous vegetables are eliminated. Large quantities of raw fruits and vegetables are also avoided due to their laxative effect. Pepper and chili powder are limited in amount or avoided completely because they are mucosal irritants. Methylcellulose is a commercial source of fiber. See Table 6-3 for an example of a high-fiber diet.

NURSING IMPLICATIONS

- Patient education is essential because diverticular disease was formerly treated with a low-residue diet.
- High-residue foods are not synonymous with high-fiber foods. Some nonfibrous foods, such as milk, leave residue in the intestine.
- Pressure within the lumen of the colon may rise when the patient is given neostigmine or morphine. Meperidine (Demerol) does not cause as much of a rise in pressure as does morphine and is the preferred narcotic for patients with diverticular disease (McKechnie, 1976).

Dumping Syndrome

PATHOPHYSIOLOGY

The dumping syndrome is a complex physiologic response to the presence of undigested food in the jejunum. If two-thirds or more of the

---

TABLE 6-3
HIGH-FIBER DIET

Breakfast
  4 ounces of unstrained orange juice
  ½ cup of bran cereal with fresh strawberries and milk
  1 slice of whole-wheat toast with margarine and jam
  Coffee
Midmorning
  Apple and cheese
Lunch
  Chicken salad sandwich on whole-wheat bread with celery, lettuce, and tomato
  1 glass of milk
  Fresh pear
Dinner
  4 ounces of tomato juice
  2 ounces of meat or fish
  Baked potato with skin
  Cooked broccoli
  Salad containing lettuce, pineapple chunks, and mayonnaise
  Ice cream and oatmeal-raisin cookies

---

stomach has been removed, the food in a regular diet reaches the jejunum in 10 to 15 minutes. The food that enters the jejunum has not been subjected to the digestive processes that normally occur in the stomach. Instead of being gradually delivered to the jejunum, large amounts of food are "dumped" quickly into the small intestine.

A delayed phase of the dumping syndrome occurs 2 to 3 hours after food intake as a result of hypoglycemia. Hypoglycemia occurs because the ingestion of sugar causes a rapid rise in the blood level of glucose, which, in turn, stimulates the release of insulin. The insulin quickly removes the glucose from the blood. This rapid removal of glucose results in hypoglycemia.

TREATMENT

The aim of treatment in the dumping syndrome is to slow gastric emptying. This goal can be accomplished by medications that slow gastric motility (cholinergic blocking agents) and by reducing the force of gravity by lying down after meals.

DIET THERAPY

The goals of diet therapy are to restore nutrition and to reduce the unpleasant symptoms of the syndrome. Patients are advised to eat frequent, small meals in preference to large meals, which would overload the reduced stomach capacity.

For absorption to take place, nutrients must be in solution; by separating fluids from meals, absorption can be slowed and symptoms of hypoglycemia reduced. Simple sugars and salty food are eliminated from the diet because they tend to draw fluid into the jejunum, causing distention of the small intestine. Simple sugars and concentrated sweets are also avoided to reduce stimulation of insulin release.

The recommended diet is usually high in protein (20%) and moderate in fat (30 to 40%), with carbohydrate supplied mainly by complex rather than simple carbohydrates. Fluids are provided between meals rather than at meal times.

NURSING IMPLICATIONS

- Counsel the patient to eat slowly, at regular intervals, and in a relaxed atmosphere.
- Caution against the ingestion of concentrated sweets.
- High-protein, unsweetened beverages may be helpful in providing nutrients and Calories.
- Some patients do not tolerate milk. This intolerance may be due to

lactase deficiency. Milk intolerance can further complicate the problem of providing adequate amounts of protein and Calories. Lean meats are usually tolerated well.

• Medications that slow gastrointestinal activity should be taken before meals.

• Cholinergic blocking agents may cause dryness of the mouth. Rinsing the mouth with water before meals may make swallowing easier.

• The importance of lying down after meals should be emphasized.

Gastritis

PATHOPHYSIOLOGY

Gastritis, inflammation of the gastric mucosa, can be caused by bacteria, viruses, food, alcohol, drugs, spices, or overeating. The mucosal response is typical of inflammation: redness, swelling, pain, and heat. The mucosa may become eroded to the point of hemorrhage. The gastric secretions become less acid and more mucoid.

TREATMENT

The treatment of gastritis involves removal of the irritating substance from the stomach and emptying of the stomach to permit the mucous lining to heal. The stomach can be emptied by vomiting or lavage. Antacids can be used to neutralize gastric secretions.

DIET THERAPY

In acute gastritis, oral feedings are usually withheld for 24 to 48 hours to rest the stomach and to avoid stimulating gastric secretions. The patient is maintained on intravenous therapy to replace fluids and electrolytes lost through vomiting and to prevent dehydration. When oral fluids are resumed, milk is often the first fluid given. A full liquid diet is then prescribed. Broths are avoided because they stimulate gastric secretions. Small, frequent feedings are recommended. The next step is a bland diet to avoid fiber and highly seasoned foods. Moderate fat intake may be permitted because fat decreases production of gastric acid and motility. Alcohol is avoided.

Chronic gastritis is treated by eliminating foods and drugs that produce symptoms. Common offenders are alcohol, caffeine, and aspirin. A bland diet may be helpful.

NURSING IMPLICATIONS

- Ice can be kept in the mouth when oral feeding is withheld, if the physician approves.
- When antacids are used, watch for constipation as a result of aluminum and calcium agents and for diarrhea as a result of magnesium agents.
- Assess the vitamin B_{12} status of patients with chronic gastritis; atrophy of gastric glands interferes with the absorption of vitamin B_{12}.

Hiatal Hernia

PATHOPHYSIOLOGY

Hiatal hernia occurs when congenital or acquired weakness of the diaphragm permits part of the stomach to herniate through the esophageal hiatus of the diaphragm, causing reflux and esophagitis.

TREATMENT

The aims of treatment are to reduce reflux and to neutralize the gastric acid to minimize irritation of the esophagus. Drug therapy options consist of cholinergic blocking agents to slow gastric emptying and antacids to neutralize gastric secretions. Anything that increases intraabdominal pressure can foster herniation of part of the stomach through the hiatus. Examples are obesity, chronic cough, straining at stool, and tight-fitting clothing. In addition to avoiding or treating these causes, the patient is advised to avoid reclining positions or physical activity after eating. The head of the bed should be elevated to reduce esophageal reflux during sleep.

Surgical correction is available for severe cases or those in which medical management fails to provide adequate relief of symptoms.

DIET THERAPY

The dietary treatment of hiatal hernia is similar to that of esophagitis. Six small feedings of a bland, fiber-restricted diet are prescribed to prevent gastric distention. Most fluid intake should be taken between meals, and fluids permitted at mealtime should be sipped.

Foods that reduce lower esophageal pressure, such as coffee and chocolate, are avoided. Fat intake is controlled because fatty meals decrease lower esophageal pressure. Fluids that irritate the esophageal mucosa, such as orange, grapefruit, and tomato juices, are eliminated from the diet. Alcohol is avoided.

NURSING IMPLICATIONS

- Patients should avoid eating within 2 hours of bedtime. Arrange the meal pattern to prevent early morning hypoglycemia, with adequate protein intake in the last meal of the day.
- Provide laxative foods to prevent constipation, which leads to straining at defecation and increased intraabdominal pressure.
- Encourage fluid intake between meals to help prevent constipation.
- Evaluate food intake for adequacy of vitamin C in the absence of citrus fruit and tomato juices.

Ileostomy

PATHOPHYSIOLOGY

An ileostomy, a surgical operation to bring the ileum through the abdominal wall, is frequently performed for intractable cases of ulcerative colitis, Crohn's disease, and carcinoma of the colon. Because an ileostomy constantly drains liquid intestinal contents, absorption of fat and vitamin B_{12} may be reduced. Losses of sodium and potassium are increased.

DIET THERAPY

The immediate postoperative dietary considerations for a patient who has had an ileostomy are discussed in Chapter 9. Ideally, the patient resumes a regular diet with minor adaptations. High-fiber foods are eliminated, and hard-to-digest kernels and seeds are avoided. Such foods as celery, corn, pineapples, turnips, beans, cabbage, onions, prunes, poppy and caraway seeds, coconuts, and popcorn are usually eliminated from the diet. Individual evaluation of the effects of other foods may result in other deletions. Adequate fluid intake is essential to replace losses in the liquid ileostomy drainage and to make up for the lack of reabsorption of fluid in the large intestine.

NURSING IMPLICATIONS

- Encourage adequate intake of fluids, especially when perspiration further increases fluid losses.

- Sodium losses can be replaced by adding salt to foods. Orange juice and bananas are good sources of potassium.
- Discourage limitation of fluid intake as a means of thickening drainage because it is ineffective and leads to dehydration.
- Diphenosylate (Lomotil) taken orally acts as a stool-thickener and deodorant (Brunner, 1976) and it may be a helpful addition to the treatment regimen if the physician permits.
- Parsley and spinach act as intestinal deodorizers. Chlorophyll and bismuth subgallate are medications that serve the same purpose.

Lactase Deficiency (Lactose Intolerance)

PATHOPHYSIOLOGY

Lactose is a disaccharide found in milk. It is hydrolyzed by the enzyme lactase into the monosaccharides glucose and galactose, which are then absorbed. With lactase deficiency, varying amounts of unhydrolyzed lactose remain in the small intestine. Lactose draws water into the intestinal lumen, creating symptoms of cramping and bloating. The unabsorbed lactose passes into the large intestine, where it is metabolized by bacteria and draws more water toward itself. This phenomenon causes continued cramping, bloating, and diarrhea.

Lactose intolerance may be present at birth, develop with maturity, or occur after damage to the small intestine. Causes of secondary lactose intolerance include gastrointestinal infections in children, antibiotic therapy, celiac disease, cystic fibrosis, ileitis, colitis, and loss of jejunal surface after subtotal gastrectomy (Newcomer, 1979).

TREATMENT

The treatment of lactase deficiency is to limit the intake of lactose to a patient's tolerance level. Lactose-hydrolyzed milk is available; it is produced by the addition of lactase derived from yeast. Lact-Aid is a commercial preparation that can be added to milk, converting lactose into saccharides that can be absorbed.

DIET THERAPY

An infant with lactase deficiency is given a soybean, meat-based, or carbohydrate-free formula. Any of the following can be used:

CHO-Free
Isomil

MBF
Nutramigen
ProSobee
Sobee

Vitamin and mineral supplementation may be necessary for the infant, and intake of calcium must be carefully evaluated.

A lactose-free diet is prescribed for patients who are unable to ingest any lactose without distress. All milk and dairy products are eliminated from the diet. Other possible sources of milk, such as breads, cakes, margarines, and processed foods, must be carefully examined to confirm that they contain no milk before they can be used. Homemade products that contain no milk or dairy products can be used safely. Organ meats are also eliminated from the diet.

Patients limit their intake of milk to fit their individual tolerance, but most can manage 4 to 8 ounces of milk per day if they drink it with meals. This combination allows for a more gradual entry of lactose into the jejunum for hydrolysis.

Fermented milk products, such as yogurt, are tolerated by some patients. Cottage cheese and aged cheddar cheese are naturally low in lactose. Lactose is used in the creaming process of some soft, smooth cheeses, however, and such cheeses should be avoided.

Cooking foods does not alter lactose. Lact-Aid-treated milk can be used in general food preparation.

NURSING IMPLICATIONS

- Patients on lactose-free diets must avoid all sources of lactose. Labels should be examined for obscure sources of milk and milk products.
- Lactose is used as a filler in some pharmaceutical products. Identification of drugs that contain lactose requires the assistance of a pharmacist; nursing drug references do not include this information.
- Lactose may be used as a processing agent in fruits, vegetables, and seasonings.
- Some foods labeled "nondairy" contain milk.
- A source of milk-free commercial products is kosher foods. The label "pareve" indicates kosher foods. All kosher meat products do not contain milk since Jewish law prohibits the eating of meat and milk in the same meal. Other processed meats may contain dry milk solids as fillers.
- Strict curtailment of milk intake can result in calcium deficiency. Cheese can become an adequate source of calcium if it is tolerated.

Food must be evaluated for calcium content and supplemented as indicated.

- Breast milk contains more lactose than does cow's milk, so breast feeding is contraindicated in infants with congenital lactose intolerance.

Peptic Ulcer

PATHOPHYSIOLOGY

A peptic ulcer is an erosion of the mucous membrane of the stomach, pylorus, or duodenum. An ulcer may extend through the muscle layers to the peritoneum. Peptic ulcers occur only in areas of the gastrointestinal tract that are in contact with hydrochloric acid and pepsin. Peptic ulcers develop because of increased acidity of gastric juices, increased secretion of gastric juices, or decreased protection of the mucosal lining due to decreased secretion of mucus and buffering action.

TREATMENT

The goals of treatment are to decrease gastric acidity, to decrease pyloroduodenal motility, and to increase the resistance of the mucosa to hydrochloric acid and pepsin. Treatment attempts to relieve pain, to heal the erosion, and to prevent recurrences. The therapy usually includes rest, antacids, and anticholinergic medications. Treatment also includes the elimination or control of predisposing factors, including excessive smoking, excessive intake of coffee and colas, overuse of aspirin, irregular meals, hurried meals, and stress.

DIET THERAPY

The traditional dietary modifications for ulcer treatment have not been supported by research. The latest diets used in ulcer therapy contain minimal food restrictions and emphasize, instead, the size and regularity of feedings. The Sippy diet has fallen into disfavor. This diet consists of hourly milk and cream feedings, with antacids administered on the half-hours. Milk and cream were thought to neutralize acid and to coat and protect the mucosa. Milk, however, stimulates secretion of acids because of its protein and calcium content.

Patients with ulcers used to progress from milk and cream to soft creamed foods to a bland diet. Roughage was eliminated from the diet of such patients because it was believed to irritate the mucosa. Research has shown that roughage does not delay ulcer healing (McKechnie, 1978). It has even been suggested that fiber might provide protection for the mucosa through its buffering action. Spices were routinely omitted from ulcer diets but present data suggest that normal amounts do not delay ulcer healing (McKechnie, 1978). Pepper, chili powder, mustard, and nutmeg are spices that patients with ulcers should still avoid.

The most acidic foods were also eliminated from the diets of patients with ulcers, but even the most acidic foods, namely, lime juice, egg whites, and graham crackers, are not as acid as gastric juice (pH 1.6). Orange and grapefruit juices (pH 3.2 to 3.6) are eliminated from the diet only if oral or esophageal lesions are present. Diluting these juices does not make them acceptable in these instances.

The present-day diet for patients with ulcers is usually an individualized modification of a regular diet. Such patients are taught that eating small meals at regular times is more important than following a rigid diet. Some food restrictions have been supported by research and continue to be accepted. Alcohol is avoided because it damages the mucosa. Concentrated meat soups and extracts stimulate secretion of gastric juices and are avoided. Coffee (regular and decaffeinated), tea, and colas also increase secretion of gastric juices and should be omitted from the diets of such patients. Patients should avoid any food that causes them discomfort.

Food acts as a buffer and protects the mucosa; frequent feedings keep food in the stomach and increase the protection of the stomach lining. Distention increases secretion of gastric juices, so meals should be kept small. Regularity of meals prevents periods in which there is no food to buffer the gastric acid.

NURSING IMPLICATIONS

- Patients who are accustomed to traditional diets may have difficulty accepting the liberalized diet. Explain the rationale for the changes.
- Evaluate the diet for adequacy of essential nutrients after individual changes have been incorporated.
- Stress the importance of laxative foods if constipating antacids are prescribed.
- Bedtime feedings may be omitted if they cause pain during the night. A bedtime dose of a cholinergic blocking agent may be helpful in delaying gastric emptying (Brunner, 1976).

Regional Enteritis (Crohn's Disease)

PATHOPHYSIOLOGY

Regional enteritis is a chronic inflammatory process that can occur anywhere in the gastrointestinal tract. Granulomas formed as the result of inflammation thicken the walls of the involved areas and reduce the lumen of the intestine. Peristaltic waves stimulated by intake of food cause cramping pain. Chronic diarrhea results from ulcers and inflammatory edema.

TREATMENT

Acute attacks of diarrhea are treated by fluid and electrolyte replacement. Antidiarrheal agents or sulfasalazine (Azulfidine) may be used. Corticosteroids that are frequently used in other inflammatory conditions are ineffective. Surgical resection or bypass may be used in patients with hemorrhage.

DIET THERAPY

A low-residue diet that is high in Calories, animal proteins, and vitamins is usually prescribed. Reduced intake of residue is recommended because residue causes pain in the area of constricted lumen; reduced intake of residue lessens mechanical irritation and provides rest. The increased intake of Calories, high-biologic-value proteins, and vitamins promotes healing and corrects the malnutrition that results from reduced intake of food and from diarrheal losses. See Table 6-4 for an example of a minimal-residue diet.

Intake of fat can be limited if steatorrhea is present. Medium-chain triglycerides may be used as a source of absorbable fat and Calories. Increased amounts of vitamins C and B_{12} are needed for healing and blood building. Parenteral vitamin C can be used if absorption is faulty. Iron intake should be increased to replace blood losses and correct anemia.

Elemental diet formulas may be used. These formulas are easy to digest and absorb and leave a minimal amount of residue to be excreted. Various products are available that differ in their sources of protein, carbohydrate, and fat. All these products meet the RDAs for vitamins and minerals if sufficient amounts are used. Some contain medium-chain triglycerides that can be used in the presence of steatorrhea. Lactose-free formulas are available if lactose intolerance is present.

Total parenteral nutrition can also be used if complete rest of the intestine is necessary. The solution used is designed to meet the individual needs of the patient.

NURSING IMPLICATIONS

- Patients need encouragement to eat because they recognize the relationship between food intake and discomfort.
- Milk and milk products are usually omitted from the diet due to their contribution of residue and lactose.

TABLE 6-4
MINIMAL-RESIDUE DIET

Breakfast
  4 ounces of orange juice
  ½ cup of cornflakes with 3 ounces of milk
  1 hard-boiled egg
  1 slice of white toast with margarine and jelly
  1 cup of black coffee
Lunch
  1 cup of chicken broth
  4 ounces of sliced chicken
  ½ cup of mashed potato
  5 stalks of cooked asparagus
  Plain cake
  Cooked apricots
  1 cup of tea
Dinner
  4 ounces of ground lamb
  1 baked potato without skin
  ½ cup of cooked beets
  ½ cup of green beans
  1 slice of white bread
  Plain cookies
  Ice cream

• When sulfasalazine (Azulfidine) therapy is used, fluids should be increased to 2,500 milliliters per day.
• Seasonings are usually poorly tolerated and should be avoided.
• Intake of potassium should be increased during periods of diarrhea.
• Elemental diets are apt to be unpalatable and poorly accepted. Fruit juices can be added to improve taste.
• The recommendation to serve elemental formulas chilled or over ice must be evaluated in relation to the poor tolerance of chilled foods.

Spastic Colon (Irritable Bowel Syndrome)

PATHOPHYSIOLOGY

Spastic colon is a functional disorder in which the nerve endings of the bowel are stimulated excessively, causing irregular and uncoordinated motility, which results in constipation and diarrhea. Stress appears to be a strong contributing factor. Spastic colon has also been related to excessive use of laxatives, tobacco, alcohol, tea, and coffee. It can follow gastrointestinal upset and antibiotic therapy. It appears to be associated with poor health habits, such as lack of regularity in rest, fluid intake, and bowel evacuation.

TREATMENT

The treatment of spastic colon is designed to help the patient cope with stress and to develop good health habits.

DIET THERAPY

The recommended diet is a regular diet with added fiber. Treatment may need to start with a low-residue diet to which fiber is added gradually. An elemental diet may be necessary in patients with acute symptoms.

NURSING IMPLICATIONS

- Fiber should be added gradually to prevent discomfort.
- Increased intake of fluid is essential with a high-fiber diet.
- Planning a regular time for bowel evacuation is important.
- Counseling about how to cope with stress may be helpful.

Tropical Sprue

PATHOPHYSIOLOGY

The villi of the small intestinal mucosa become blunted or obliterated in tropical sprue. This change results in a reduction of the absorptive area and malabsorption of certain nutrients.

TREATMENT

The treatment of tropical sprue is folic acid. Tropical sprue does not respond to a gluten-free diet. Fat-soluble vitamins and iron are also prescribed to correct the deficiencies that are usually present.

DIET THERAPY

A regular diet with vitamin B_{12} and folic acid sources is usually prescribed. Sufficient amounts of Calories, protein, iron, and vitamins are included. In the early phase of treatment, a high-protein, low-carbohydrate, low-fat diet may be used until absorption improves. The carbohydrate component of the diet should consist of simple sugars and nonstarchy vegetables. The fat component should include easy-to-digest fats, which may be most easily provided by the use of medium-chain triglycerides.

NURSING IMPLICATIONS

- Patients may need help in differentiating between tropical and non-tropical sprue and may need to know why they are allowed gluten.
- Lactase deficiency may occur with tropical sprue.
- Good sources of folic acid include liver, kidney, yeast, leafy green vegetables, lean beef, eggs, and whole grains.
- Good sources of vitamin B_{12} are meats, poultry, fish, dairy products, and eggs.

Ulcerative Colitis

PATHOPHYSIOLOGY

In ulcerative colitis, there is widespread ulceration, inflammation, and loss of epithelium in the colon. This disease, which has periods of exacerbations and remissions, follows an upward path from the rectum and can eventually involve the entire colon.

TREATMENT

The treatment of ulcerative colitis includes rest, sedation, and antidiarrheal medications. Antibacterial drugs such as sulfasalazine (Azulfidine) may be used for secondary infections of the ulcerated areas. Corticosteroid therapy may also be used. Surgical removal of the colon with an ileostomy may be indicated if medical treatment fails.

DIET THERAPY

The aim of diet therapy is to restore the patient to normal nutritional status by preventing further losses and by correcting deficiencies that have occurred. An elemental formula diet may be used initially. A bland, high-protein (125 to 150 grams), high-Calorie (2,500 to 3,500 kcal), low-residue diet may also be used.

Dairy products are usually eliminated from the diet because secondary lactose intolerance is likely to be present. Milk is also a medium-residue food. Intravenous fluids and electrolytes may be used to correct losses due to diarrhea.

NURSING IMPLICATIONS

- Lactose-free elemental diets should be prescribed if lactose intolerance is an associated problem.
- Avoid foods that the patient identifies as aggravating diarrhea.
- Anorexia is a symptom of ulcerative colitis. Every nursing strategy that makes meals attractive and mealtimes pleasant should be used.
- The diet should contain a minimum of undigestible carbohydrate and no tough meats.
- Frequent, small meals may increase total nutritional intake.
- Eating stimulates peristalsis, and the patient may need to defecate at mealtime. When the patient has to defecate, the food should be removed and returned only when the patient and environment are ready. Every effort should be made to have the food at the proper temperature when the tray is returned.
- Iced or carbonated beverages may stimulate peristalsis and should be avoided.
- Sodium and fluid restriction may be prescribed for patients with fluid retention due to corticosteroid therapy.
- Fluid retention may be mistaken for improved nutrition when weight gain occurs.
- Fluid intake to at least 2,500 milliliters per day is an important adjunct to sulfasalazine (Azulfidine) therapy.

Gallbladder Disease

PATHOPHYSIOLOGY

Cholelithiasis is the formation of stones in the gallbladder. Such stones are usually composed of cholesterol, calcium, bilirubin, and inorganic salts. The stones may obstruct the bile passages, causing biliary colic. Cholecystitis is inflammation of the gallbladder. The presence of fat in the small intestine stimulates the gallbladder to contract and release bile. When stones or inflammation is present, this contraction causes pain.

TREATMENT

The treatment of gallbladder disease involves relief of symptoms and removal of the obstruction. Chenodeoxycholic acid and lithium dissolve small stones and prevent new stones from forming if taken daily for 6 months. Surgical removal of stones or the gallbladder is the treatment of acute obstruction or chronic inflammation.

DIET THERAPY

The dietary treatment of gallbladder disease is related to restriction of fat intake to prevent gallbladder contraction and pain. In acute gallbladder attacks, intravenous fluids and electrolytes may be used to replace losses from vomiting and to maintain the gallbladder at rest. A fat-free diet may be permitted; skim milk is used as the protein source, and fruit juices and gelatin are given as sources of carbohydrate.

The diet usually progresses to one that contains plain foods and avoids rich, fatty, and gas-forming foods. Condiments and highly seasoned foods are also eliminated from the diet since they cause distention and increase peristalsis, which irritates the gallbladder. Intake of fat is restricted. Milk and butter are usually tolerated.

Chronic gallbladder disease is usually treated with a low-fat diet. Fat is usually limited to one-half of the total Calories; some fat is necessary to stimulate gallbladder drainage. Protein intake is normal, and the carbohydrate intake is normal or reduced if weight loss is desirable. Increased intake of carbohydrate aids in the resolution of jaundice.

After surgical removal of the gallbladder, intake of fat is restricted for a few months, then gradually increased to the amount tolerated by the patient. See Table 6-5 for an example of a low-fat diet.

TABLE 6-5
LOW-FAT DIET

Breakfast
  4 ounces of orange juice
  ½ cup of any cereal, except granola-type that contains coconut and nuts
  4 ounces of skim milk
  1 slice of toast with jelly
  1 cup of black coffee
Lunch
  6 ounces of tomato juice
  4 ounces of sliced chicken
  Lettuce and tomato salad with lemon juice or vinegar
  Whole-wheat crackers
  8 ounces of skim milk
  Fresh fruit
Dinner
  4 ounces of clear broth
  4 ounces of baked fish
  4 stalks of broccoli with lemon juice
  ½ cup of parslied carrots
  ½ cup of tapioca pudding, made with skim milk
  Angel cake
  Black coffee or tea with lemon

NURSING IMPLICATIONS

- Patients who have suffered from gallbladder disease for any period are usually well aware of the foods that cause them discomfort. Input from the patient in planning the diet will ensure that such foods are avoided and that alternative sources of essential nutrients are included.
- If bile drainage is collected and refed to the patient as part of the treatment regimen, it should be strained, chilled, and served in apple or grape juice. Reference to the source of bile should be avoided.
- Evaluate the diet for adequacy of intake of fat-soluble vitamins.
- Provide guidance in the methods of food preparation. Frying of foods should be avoided.

Pancreatitis

PATHOPHYSIOLOGY

Inflammation of the pancreas (pancreatitis) is related to many etiologic factors that result in obstruction of the pancreatic secretions and their accumulation in the pancreas. Because these pancreatic juices contain proteolytic enzymes, autodigestion and destruction of the pancreatic cells can occur.

TREATMENT

Edematous pancreatitis is a self-limiting disease; treatment is supportive. Analgesia is used to relieve pain until symptoms subside. Hemorrhagic pancreatitis is a medical emergency, and treatment is directed toward the prevention or treatment of shock and renal shutdown. Secretion of pancreatic juices is inhibited by cholinergic blocking agents, and antacids are used to neutralize gastric juices. Chronic pancreatitis is treated by analgesia and oral replacement of pancreatic enzymes.

DIET THERAPY

The aim of dietary treatment in pancreatitis is to inhibit the activation and secretion of pancreatic enzymes. Both food and alcohol stimulate pancreatic secretions. Fat stimulates the flow of bile, which can regurgitate into the pancreatic ducts and cause irritation.

In severe pancreatitis, the patient is not given anything by mouth because the absence of food inhibits secretion of pancreatic juices. The use of nasogastric suction further reduces the amount of pancreatic secretions. Intravenous feedings or total parenteral nutrition are used during the nothing-by-mouth phase of treatment. The initial oral diet is usually clear liquids; amino acids and predigested fat can be added gradually to the diet. Medium-chain triglycerides are usually well tolerated as a source of fat and Calories. Gradually, the patient progresses to six small, bland meals that are low in fat and easy to digest and that contain foods that will not stimulate the pancreas. Chronic pancreatitis also necessitates the use of a diet that reduces pancreatic stimuli. Fat digestion is assisted by the use of pancreatic enzymes given by mouth with food.

NURSING IMPLICATIONS

- Alcohol is completely eliminated from the diet because it is frequently involved in the causation of pancreatitis and is known to increase the resistance of the sphincter of Oddi and increase obstruction to flow of pancreatic enzymes.
- Caffeine is also avoided. Coffee, tea, cocoa, and cola beverages are common dietary sources of caffeine.
- Hypocalcemia may be an associated problem because calcium may be deposited in the areas of fat necrosis in the pancreas. Assess the patient for signs of tetany.
- Evaluate the patient for signs of diabetes mellitus; some islet involvement may occur.
- Pancreatin (pancreatic enzyme) is available in granule or tablet form. Because pancreatin contains enzymes, it must be administered in a manner that prevents enzyme destruction. Capsules and tablets should be swallowed whole. These medications should not be given with hot foods or liquids because the heat may destroy the protective coating.
- Pancreatin should be taken only with meals.

Hepatitis

PATHOPHYSIOLOGY

Inflammation of the liver can result in destruction of liver cells. The liver is normally capable of regeneration of destroyed cells. Excessive destruction of liver tissue interferes with the liver's varied and extensive functions, which include:

- Secretion and excretion of bile
- Multiple conversions of carbohydrates, proteins, and fats
- Production, storage, and release of glucose

- Conversion of ammonia to urea
- Synthesis of albumin
- Storage of vitamins and iron
- Detoxification of drugs and other foreign substances
- Production of prothrombin and fibrinogen for blood clotting
- Storage and filtration of blood

TREATMENT

The aims of treatment are to prevent further injury to the liver and to provide rest to allow the liver to regenerate cells. Removal of causative agents, such as alcohol or drugs, is indicated. Symptomatic treatment is related to specific problems that arise when the liver is unable to carry out some of its functions.

DIET THERAPY

In patients with vomiting, intravenous glucose is used to provide Calories. A 5 to 10% solution of glucose may be used. Amino acids may be given intravenously as a source of proteins; plasma or albumin may also be used.

A concentrated liquid formula can be used orally or through a feeding tube to provide a high-Calorie (3,000 to 4,000 kcal) diet. The usual components of the diet include generous intake of carbohydrate (300 to 400 grams) to promote synthesis and storage of glycogen and to spare protein for repair of liver tissue. High intake of protein (1.5 to 2 grams per kilogram of body weight) is prescribed for regeneration of tissue. The intake of fat need not be restricted if adequate amounts of carbohydrates and proteins are provided. Fat increases both the palatability and caloric value of the diet. Vitamin B supplementation, particularly with thiamine, which aids in the metabolism of carbohydrates, proteins, fats, and vitamin B_{12}, normally stored in the liver, is indicated. Vitamin K is given to counteract bleeding tendencies.

Progression is to an oral diet of frequent, small feedings of the above components. High-Calorie feedings between meals are needed to meet the desired intake without excessive food volume at any one time. Dry skim milk can be added to foods and beverages to increase intake of proteins and Calories. The liberal use of butter and margarine also increases caloric intake.

NURSING IMPLICATIONS

- Alcohol is eliminated from the diet because of its toxic effect on the liver. Abstinence for 4 to 6 months after recovery is usually recommended.

• Drugs must be used with caution in patients with hepatitis. Nursing measures to promote comfort and induce rest may reduce the need for sedatives. Warm milk beverages at bedtime may promote sleep.

Cirrhosis

PATHOPHYSIOLOGY

When the liver is unable to regenerate cells after their destruction, the cells are replaced by fibrous, nonfunctioning connective tissue. Cirrhosis is the final stage of many types of liver injury, including alcoholism and toxic and viral hepatitides.

TREATMENT

The aims of treatment in cirrhosis are to support residual liver function and to prevent further cell destruction. Alcohol or other responsible toxins are eliminated from the diet. Infections are prevented, treated, or controlled. Supportive treatment is provided for disabling symptoms, such as ascites, esophageal varices, and renal failure.

DIET THERAPY

A patient whose cirrhosis is related to alcoholism usually has a long history of poor nutrition. Adequate intake of food has been replaced by alcohol, which interferes with the absorption of thiamine, vitamin B_{12}, folic acid, and vitamin C. As the absorption of these vitamins decreases, the need for B vitamins to metabolize the alcohol increases. Magnesium deficiency is often an associated problem because alcohol increases excretion of magnesium.

A high-Calorie, high-protein, high-carbohydrate diet is the usual prescription. Intake of protein should consist of high-biologic-value proteins and should be rich in the amino acids methionine and choline. Methionine and choline metabolize fat in the liver and reduce fatty infiltration of the organ. Good sources of methionine and choline include egg yolk, legumes, organ meats, milk, muscle meats, and whole grain. Intake of protein is balanced between increased need for liver regeneration and limitation to avoid precipitation of hepatic coma. Moderate intake of fat is permitted in patients in whom intake of proteins and carbohydrates is adequate. Medium-chain triglycerides may be used to supply fat in the diet; however, they should not be used in advanced cases of cirrhosis. Intake of fat is also reduced in the presence of steatorrhea, which accompanies cirrhosis in about one-half of cases.

Hepatic-Aid, a mixture of amino acids, carbohydrates, and fats, is used as a nitrogen and Calorie supplement for patients with severe hepatic insufficiency secondary to cirrhosis. Hepatic-Aid must be supplemented with vitamins, minerals, and electrolytes because it is nutritionally incomplete. Supplied as a powder that is reconstituted before use, Hepatic-Aid can be given orally or by tube feeding. When given by mouth, it should be sipped slowly; however, it is unpalatable and is frequently given by tube.

The presence of ascites may dictate the need to limit intake of sodium and fluid. Low-sodium milk may be used, but protein intake must be carefully planned because eggs and meats are also high in sodium.

NURSING IMPLICATIONS

- Anorexia, nausea, vomiting, and diarrhea may interfere with the diet plan.
- Patients with advanced cirrhosis tend to have a better appetite in the morning. Plan a big breakfast.
- The dietary intake must be adjusted to the changing status of the patient's condition.
- Frequent, small meals may be less distressing in patients with ascites. Large meals increase portal pressure.
- Tube feedings are helpful in increasing intake but must be avoided in patients with esophageal varices.
- Coarse or fibrous foods are avoided when esophageal varices are present because they are mechanical irritants. Chemical irritation of varices is reduced by avoiding coffee, tea, pepper, and chili powder. All food should be well chewed.
- Liquid diet formulas that contain medium-chain triglycerides are not too palatable and are best accepted when served in small, chilled servings.
- Appetites tend to improve as deficiencies are corrected and the appropriate nutrients consumed.
- The addition of honey, vanilla, or maple flavoring may increase the palatability of low-sodium milk.

Hepatic Coma: Hepatic Encephalopathy

PATHOPHYSIOLOGY

Hepatic coma is a stupor that results from cerebral damage due to degeneration of liver cells.

Blood levels of ammonia rise when there is severe liver damage or when blood bypasses the liver through collateral circulation or surgical shunts. The liver is unable to convert ammonia to urea in these situations. Elevated serum levels of ammonia have a toxic effect on brain cells, producing central nervous system and psychiatric disturbances.

TREATMENT

The aim of treatment is to reduce the protein concentration in the intestine. Protein is the precursor of ammonia. Intake of proteins and bleeding lead to the appearance of protein in the intestines. Ammonia is also produced by bacterial action within the intestines. Treatment consists of antibiotic therapy to destroy intestinal bacteria, lactulose to decrease formation of ammonia, levodopa to relieve psychiatric symptoms, and enemas to remove blood and protein from the bowel.

DIET THERAPY

Intake of protein may be eliminated or severely restricted, depending on the serum level of ammonia. Protein restriction is imposed for as short a period as possible because the protein is needed for regeneration of liver cells. Intake of protein is gradually increased as the patient improves. The serum level of ammonia is used as the criterion for increasing the protein intake. Foods that have a dramatic influence on the serum level of ammonia are avoided. Examples are cheeses, meats, and vegetables. Lactulose (a five-carbon sugar) or neomycin may be used to decrease absorption of ammonia.

NURSING IMPLICATIONS

- Milk and eggs produce less ammonia than do meats.
- Thirty to 40 grams of high-biologic-value proteins are needed every day for a positive nitrogen balance in an otherwise adequate diet.
- Tube feedings or parenteral nutrition is necessary when the patient is in coma; intake of proteins can be appropriately controlled in these forms of nutrition.
- The proteins with the most ammoniagenic potential are the group A amino acids, most of which are nonessential amino acids.

References

Blackburn, G., Williams, L., Biotrian, B. New approaches to the management of severe acute pancreatitis. *The American Journal of Surgery*, January 1976, *131*, 1.

Broitman, S., & Zamcheck, N. Nutrition in diseases of the intestines. In R. Goodhart & M. Shils (Eds.), *Modern nutrition in health and disease* (6th ed.). Philadelphia: Lea & Febiger, 1980.

Brunner, L. What to do (and what to teach your patient) about peptic ulcer. *Nursing 76*, November 1976, *6*, 11.

Brunner, L., & Suddarth, D. *Textbook of medical-surgical nursing* (4th ed.). Philadelphia: J. B. Lippincott Company, 1980.

Castell, D., & Frank, B. How to treat heartburn with diet therapy. *Nutrition Today*, May/June 1979, *14*, 3.

Davidson, C. Nutrition in disease of the liver. In R. Goodhart & M. Shils (Eds.), *Modern nutrition in health and disease* (6th ed.). Philadelphia: Lea & Febiger, 1980.

Dhar, P., Zamcheck, N., & Broitman, S. Nutrition in diseases of the pancreas. In R. Goodhart & M. Shils (Eds.), *Modern Nutrition in health and disease* (6th ed.). Philadelphia: Lea & Febiger, 1980.

Fein, H. Nutrition in diseases of the stomach, including related areas in the esophagus and duodenum. In R. Goodhart & M. Shils (Eds.), *Modern nutrition in health and disease* (6th ed.). Philadelphia: Lea & Febiger, 1980.

Greenburg, J. Why your hospitalized patient won't eat. *Consultant*, September 1979, *19*, 9.

Heaton, K. W. The real value of fiber. *Consultant*, August 1979, *19*, 8.

Howe, P. *Basic Nutrition in health and disease* (6th ed.). Philadelphia: W. B. Saunders Company, 1976.

Katz, J. Who needs a milk-free or gluten-free diet—And why. *Consultant*, July 1977, *17*, 7.

Krause, M., & Mahan, L. *Food, nutrition and diet therapy* (6th ed.). Philadelphia: W. B. Saunders Company, 1979.

Luckmann, J., & Sorensen, K. *Medical-surgical nursing: A psychophysiologic approach* (2nd ed.). Philadelphia: W. B. Saunders Company, 1980.

Luke, B. *Case studies in therapeutic nutrition*. Boston: Little, Brown & Company, 1977.

Massachusetts General Hospital Dietary Department. *Diet manual*. Boston: Little, Brown & Company, 1976.

Mayer, J. *Health*. New York: D. Van Nostrand Company, 1974.

McKechnie, J. Diverticular disease and diet. *Consultant*, July 1976, *16*, 7.

McKechnie, J. Outdated and updated diets for G.I. disease. *Consultant*, September 1978, *18*, 9.

Mitchell, H., Rynbergen, H., Anderson, L., et al. *Nutrition in health and disease* (16th ed.). Philadelphia: J. B. Lippincott Company, 1976.

Murray, C., Herbold, N., & Howard, R. The gastrointestinal system. In R. Howard & N. Herbold, *Nutrition in clinical care*. New York: McGraw-Hill Book Company, 1978.

Myer, S. The chronic threat of Crohn's disease. *RN*, November 1978, *41*, 11.

Newcomer, A. Lactase deficiency. *Contemporary Nutrition*, April 1979, *4*, 4.

Robinson, C., & Lawler, M. *Normal and therapeutic nutrition* (15th ed.). New York: Macmillan Publishing Company, 1977.

Rosenberg, F. Lactose intolerance. *American Journal of Nursing*, May 1977, *77*, 5.

Thiele, V. *Clinical nutrition*. St. Louis: C. V. Mosby Company, 1976.

7
Diet Therapy in Blood Conditions

The body depends on food intake to provide the materials needed for red blood cell production (erythropoiesis). A well-balanced diet provides the following essential nutrients for the manufacture of red blood cells:

- Iron, vitamin B_6 (pyridoxine), and copper for synthesis of hemoglobin
- Folic acid and vitamin B_{12} (cyanocobalamin) for maturation of red blood cells
- Protein for globulin formation
- Vitamin C (ascorbic acid) to aid in absorption of iron

Iron Deficiency Anemia

PATHOPHYSIOLOGY

Iron deficiency anemia occurs as a result of inadequate intake or impaired absorption of iron, blood loss, or repeated pregnancies. When iron deficiency anemia occurs as the result of poor diet or interference with absorption, it may take years to produce symptoms in an adult with normal body stores of iron. This delay is the result of the body's limited excretion of iron. Infants, 6 to 12 months of age, who have little stored iron would suffer from iron deficiency anemia more quickly. Other people of any age with minimal stores of iron or superimposed blood loss would exhibit symptoms in a shorter period on an iron-deficient diet.

ʻThe function of iron in the body is to enter into the formation of hemoglobin. Hemoglobin is intimately involved in the transport of oxygen to all body cells. Iron is also needed to manufacture enzymes that

100

control cellular oxidation. About 90% of the body's iron is reused; dietary intake has to replace only the minimal daily losses that occur through the sweat, urine, and feces. In addition to the iron lost in the sweat, urine, and feces, a menstruating woman loses an average of 30 milligrams of iron per menstrual period.

Iron is poorly absorbed in the body, and much of the iron ingested is excreted unabsorbed. A healthy adult absorbs only about 10% of the dietary intake. Because iron becomes more soluble in an acid medium, an ample secretion of hydrochloric acid in the stomach favors absorption of iron in the duodenum and jejunum. A small amount of iron is absorbed in the stomach. Iron is absorbed only in the ferrous state. When iron in excess of the body's needs is absorbed, it can be stored. The major storage areas are the liver, bone marrow, and spleen.

The body has no mechanism for the excretion of excess iron. The rate of absorption varies in relation to need. An iron-deficient person absorbs more iron than does a person with adequate iron stores.

TREATMENT

The most efficient and effective treatment of iron deficiency anemia is to provide iron by means of drug therapy. Oral iron should be the ferrous salt for the best absorption. Parenteral iron preparations are available when oral therapy is inappropriate or ineffective.

DIET THERAPY

Diet therapy can be an important adjunct to the medication. Diet therapy also provides information on food habits that could be effective in preventing recurrences once the drug regimen is discontinued. A well-balanced diet should provide sufficient iron for most people. However, during certain periods of life, iron requirements are increased, and the diet needs to be altered appropriately. See Table 7-1 for the iron requirements at various ages.

The diet of an adult American is estimated to provide 12 to 18 milligrams of iron per day on the average. The populations at risk for iron deficiency anemia are:

Infants, especially those from 6 to 12 months of age

Adolescent girls

Menstruating women

Pregnant women

An infant's diet is composed primarily of milk or a milklike formula, with the gradual addition of solid foods. Pediatricians vary in their directions for the solid food additions to the diet. Cereals and fruits tend to be

TABLE 7-1
DAILY DIETARY REQUIREMENTS FOR IRON
(ASSUMING 10% ABSORPTION)

Infants	5–15 milligrams
Children	4–10 milligrams
Adolescent girls	10–27 milligrams
Adolescent boys	10–20 milligrams
Men	6.5–13 milligrams
Menstruating women	7–23 milligrams
Nonmenstruating women	6–9 milligrams
Pregnant women	16.5–35 milligrams[a]

[a]The requirement for pregnant women cannot be met by diet alone; iron supplementation is indicated.

early choices. Mothers vary in their ability to follow the dietary instructions because of their limited understanding or limited budget. Consequently, the amount of dietary iron that infants receive varies considerably. An infant's diet should be carefully assessed, and emphasis should be placed on the use of iron-rich foods or enriched foods and formulas. (See Chapter 21 for more detail on the dietary needs in infancy.)

Adolescent girls are apt to become iron-deficient due to a combination of inadequate diet and menstrual losses. Many teenage girls resort to fad or "quickie" diets in an attempt to attain or maintain a slim figure. The food selections of the adolescent outside the home are not apt to contain iron-rich foods.

Pregnancy places a heavy requirement for iron on the maternal diet. The iron requirements in pregnancy cannot be met by diet alone, and supplemental iron is needed. However, a woman who begins pregnancy with an adequate body supply of iron and continues to eat iron-rich foods not only needs less supplemental iron but is maintaining good habits for after delivery.

A woman could lose iron in the menstrual discharge for roughly 30 years. Pregnancy, although curtailing menses, does not reduce iron needs but, in fact, increases them greatly. The importance of an iron-rich diet for women seems obvious. Thirty years of supplemental iron is not only expensive but also unnecessary. These years of a woman's life are also years when the demands on her energy and vitality are great; she cannot afford the fatigue and listlessness of even borderline iron deficiency anemia. Even though iron in its ferrous form is not an expensive drug, the cost of a 30-year supply could be considerable. The price of some of the multivitamin and mineral supplements, particularly those advertised especially for menstruating women, is a great deal more than that of a simple iron medication. Diet therapy can be used as a supportive measure during drug therapy and prophylactically during periods of increased need.

The rich food sources of iron tend to have a distinct flavor and are not staples in the North American diet. Liver, the most touted source, is disliked by many people because of its flavor, texture, aroma, or association. Parsley and molasses are usually dismissed as impractical sources because of the limited amounts used in the average diet. Legumes are not used to the degree that their nutritional qualities merit (see Table 7-2).

Planning an iron-rich diet that would be acceptable to most people or, better still, most families is a challenge. The starting point should be an assessment of present food intake, including a list of food likes and aversions. The cultural background and economic status of the family influence the diet. The diet should then be revised to increase the iron intake to the desired level. If liver is acceptable to the family, increased use could be suggested. Gourmet recipes are available, and variety in preparation could double the weekly intake of liver without changing the family's habits unduly. However, if liver and other organ meats are never eaten by the family, it is useless to suggest them; other foods should be selected to increase the iron in the diet.*

A traditional New England favorite, baked beans and brown bread, is rich in iron. One-half cup of beans prepared with molasses and pork contains 2.3 milligrams of iron; two slices of brown bread contain 1.9 milligrams of iron. Slow cooking in an iron pot could increase the iron content of the beans, and raisins could be added to the brown bread. The enrichment of flour, breads, and cereals is another aid in the selection of iron-rich foods. The homemaker who enjoys cooking can find many ways of increasing the iron content of foods: the substitution of molasses for sugar, the addition of parsley to soups, sauces, salads, vegetables, and casseroles, and the use of iron cookware.

TABLE 7-2
FOODS WITH HIGH IRON CONTENT

Food	Milligrams of Iron per 100 Grams
3½ ounces of calf's liver	14.2
3½ ounces of beef kidney	13.1
5 large clams	7.5
⅝ cup of chopped parsley	6.0
5 tablespoons of molasses	4.5
8 large, uncooked prunes	4.4
⅝ cup of raisins	3.5
½ cup of dried beans cooked	2.7
½ cup of dried peas cooked	1.7

*The most highly bioavailable food sources of iron include lean red meats, leafy, deep-green vegetables, whole grains, and enriched breads and cereals.

Parsley, used mainly for decoration, is often left uneaten. Parsley imparts such a mild flavor to foods that it could be used liberally to increase the iron content of the family diet. Spaghetti sauce and pizza are two favorites that could be used as vehicles for parsley. A recent prize-winning recipe for zucchini pie has one-half cup of parsley as one of the ingredients. In terms of economy, parsley plants grown on the windowsill provide an inexpensive, readily available source of iron.

The simple act of cooking foods in larger pieces in smaller amounts of water reduces the amount of iron lost in food preparation. Steaming foods is an ideal way to conserve iron and other nutrients. The use of fruit pulp, meat drippings, and unpeeled potatoes conserves some of the iron usually lost from these foods.

The use of iron cookware can have a substantial impact on the iron content of foods, especially acid foods that are cooked for long periods. The iron content of 100 grams of spaghetti sauce cooked for 3 hours in a glass container is 3 milligrams, as compared to 87.5 milligrams when the same sauce is cooked in an iron pan. Other foods cooked for shorter periods show smaller increases, but all have at least double their original iron content. Scrambled eggs show a 40% increase in iron content when prepared in an iron skillet. The initial cost of investing in an iron skillet and Dutch oven for the family seeking sources of iron would seem worthwhile. See Table 7-3 for an example of a diet that uses some alternative sources of iron.

NURSING IMPLICATIONS

- Patients undergoing iron therapy should be instructed to expect changes in the color of their stools. The usual bowel movements are described as tarry or black.
- Iron is more soluble in acid; optimal absorption occurs when the stomach is empty. However, gastric irritation is a common side effect of iron therapy that can be alleviated by taking the medication with meals. A gradual increase in dosage until the prescribed amount is given can also be helpful in alleviating gastric irritation.
- A diet high in bulk reduces iron absorption.
- Low gastric acidity as a result of achlorhydria or a high alkaline intake (antacids) reduces iron absorption. Older people tend to have achlorhydria.
- Ingestion of clay (geophagia) reduces absorption of iron. Clay and starch are intentionally ingested during pregnancy in some areas and in some cultures.
- Phosphates, oxylates, phylates, and cellulose inhibit iron absorption. However, when there is adequate calcium in the diet to unite with

TABLE 7-3

AN EXAMPLE OF AN IRON-RICH DIET THAT EXCLUDES SOME OF THE RICHEST
SOURCES OF IRON

Diet	Iron Content in Milligrams
Breakfast	
Orange juice, including pulp[a]	0.04
Enriched cereal with strawberries[a]	2.2
½ cup of milk for cereal	0.1
Scrambled eggs, cooked in iron skillet	4.1
Lunch	
½ grapefruit[a]	0.4
Tuna salad sandwich on whole-wheat bread (1 tablespoon of parsley in salad)	2.4
Oatmeal cookies (made with molasses and raisins)	1.2
1 cup of milk	0.2
Dinner	
½ cup of tomato juice[a]	0.9
90 grams of beef	2.7
2 large stalks broccoli	1.5
Baked potato with 1 ounce of cheese and 1 tablespoonful parsley	1.2
Lettuce and tomato salad with mayonnaise[a]	2.5
Whole wheat roll	0.5
Gingerbread	1.6
Total iron content	21.5

[a]A source of ascorbic acid is included at every meal to aid in the absorption of iron.

phosphates, oxylates, phylates, and cellulose, more iron will be absorbed. The amount of iron in a food is not the only indicator of its
value as a source of iron. Spinach, which was formerly considered a
good source of iron, is no longer as highly recommended because it
contains oxalates that inhibit iron absorption.

• Ascorbic acid promotes absorption of iron by reducing ferric salts to
ferrous salts. Ferrous salts are the only form in which the body can
absorb iron.

• Iron-poor foods have a noticeable lack of pigment; iron salts are colored and impart their color to the foods that contain them. For example, there is a distinct contrast between the color of iron-poor milk
and the color of iron-rich liver.

• The body has no physiologic mechanism for excreting excess iron.
Iron medications should be kept out of the reach of children. The
indiscriminate use of over-the-counter preparations that contain iron
and iron-enriched foods should be avoided. Iron poisoning is the

fourth most common type of poisoning. Relatively small amounts of iron can be lethal to young children.
- Oral iron medications interfere with the absorption of tetracycline antibiotics. Instruct patients who are taking both medications to separate their administration times as much as possible.

Pernicious Anemia

PATHOPHYSIOLOGY

Pernicious anemia is the result of the absence of intrinsic factor, a mucoprotein enzyme secreted by the stomach. Intrinsic factor must be present for vitamin B_{12} (extrinsic factor) to be absorbed from ingested food. Vitamin B_{12} is needed for red blood cell maturation; in its absence, red blood cells do not mature and anemia develops.

TREATMENT

The treatment of pernicious anemia is intramuscular or subcutaneous injections of vitamin B_{12} (cyanocobalamin) for life. Daily injections are required early in the treatment regimen, but after initial therapy, the disease can usually be kept in remission by injections given six to eight times per year. Because some vitamin B_{12} (about 1%) is absorbed by diffusion in the absence of intrinsic factor, it is possible to treat pernicious anemia with large doses of oral vitamin B_{12}. This observation explains the success of an early treatment that consisted of large quantities of raw and cooked liver.

DIET THERAPY

The availability and effectiveness of oral and parenteral vitamin B_{12} make diet as the sole treatment of pernicious anemia of historical interest only. The diet was unpleasant and unpalatable; drug therapy is simple and necessitates relatively infrequent administration, so there is no reason to treat the disease by diet alone. Diet therapy can play a supportive part in the treatment of pernicious anemia. When the body begins to build red blood cells in response to vitamin B_{12} therapy, it will need dietary sources of other nutrients required for erythropoiesis. These nutrients include proteins, iron, vitamin C, copper, and folic acid.

Glossitis is a symptom of pernicious anemia that causes a smooth, red, beefy tongue and sore mouth. Glossitis decreases the desire to eat. Soft, bland food or a bland liquid diet can be helpful in maintaining nutrition until this symptom responds to drug therapy.

NURSING IMPLICATIONS

- Pernicious anemia develops after a total gastrectomy unless vitamin B_{12} is administered. Some (15%) patients with partial gastrectomies and gastrojejunostomies also suffer from pernicious anemia unless they are given vitamin B_{12}.
- Vegetarian diets, if strictly followed, can lead to vitamin B_{12} deficiency because vitamin B_{12} is found only in foods of animal origin.

Folic Acid Deficiency Anemia

PATHOPHYSIOLOGY

Folic acid is needed for the synthesis of DNA and the maturation of red blood cells. Folic acid deficiency can result from an inadequate diet. It is also frequently seen in chronic alcoholism because high blood levels of alcohol block the response of the bone marrow to folic acid and interfere with the formation of red blood cells.

TREATMENT

The treatment of folic acid deficiency anemia involves supplying folic acid daily by drug therapy until the deficiency is corrected.

DIET THERAPY

Patients with folic acid deficiency anemia need a diet rich in all the other nutrients needed for the production of red blood cells. A diet that includes proteins, iron, copper, vitamin C, and vitamin B_{12} supports drug therapy with folic acid. If the folic acid deficiency is related to a faulty diet, the patient needs instruction in diet planning to prevent recurrences. The ingestion of one fresh fruit or one raw vegetable daily would prevent folic acid deficiency, but these foods may not be available to many people. Less expensive sources of folic acid include fish, legumes, and whole grains. Prolonged cooking destroys much of the folic acid in foods. Vitamin C promotes absorption of folic acid. Patients with folic acid deficiency anemia also have sore mouths and tongues; the use of soft, bland solids or liquids is recommended until this symptom responds to therapy.

NURSING IMPLICATIONS

- Folic acid deficiency anemia may occur in conjunction with malabsorption syndromes.

- Drugs, such as primidone, phenytoin, and phenobarbital, used in long-term anticonvulsant therapy, interfere with the body's use of folic acid.
- Folic acid antagonists, purine analogues, and pyrimidine analogues, used in the treatment of cancer, affect the body's use of folic acid.
- Some oral contraceptives affect folic acid metabolism.
- Folic acid deficiency is common in the third trimester of pregnancy because the need for folic acid increases to six times the usual amount required.
- Most multivitamin preparations do not contain folic acid.

Protein Deficiency Anemia

PATHOPHYSIOLOGY

Protein is required for the production of hemoglobin and red blood cells, as well as for growth and repair of all body cells. When intake of protein falls, the body may decrease production of red blood cells to free protein for more essential processes. Decreased production of red blood cells leads to anemia. Protein deficiency anemia due to inadequate intake of protein rarely occurs as an isolated deficiency; there are usually several deficiencies in the nutrients needed for erythropoiesis.

TREATMENT

A normal, well-balanced diet with emphasis on high-quality proteins is the usual treatment. Patients who have been deprived of protein for long periods need to be reintroduced to a protein-rich diet gradually. Iron, vitamin B_{12}, and folic acid may be given by drug therapy to correct concurrent deficiencies and support production of red blood cells.

DIET THERAPY

The dietary treatment of protein deficiency anemia is gradual ingestion of a well-balanced diet rich in high-quality proteins. The usual recommendation for daily protein intake is 1.5 to 2 grams per kilogram of body weight. Good sources of protein include:

Milk
Meat
Poultry
Eggs

Fish
Soybeans
Dried peas and beans
Cheese

NURSING IMPLICATIONS

- Protein foods tend to be expensive; patients may need assistance in selecting low-cost protein sources. Two tablespoons of peanut butter provide 8 grams of protein and 0.6 milligram of iron.
- Nonfat dry milk, a less expensive source of protein than fresh whole milk, can be added to skim milk, puddings, and casseroles to increase protein content.
- Less expensive cuts of meat contain as much protein as do more expensive cuts.
- Textured vegetable protein is being processed to resemble ground beef, ham, bacon, chicken, and turkey.
- Protein deficiency anemia may occur in conditions in which the body loses protein in abnormal amounts, as in nephrosis.
- Protein deficiency leads to nutritional edema, which may mask signs of poor nutrition.

Acute and Chronic Blood Loss

PATHOPHYSIOLOGY

Blood loss, whether due to sudden hemorrhage or slow seepage, represents a loss of red blood cells from the body. When a sufficient amount of blood is lost, anemia develops.

TREATMENT

The treatment of blood loss involves control of bleeding, management of the underlying cause, and replacement of lost blood. Blood or packed red blood cells may be transfused. In less severe losses, iron, vitamin B_{12}, and folic acid may be given to assist the body in replacing red blood cells.

DIET THERAPY

A diet rich in the nutrients needed for erythropoiesis is desirable to supplement drug therapy. Iron, protein, vitamin B_{12}, folic acid, and copper sources should be included in a diet that is compatible with the patient's diagnosis (reason for blood loss) and tastes.

NURSING IMPLICATIONS

- Anemia in a postmenopausal woman or adult man should alert the health team to the possibility of occult blood loss.
- Blood donors lose 250 milligrams of iron with every pint donated. To replace this loss, donors should increase their daily iron intake by 0.7 milligram for a year. People who donate blood more frequently should make sure that their iron intake is above average for their age and sex.

Copper Deficiency Anemia

Although copper is essential in the formation of hemoglobin, the amount needed is minute. Copper deficiency is an unusual occurrence in a person who has a well-balanced diet. Good sources of copper are similar to good sources of iron and include:

Oysters
Liver
Nuts
Dried legumes
Raisins

Milk and milk products are extremely poor sources of copper; copper deficiency may occur in infants maintained exclusively on milk diets for extended periods.

References

Beutler, E. Iron. In R. Goodhart & M. Shils (Eds.), *Modern nutrition in health and disease* (6th ed.). Philadelphia: Lea & Febiger, 1980.

Flynn, K. Iron deficiency anemia among elderly. *Nurse Practitioner*, November/December 1978, *3*, 6.

Herbert, V., Coleman, N., & Jacob, E. Folic acid and vitamin B_{12}. In R. Goodhart & M. Shils (Eds.), *Modern nutrition in health and disease* (6th ed.). Philadelphia: Lea & Febiger, 1980.

Hine, J. Minerals. In R. Howard & N. Herbold, *Nutrition in clinical care*. New York: McGraw-Hill Book Company, 1978.

Howe, P. *Basic nutrition in health and disease* (6th ed.). Philadelphia: W. B. Saunders Company, 1976.

Krause, M., & Mahan, L. *Food, nutrition and diet therapy* (6th ed.). Philadelphia: W. B. Saunders Company, 1979.

Kreutler, P. Vitamins. In R. Howard & N. Herbold, *Nutrition in clinical care.* New York: McGraw-Hill Book Company, 1978.

Mitchel, H., Rynberger, H., Anderson, L., et al. *Nutrition in health and disease* (16th ed.). Philadelphia: J. B. Lippincott Company, 1976.

Williams, S. *Nutrition and diet therapy* (3rd ed.). St. Louis: C. V. Mosby Company, 1977.

8

Diet Therapy
in Cardiovascular
Disorders

The role of diet in the prevention of cardiovascular disorders remains controversial. Authorities on one side of the controversy point to the relationships between high serum levels of cholesterol and increased incidence of atherosclerosis, coronary artery disease, hypertension, and cerebrovascular accidents. Authorities on the other side claim that there is a lack of conclusive evidence of the role of diet, that diet is only one of many risk factors. These experts believe that recommendations should be made for individuals rather than for the general population.

Nurses are not charged with the responsibility for prescribing treatment but should be able to support the dietary regimens that have been prescribed for their patients. Nurses will need information regarding the rationale for altering food intake to promote health.

The following facts and theories are included to help nurses support dietary prescriptions and to discuss the possible role of diet in the prevention of cardiovascular disorders honestly and knowledgeably.

The Facts

- Heart disease is the leading cause of death in the United States.
- No single factor is the absolute cause of atherosclerosis and coronary artery disease.
- Atheromatous plaques begin as accumulations of lipid materials in the intima of blood vessels. This lipid material consists of free cholesterol, cholesterol esters, and triglycerides.
- Atherosclerosis sets the stage for heart disease; however, many people with atherosclerosis do not suffer from heart disease.

112

- An elevated serum level of cholesterol is a major risk factor in the development of cardiovascular disorders.
- Serum levels of cholesterol can be altered by diet.
- The body manufactures cholesterol.
- Cholesterol is needed by the body for the production of steroid hormones.
- Saturated fats in the diet tend to increase serum levels of cholesterol.
- Polyunsaturated fats in the diet tend to decrease serum levels of cholesterol.
- Excessive intake of simple sugars and alcohol frequently contributes to elevated serum levels of triglycerides.
- Throughout the world, people who subsist on diets rich in saturated fats have higher cholesterol levels and a greater incidence of heart disease than do those whose diets are not rich in animal fats, eggs, and dairy products. This relationship cannot be explained on the basis of race, climate, or geographic considerations (O'Malley et al., 1978).

The Theories

- Habitual consumption of foods that are high in cholesterol and saturated fats is a key factor in the development of coronary artery disease.
- Lowering serum levels of cholesterol decreases the risk for coronary artery disease.
- There is insufficient evidence to support therapeutic diets for everyone to reduce the risk for heart disease. There is controversy about the advisability of altering the diets of infants, children, pregnant women, and the elderly.
- In one study, children who consistently consumed foods that are high in polyunsaturated fats showed a high incidence of gallbladder disease when they reached adulthood (Gotto, 1977).

Hyperlipoproteinemia

PATHOPHYSIOLOGY

Hyperlipoproteinemia is characterized by increased levels of lipids attached to serum proteins. Lipoproteins are combinations of proteins and triglycerides, phospholipids, and cholesterol. The function of lipoproteins is to transport insoluble lipids in an aqueous medium. Alterations of lipid metabolism result in elevated serum levels of cholesterol or triglycerides or both. This increase may occur as a primary or secondary disorder. Primary hyperlipoproteinemia is occasionally an inherited disorder and may result in premature atherosclerosis in children and adults. Severe hyperglyceridemia may result in recurrent abdominal pain and acute pancreatitis.

Frederickson et al. (1967) have classified hyperlipoproteinemia into five types, which differ in their characteristics and management.

Type I Hyperlipoproteinemia: Hyperchylomicronemia

PATHOPHYSIOLOGY

Type I, which is usually a rare familial disorder, is characterized by an inability to clear chylomicrons (dietary fat) from the blood. Plasma levels of cholesterol may be normal or elevated; triglyceride levels are very high.

TREATMENT

The only treatment at the present time is dietary intervention. Drug therapy is ineffective.

DIET THERAPY

The diet for children who are less than 12 years of age is restricted to 10 to 15 grams of fat per day. The adult diet is a low-fat diet in which fat is limited to 25 to 35 grams per day. Intake of cholesterol is not restricted, and the ratio of polyunsaturated fats to saturated fats is not considered important. Intake of proteins and carbohydrates is not limited, and intake of carbohydrates must be increased to provide an adequate amount of Calories. Alcohol is not recommended.

To limit the intake of fat to the level permitted, the fat content of all foods ingested must be considered. Meat, for example, is calculated as 8 grams of protein and 3 grams of fat for each ounce. Five ounces of meat per day is usually permitted. This allowance can be increased to 7 ounces daily if beef, lamb, and pork are limited to three 3-ounce servings per week, with poultry and fish making up the remainder of the allowance.

All butter, margarine, oils, and shortenings are eliminated from the diet, as are any baked products that contain them. Nuts are also eliminated from the diet, and intake of dairy products that contain fat is restricted. Medium-chain triglycerides may be permitted by the physician since these fatty acids do not lead to formation of chylomicrons and improve the palatability of the diet. See Table 8-1 for an example of a diet

TABLE 8-1
EXAMPLE OF A MENU FOR A CHILD WITH TYPE I HYPERLIPOPROTEINEMIA
(4 to 6 YEARS OF AGE, 35 to 40 POUNDS, 1,400 to 1,600 CALORIES

Daily Food Plan	Menu Pattern
1 quart of skim milk	Breakfast
2 ounces of cooked poultry, fish, or lean, trimmed meat	Citrus fruit or juice
4 servings of vegetable and fruit	Cereal
4 or more servings of bread or cereal	Toast
1 or more servings of potato, rice, etc.	Jelly and sugar
Allowed desserts and sweets	Skim milk
	Lunch
	1 ounce of cooked poultry, fish, or lean meat
	Potato or substitute
	Vegetable
	Bread
	Jelly and sugar
	Allowed dessert
	Skim milk
	Dinner
	1 ounce of cooked poultry, fish, or lean meat
	Vegetable, raw or cooked
	Bread
	Jelly and sugar
	Fruit
	Skim milk
	Between-meal snack
	Skim milk
	Allowed dessert
	Bread with jam or jelly

Source: From *The dietary management of hyperlipoproteinemia—A handbook for physicians and dietitians*, National Heart, Lung, and Blood Institute, 1978.

for a child with Type I hyperlipoproteinemia. See Table 8-2 for an example of a menu for an adult with Type I hyperlipoproteinemia.

NURSING IMPLICATIONS

- A very-low-fat diet lacks palatability and tends to be dry. The use of medium-chain triglycerides in the preparation of meats, sauces, and dressings may improve taste and compliance with the diet.
- Low-grade meats, which contain less fat marbling, are lower in fat content. All visible fat should be trimmed from meats before cooking.

TABLE 8-2
EXAMPLE OF A MENU FOR AN ADULT WITH TYPE I HYPERLIPOPROTEINEMIA
(1,700 to 2,000 CALORIES)

Daily Food Plan	Menu Pattern
1 quart of skim milk	Breakfast
5 ounces of cooked poultry, fish, or lean, trimmed meat	Citrus fruit or juice
	Cereal
5 servings of vegetable and fruit	Toast
6 or more servings of bread or cereal	Jelly and sugar
1 or more servings of potato, rice, etc.	Skim milk
Allowed desserts	Coffee or tea, if desired
Sugar, sweets	Lunch
	2 ounches of cooked poultry, fish, or lean meat
	Potato, rice, spaghetti, or noodles
	Vegetable
	Bread
	Jelly and sugar
	Fruit
	Allowed dessert
	Skim milk
	Dinner
	3 ounces of cooked poultry, fish, or lean meat
	Potato, rice, or noodles
	Vegetable
	Bread
	Jelly and sugar
	Allowed dessert
	Between-meal snack
	Skim milk
	Fruit or allowed dessert
	Bread with jam or jelly

Source: From *The dietary management of hyperlipoproteinemia—A handbook for physicians and dietitians,* National Heart, Lung, and Blood Institute, 1978.

- Meats should be cooked without added fats (except medium-chain tri-glycerides) on a rack to permit fat to drain away from the portion to be eaten.
- Homemade breads, cakes, and cookies can be made without fat (or with medium-chain triglycerides) and with the skim milk and egg allowance from the diet.
- Hamburger should be ground to order or ground at home from lean, well-trimmed cuts of beef.
- Intake should be evaluated for adequacy of iron and fat-soluble vitamins.

Type IIa Hyperlipoproteinemia: Hypercholesterolemia

PATHOPHYSIOLOGY

This type of disorder of the blood lipids occurs in all age groups. The serum levels of beta-lipoproteins are markedly increased. The triglyceride levels are normal, and the plasma is clear. Type IIa is frequently familial and is characterized by the development of xanthomas (deposits of cholesterol in the skin and tendons over the elbows and knees) and early onset of vascular disease. Type IIa hyperlipoproteinemia may develop secondary to excessive intake of cholesterol in the diet, myxedema, nephrosis, or liver disease.

TREATMENT

The aim of treatment is to lower the serum level of cholesterol by means of drugs and dietary intervention.

DIET THERAPY

The diet prescription for Type IIa includes limiting intake of cholesterol to as low a level as possible and decreasing intake of saturated fats while increasing intake of polyunsaturated fats. To reduce intake of cholesterol, egg yolks, organ meats, and most dairy products are eliminated from the diet, with meat remaining the major source of cholesterol. Intake of carbohydrates and proteins is not restricted. Alcohol may be used in moderation. Intake of polyunsaturated fatty acids is increased by the use of safflower, sunflower, and corn oils and soft margarines made from these oils at a ratio of 1 teaspoon of polyunsaturated fat for every ounce of cooked meat.

Beef, lamb, and pork are limited to three 3-ounce servings per week. Fish, chicken, veal, and turkey should be used for the remainder of the meat allotment. Skim milk and skim milk products should replace whole milk as a beverage and in cooking. Shellfish, with the exception of shrimp, may be used in the diet. The prescribed diet is adequate in all nutrients, except iron. See Tables 8-3 and 8-4 for examples of diets for children and adults with Type IIa hyperlipoproteinemia.

NURSING IMPLICATIONS

- Remind patients that cholesterol is found in meat and animal products. Foods of plant origin normally contain no cholesterol, unless it has been added in processing.

TABLE 8-3
EXAMPLE OF A MENU FOR CHILD WITH TYPE IIa HYPERLIPOPROTEINEMIA
(4 to 6 YEARS OF AGE, 35 to 40 POUNDS, 1,400 to 1,600 calories)

Daily Food Plan	Menu Pattern
1 quart of skim milk	Breakfast
Cooked poultry, fish, or lean, trimmed meat	Citrus fruit or juice
4 servings of vegetables and fruit, including	Cereal
1 serving of citrus fruit[a]	Toast
1 serving of dark green or deep yellow vegetable[b]	Allowed fat
	Jelly and sugar
4 or more servings of whole-grain or enriched bread or cereal[c]	Skim milk
	Lunch
1 or more servings of potato, rice, etc.	Cooked poultry, fish, or lean, trimmed meat
Allowed fat	
Allowed desserts	Potato or substitute
Sugars and sweets	Vegetable
	Bread
	Allowed fat
	Allowed dessert
	Skim milk
	Dinner
	Cooked poultry, fish, or lean, trimmed meat
	Vegetable, raw or cooked
	Bread
	Allowed fat
	Fruit
	Skim milk
	Between-meal snack
	Skim milk
	Fruit or allowed dessert
	Bread
	Allowed fat

Source: From *The dietary management of hyperlipoproteinemia—A handbook for physicians and dietitians,* National Heart, Lung, and Blood Institute, 1978.
[a]One serving of citrus fruit is recommended daily to provide adequate vitamin C.
[b]One dark-green or deep-yellow vegetable is recommended daily to provide adequate vitamin A.
[c]Enriched cereal or bread should be included in the diet to provide adequate vitamin B complex and iron.

- Many food labels contain information about cholesterol or indicate sources for obtaining such information. All labels should be checked and foods investigated for cholesterol content before use.
- Coconut and palm oils, although vegetable products, are sources of saturated fats. Be sure that the patient understands that he or she must specifically check for the special oils (safflower, sunflower, corn) and not accept the label "vegetable oils."

TABLE 8-4

EXAMPLE OF A MENU FOR AN ADULT WITH TYPE IIa HYPERLIPOPROTEINEMIA
(1,700 to 2,000 CALORIES)

Daily Food Plan	Menu Pattern
1 pint of more of skim milk	Breakfast
Cooked poultry, fish, or lean, trimmed meat	Citrus fruit or juice
5 servings of vegetable and fruit, including	Cereal
1 serving of citrus fruit[a]	Toast
1 serving of dark green or deep yellow vegetable[b]	Allowed fat
	Jelly and sugar
7 or more servings of whole-grain or enriched bread or cereal[c]	Skim milk
1 or more servings of potato, rice, etc.	Coffee or tea if desired
Allowed fat	Lunch
Allowed desserts and sweets	Poultry, fish, or lean meat
	Potato or substitute
	Vegetable
	Bread
	Allowed fat
	Fruit or allowed dessert
	Skim milk
	Dinner
	Poultry, fish, or lean meat
	Potato or substitute
	Vegetable
	Bread
	Allowed fat
	Fruit or allowed dessert
	Skim milk
	Between-meal snack
	Fruit
	Skim milk

Source: From *The dietary management of hyperlipoproteinemia—A handbook for physicians and dietitians*, National Heart, Lung, and Blood Institute, 1978.

[a]One serving of citrus fruit is recommended daily to provide adequate vitamin C.
[b]One dark-green or deep-yellow vegetable is recommended daily to provide adequate vitamin A.
[c]Enriched cereal or bread should be included in the diet to provide adequate vitamin B complex and iron.

- The meat selected for use in the diet should be nonmarbled and well trimmed. Cooking methods that drain the fat from the meat should be used. Skin should be removed from poultry before cooking, if possible, and should not be eaten if not removed when preparing the food.
- Gravies should be avoided, unless all fat has been removed from the meat drippings in their preparation. A substitute for gravy can be made by thickening bouillon.

- Homemade baked products that contain skim milk, egg whites, and special oils can increase the variety of foods permitted on the diet.
- Check the diet for adequacy of iron intake.

Types IIb and III Hyperlipoproteinemia: Hypercholesterolemia with Endogenous Hyperglyceridemia

PATHOPHYSIOLOGY

Type IIb is a common pattern showing elevated serum levels of cholesterol and triglycerides. It may be a familial disorder. Type III is much less common and is characterized by very high elevations of serum levels of cholesterol and triglycerides and by the development of xanthomas and tuberous lesions. Type III is a familial disorder and is associated with premature coronary artery and peripheral vascular disease.

TREATMENT

The treatment of Types IIb and III hyperlipoproteinemia involves dietary intervention with drug therapy added if diet alone fails to lower the serum levels of cholesterol and triglycerides.

DIET THERAPY

The dietary treatment of Types IIb and III hyperlipoproteinemia includes reduced intake of Calories until appropriate body weight is reached, after which the intake of Calories is stabilized to maintain ideal body weight. The diet in both phases consists of controlled intake of cholesterol and triglycerides. The dietary regimen is implemented by dividing the caloric allowance into approximately 40% carbohydrate, 40% fat, and 20% protein. The fat allowance should not exceed 2 grams per kilogram of ideal body weight. Polyunsaturated fats are used in place of saturated fats. Intake of cholesterol should be as low as possible, with meat being the major dietary source. Egg yolks, organ meats, and shrimp are excluded from the diet.

No more than 4 grams of carbohydrate per kilogram of desired body weight is permitted. Starches are preferred to concentrated sweets as carbohydrate sources. The protein allowance is high, with 1.5 to 2 grams per kilogram of ideal body weight recommended. The physician may permit two servings of alcohol to be substituted for carbohydrate foods. One ounce of whiskey, rum, gin, or vodka equals 1 slice of bread.

NURSING IMPLICATIONS

- Check the diet for adequacy of iron intake. Limited intake of meat may result in inadequate iron intake.
- Whole-grain breads and cereals or enriched breads and cereals increase the amount of iron in the diet.
- Alcohol is high in Calories and provides little nutrition. It is also responsible for a rise in serum levels of triglycerides.
- Excessive consumption of sugar has been linked to elevated serum levels of triglycerides. Desserts should be simple, prepared without egg yolks and with skim milk. Although two daily servings of allowed desserts are usually permitted, unsweetened fruit is a better dessert choice.
- See Nursing Implications for Types I and II for suggestions related to polyunsaturated fats and cholesterol.

Type IV Hyperlipoproteinemia: Endogenous Hyperglyceridemia

PATHOPHYSIOLOGY

Type IV is characterized by an increase in the prebeta (very low density) lipoproteins. Serum levels of triglycerides may be slightly to grossly elevated. Serum levels of cholesterol may be normal to elevated. Cholesterol levels tend to rise in direct proportion to triglyceride levels. Many patients with Type IV hyperlipoproteinemia have abnormal glucose tolerance and increased serum levels of uric acid. A Type IV pattern is frequently associated with diabetes mellitus and obesity.

TREATMENT

The treatment of Type IV hyperlipoproteinemia is dietary intervention. Clofibrate (Atromid-S), an antilipidemic agent, is sometimes used.

DIET THERAPY

The dietary regimen is aimed at weight reduction in the overweight patient. Obesity exaggerates the condition, and weight loss usually reduces serum levels of triglycerides. Caloric intake is calculated to achieve and then maintain appropriate body weight.

Intake of carbohydrates is controlled. About 45% of the Calories may be derived from carbohydrate foods as long as the intake does not exceed 5 grams per kilogram of ideal body weight. Concentrated sweets are restricted. Fat intake is limited only because of the need for weight reduction. Polyunsaturated fats are preferred to saturated fats. Intake of cholesterol is only moderately restricted. Intake of proteins is of concern only in relation to caloric intake. Alcohol may be used if the physician permits. The amount of alcohol should be limited to two servings daily and must be substituted for carbohydrates.

The diet for Type IV hyperlipoproteinemia is relatively free, and restrictions are placed only on carbohydrate foods. If the patient's triglyceride levels do not fall during diet therapy, the more controlled diet used in Type III hyperlipoproteinemia may be substituted, or drug therapy may be added to the dietary regimen.

NURSING IMPLICATIONS

- Regular weight measurements are important. Encourage the patient to establish regular weighing times and to seek counsel if weight loss is not achieved or maintained.
- Excessive intake of sugar may result in elevated serum levels of triglycerides and should be avoided.
- Excessive consumption of alcohol is also thought to increase triglyceride levels.

Type V Hyperlipoproteinemia: Mixed Hyperglyceridemia

PATHOPHYSIOLOGY

Type V hyperlipoproteinemia is characterized by increased levels of chylomicrons and prebeta-lipoproteins in the plasma. Type V is referred to as a "mixed" hyperglyceridemia since the chylomicrons are exogenous and the prebeta-lipoproteins are endogenous. Type V patterns are usually secondary to metabolic disorders, such as diabetes mellitus, nephrosis, and pancreatitis. A familial Type V pattern is usually manifested after the second decade of life. Triglyceride and cholesterol levels are usually elevated, with triglyceride levels grossly elevated and cholesterol levels moderately elevated. Abnormal glucose tolerance and elevated serum levels of uric acid are frequently associated with Type V patterns.

TREATMENT

The treatment of Type V hyperlipoproteinemia is dietary intervention.

DIET THERAPY

The dietary treatment of Type V is reduction of body weight to an ideal level and maintenance of weight at that level. At the same time, intake of foods that may increase triglyceride and cholesterol levels is limited. Fat is restricted to 30% of the caloric intake, with cholesterol moderately restricted. A low-fat diet is desirable. Carbohydrates may contribute 50% of the Calories, although they should not exceed 5 grams per kilogram of ideal body weight. Alcohol is not permitted in a Type V diet. Protein is allowed in levels of 1.5 to 2 grams per kilogram, a high-protein diet.

The diet must be compatible with the patient's underlying metabolic disorder. For example, a patient with pancreatitis may not be able to tolerate the fat content of the diet, and the diet for Type I hyperlipoproteinemia may have to be substituted.

NURSING IMPLICATIONS

- Weight should be carefully monitored, and weight gain or failure to lose during the weight reduction phase should be investigated.
- Alcohol is not permitted because it may be associated with elevated triglyceride levels and abdominal pain.

Atherosclerosis

PATHOPHYSIOLOGY

As aging progresses, deposits of lipid and fibrous materials accumulate in the intima of the medium-sized and large arteries. The lesions start as fatty streaks and may progress to plaques composed of fibrous tissue, cholesterol and other lipids, and calcium. The deposits narrow the lumen of the vessels and reduce or obstruct blood flow. Thrombi, emboli, angina, and intermittent claudication can result from this interference to blood flow.

Atherosclerotic cardiovascular disease has been linked by studies to:

Increased age
Male sex
Diabetes mellitus
Cigarette smoking
Elevated blood pressure
Elevated serum levels of cholesterol

These risk factors are related to premature development of atherosclerosis (Taylor & Raizner, 1978).

TREATMENT

The treatment depends on the damage done to the body by the various manifestations of atherosclerosis. Surgical removal of plaque has been attempted to prevent blockage of major vessels. Surgical bypasses or replacement of blocked vessels has also been performed. Drugs that reduce serum levels of cholesterol have been used in an attempt to forestall the atherosclerotic process. Other attempts to slow the atherosclerotic process have been aimed at elimination of risk factors that can be manipulated.

DIET THERAPY

Some patients may be prescribed low-saturated-fat, low-cholesterol diets in an attempt to lower serum levels of cholesterol. Other patients may elect to lower their intake of cholesterol and saturated fats by following diets recommended by the American Heart Association and other reputable authorities.

The recommended diet is caloric control to attain and maintain ideal body weight. Cholesterol intake is limited to 300 milligrams per day. Fat intake should represent only 30% of the total Calories and should be made up of 10% polyunsaturated fats, less than 10% saturated fats, and the remainder monounsaturated fats. Carbohydrate Calories are increased to make up for reduction of fat intake. The carbohydrates should come from cereals, fruits, and vegetables and not from concentrated sweets. Restriction of sodium intake is an additional dietary measure for the many patients who are also hypertensive.

NURSING IMPLICATIONS

- Patients should be provided with a list of foods with high cholesterol content (see Table 8-5).

TABLE 8-5
FOODS HIGH IN CHOLESTEROL

Organ meats
Egg yolks
Cheese: cheddar, Swiss, American
Shrimp
Beef
Lamb
Pork

- A good general guide to cholesterol content is to remember that there is no cholesterol in foods of plant origin.
- Saturated fats tend to increase serum levels of cholesterol.
- Polyunsaturated fats tend to decrease serum levels of cholesterol.
- Monounsaturated fats tend to decrease cholesterol levels minimally. See Table 8-6 for the spectrum of fat saturation.
- Saturated fats tend to be of animal origin, such as those in meats and dairy products. However, saturated fats are also present in some vegetable fats, such as coconut oil, palm oil, and cocoa butter.
- Read labels carefully. Foods that contain vegetable oils may still have high percentages of saturated fats. Examples are solid shortenings, commercial bakery products, and nondairy cream substitutes and toppings.
- The limitation of egg yolks to three per week includes eggs used in cooking and in prepared foods. The use of cholesterol-free egg substitutes in cooking may help prevent the patient from exceeding this limitation. (The sodium content of one brand of egg substitutes is twice that of fresh eggs. This observation is important for patients on sodium-controlled diets.)

TABLE 8-6
SPECTRUM OF DEGREE OF POLYUNSATURATION OF OIL

100%
95
90
85
80 Safflower oil
75
70
65 Soybean oil
60 Corn oil
55 Cottonseed oil
50
45
40
35 Peanut oil
30
25 Olive oil
20
15
10 Lard, palm oil
5 Butterfat, cocoa butter
palm kernel, coconut oil
0%

- Shrimp and organ meats are high in cholesterol and should be limited.
- Meat selections should be made primarily from fish, chicken, turkey, and veal. Beef, pork, and lamb should be consumed in limited amounts.
- Chicken and turkey skin should not be eaten; most of the fat is in the skin.
- Lean cuts of meat should be selected, and all visible fat should be removed before cooking.
- Meats should be cooked in a manner that permits fat to drip away from the meat. Fat drippings should be discarded.
- Skim milk and nonfat dry milk should replace whole milk as beverages and for cooking.
- Skim milk cheeses should be used in preference to whole milk varieties.
- Polyunsaturated oils may be substituted for butter or margarine in home recipes. One tablespoon of butter or margarine is equal to ¾ tablespoon of oil.
- Tub margarines of safflower, sunflower, or corn oil are preferable to stick margarines made from the same oils because of their higher content of polyunsaturated oils. Hydrogenation, which solidifies oils, decreases the degree of polyunsaturation.
- Reducing the intake of red meats may lead to inadequate iron intake. Encourage consumption of whole grains and enriched breads and cereals, and check for adequacy of iron intake.

Cerebrovascular Accidents

PATHOPHYSIOLOGY

Atherosclerosis of the vessels supplying the brain can lead to thrombosis of an artery, interference with blood supply to an area of the brain, ischemia and necrosis of brain tissue, and varying degrees of dysfunction related to the necrotic areas of the brain. Two other common causes of cerebrovascular accidents are embolism and hemorrhage. Embolitic cerebrovascular accidents may be related to atherosclerosis; cerebral hemorrhage is most frequently a result of hypertension.

TREATMENT

Immediately after the cerebrovascular accident, treatment is directed toward lifesaving measures. Ongoing therapy is focused on improvement of residual defects, such as hemiplegia and aphasia. Surgical intervention, such as thromboendarterectomy, embolectomy, or evacuation of hemorrhage, may be performed.

DIET THERAPY

Diet therapy in cerebrovascular accidents usually includes the use of intravenous fluids for the first 24 to 48 hours. In patients with cerebral edema, close monitoring of the intravenous flow rate is critical to prevent overhydration. Depending on the patient's progress, oral liquid feedings may be started after intravenous therapy. The presence of coma or paralysis may necessitate the use of tube feedings until the patient is able to swallow. If the patient experiences difficulty swallowing liquids, semisolid foods may be tried.

The progression is usually from a liquid diet to a soft diet that requires little or no chewing. Eventually the patient advances to a regular diet. In patients with atherosclerosis or hypertension, low-fat, low-cholesterol, or low-sodium diets are prescribed. Low-Calorie diets for weight reduction may be ordered to lower blood pressure and the work load of the heart. Obesity also makes the physical rehabilitative process more difficult.

NURSING IMPLICATIONS

- Assess the deficits related to food intake. Common residual problems related to cerebrovascular accidents include the inability to close lips, suck, chew, or swallow. Poor hand-to-mouth coordination may be evident.
- Position the patient at feeding times to allow maximal use of abilities and protection from aspiration. A hemiplegic patient usually manages best on the unaffected side. Food should be placed in the nonparalyzed side of the mouth. In testing the ability to swallow, give a small amount of water first.
- Cut food into small pieces, and encourage patients to take small bites.
- Eliminate foods that could cause choking spells, such as stringy meats, unboned fish, and crisp-cooked vegetables.
- Encourage independence by allowing patients to do whatever they are able at mealtimes. Investigate the feasibility of feeding devices that may assist patients to gaining independence.
- Provide mouth care after feedings to remove particles of food from the affected side of the mouth to prevent aspiration.
- Protect the patient from spillage in ways that preserve dignity. References to "bibs" and "babies" should be avoided.
- Provide prompt change of wet or soiled linen and clothes. Conversation with the patient during linen changes should emphasize suc-

cesses in the feeding process rather than the soiling that results from the effort.

- Attempt to learn the food habits of aphasic patients to avoid feeding them foods that they dislike. When communication is established, provide an opportunity for food choice within the prescribed diet limitations.

Myocardial Infarction

PATHOPHYSIOLOGY

Myocardial infarction is a process in which heart tissue that is deprived of a blood supply becomes necrotic. Deprivation of blood supply, ischemia, is the result of closure of a coronary artery or one of its branches due to thrombosis or obstruction of the lumen by atherosclerotic plaque.

TREATMENT

The treatment is to provide rest to reduce the work load of the heart and to decrease the burden on the damaged myocardium. Treatment also includes prevention of complications, such as shock and cardiac arrhythmias, and attempts to eliminate factors that might lead to further attacks.

DIET THERAPY

Immediately after infarction, an intravenous line is established, primarily for drug administration. The intravenous line must be carefully monitored to prevent excess circulating fluid from overburdening the damaged heart.

Clear fluids are the first oral feeding permitted. In the event of vomiting and aspiration, clear fluids are less hazardous. Approximately 1 to 1.5 liters of clear fluids per day are given for 2 days. Progression to a soft, low-Calorie, mildly sodium-restricted (2,000 milligrams per day) diet follows. Feedings are usually divided into six small meals to avoid gastric distention.

Eventually, a return to a regular or special diet is achieved. Special diets may restrict intake of sodium, Calories, cholesterol, or saturated fats. Any combination of these dietary restrictions may be used to meet individual needs. Regular diets usually are apportioned into 45% carbohydrate, 20% protein, and 35% fat.

NURSING IMPLICATIONS

- Temperature extremes in foods and beverages are avoided in the early postinfarction period because such extremes may trigger arrhythmias. Foods and fluids are served at body temperature.

- Any beverage that contains caffeine may increase the heart rate. Tea, cola, and cocoa should be avoided. Decaffeinated coffee may be used.
- Weight reduction in the overweight patient reduces the work load of the heart.
- Patients are often permitted to feed themselves 24 hours after infarction. Every effort should be made to position the patient and to arrange food and utensils to minimize fatigue.
- Egg yolks may be limited to three per week when cholesterol levels are a concern.

Congestive Heart Failure

PATHOPHYSIOLOGY

In congestive heart failure, the heart is unable to pump sufficient blood at a rate required to provide body cells with adequate amounts of oxygen and other nutrients. As a result of this failure, the vascular bed of the lungs is no longer emptied. This situation leads to the development of pulmonary vessel engorgement, pulmonary hypertension, and pulmonary edema. Blood returning to the heart from the systemic circulation cannot travel to the pulmonary circulation promptly and thus congests the systemic veins and venules, increases venous pressure, and causes edema and ascites. Atherosclerosis may increase the resistance against which the heart must pump and thus contribute to the work load of the heart and its eventual failure.

TREATMENT

The treatment of congestive heart failure is to provide rest to reduce the demands on the heart. Drug therapy is used to reinforce the heart's action by slowing the rate and strengthening the beat. A combination of rest, diuretics, and diet therapy is used to eliminate edema.

DIET THERAPY

The primary aim of diet therapy is to eliminate edema. This goal is achieved by restricting intake of sodium. The degree of restriction varies from 200 to 4,000 milligrams of sodium daily. A 250-milligram sodium diet is considered severely restricted and, because it is difficult to monitor and quite unpalatable, is usually prescribed only for hospitalized patients. Five hundred milligrams of sodium daily is considered a strict restriction, 1,000 milligrams is a moderate restriction, and 2,400 to 4,500 milligrams is a mild restriction (American Heart Association, 1978a).

The American diet contains from 6 to 15 grams of salt per day on the average; because salt is 40% sodium, this diet includes 2,400 to 6,000 milligrams of sodium per day from salt alone. By not adding salt to food, the dietary intake of sodium can be reduced to 1,600 to 2,800 milligrams per day. By eliminating salt in food preparation, sodium intake can be reduced to 1,200 to 1,600 milligrams per day.

The prescribed food intake for patients with congestive heart failure is usually divided into five or six small meals to avoid distention and elevation of the diaphragm, which would reduce vital capacity. Weight loss may be desirable, and a low-Calorie diet may be ordered. Assessing the actual degree of obesity may be difficult in the presence of edema.

The time-honored Karell diet, which consists of 800 milliliters of milk daily for 3 to 7 days, may still be prescribed for some patients with congestive heart failure. This diet has the advantage of being low in Calories, providing only 600 kcal; severely sodium restricted, providing only 500 milligrams of sodium; and limited in fluid content. Present-day concerns about the saturated fat content of whole milk have led to the substitution of skim milk and the further reduction of daily intake of Calories to 350 kcal. Even greater restriction of sodium can be obtained by the use of low-sodium milk as part of the diet. Low-sodium milk provides 12 milligrams of sodium in 240 milliliters. The Karell diet is nutritionally inadequate, and its use is usually limited to short periods.

Fluids are not usually restricted in congestive heart failure despite the presence of edema. Excessive fluid intake is not allowed, and 3,000 milliliters is usually set as the maximal daily fluid intake. In patients with refractory edema, fluid intake may be restricted. See Tables 8-7 through 8-10 for examples of sodium-restricted diets.

NURSING IMPLICATIONS

- Check trays of all patients on sodium-restricted diets to make sure that salt has not been inadvertently placed on them.
- Patients with congestive heart failure tend to have poor appetites due to a feeling of fullness related to the congestion.
- Raw fruits and vegetables and gas-forming vegetables are usually eliminated from the diet because they tend to enhance distention.
- One level teaspoon of salt contains 2,300 milligrams of sodium. Sodium chloride is 40% sodium and 60% chloride.
- Caution patients to read labels to identify other sources of sodium in foods, such as MSG (monosodium glutamate), a seasoning; sodium caseinate or sodium benzoate, preservatives used in sauces and salad dressings; and sodium propionate, a mold retardant in breads, cakes, and pasteurized cheeses.
- Investigate the sodium content of the water supply used by patients on sodium-restricted diet. Hard water contains less sodium than does water softened by ion-exchange systems.

TABLE 8-7

SEVERELY RESTRICTED SODIUM DIET, 250 MILLIGRAMS

Breakfast

  4 ounces of orange juice

  ½ cup of salt-free oatmeal

  8 ounces of low-sodium milk

  2 slices of salt-free bread with salt-free margarine

  1 teaspoon of jelly

  1 teaspoon of sugar

  Coffee

Lunch

  4 ounces of sliced breast of chicken without skin

  ½ cup of rice with herbs

  ½ cup of cooked broccoli without salt

  1 slice of salt-free bread with salt-free margarine

  ½ cup of canned pear halves

  8 ounces of low-sodium milk

Dinner

  4 ounces of roast beef prepared without salt

  1 baked potato with salt-free margarine

  ½ cup of green beans cooked without salt

  ½ cup of shredded lettuce, 1 tomato, salt-free dressing

  ½ cup of canned peaches

  1 slice of salt-free bread with salt-free margarine

  Tea with lemon

All food is prepared without seasonings containing sodium.

- Home-installed water softeners usually add sodium to the water and should not be used when sodium intake is restricted.
- Sodium is frequently used in medications, such as alkalizers, antibiotics, analgesics, and sedatives. Check the patient's medications and, if indicated, inquire about alternative nonsodium-containing substitutes.
- Toothpaste and mouthwashes may contain sodium; advise patients to rinse their mouths well after using these products.
- Frozen peas and lima beans usually contain small amounts of salt. Other frozen vegetables without sauces usually do not contain added salt.
- Chinese foods and kosher foods are usually high in sodium. Chinese foods may contain MSG or soy sauce, both of which contain large amounts of sodium. Foods may be prepared kosher style by salting to remove blood from meats, but broiling has the same effect. Meats and fish prepared kosher style by salting can be used if they are boiled in large amounts of water. The cooking water is discarded.
- Low-sodium milk is more palatable when well chilled. It can also be flavored if an acceptable flavoring is used.

TABLE 8-8
LESS SEVERELY RESTRICTED SODIUM DIET, 500 MILLIGRAMS

Breakfast
 1 banana
 1 shredded-wheat biscuit
 4 ounces of skim milk
 2 slices of low-sodium bread, toasted
 Salt-free margarine
 Jelly
 Coffee
 Sugar
Midmorning
 4 ounces of orange juice
 Salt-free crackers
Lunch
 3 ounces of chicken
 2 slices of low-sodium bread, toasted
 Salt-free margarine
 Lettuce
 1 tablespoon of special dietary mayonnaise[a]
 2 slices of canned pineapple
 Tea
Dinner
 3 ounces of roast beef
 1 baked potato
 ½ cup of cooked carrots
 ½ cup of broccoli
 Salt-free margarine
 Fruit salad (canned fruits for salad, lettuce)
 1 tablespoon of special dietary mayonnaise[a]
 1 cupcake, no icing
 Coffee or tea
Bedtime
 4 ounces of skim milk
 Salt-free crackers
All food is prepared without seasonings containing sodium.
[a]Low-sodium.

• Instant rice, instant mashed potatoes, and instant forms of cooked
  cereals are precooked with disodium phosphate and should not be
  substituted for regular rice, potatoes, or cooked cereals in a prescribed diet.
• Do not suggest the use of salt substitutes without the physician's ap-

TABLE 8-9
MODERATELY RESTRICTED SODIUM DIET, 1,000 MILLIGRAMS

Add the following to the 500-milligram sodium diet in Table 8-8:
Breakfast
 1 egg
 ¼ cup of light cream
Lunch
 8 ounces of skim milk
 ½ cantaloupe
 1 ounce of chicken
Dinner
 1 ounce of beef
 ½ cup of 10% fat ice cream
All food is prepared without seasonings containing sodium.

proval. Most salt substitutes have a potassium base that could lead to hyperkalemia if potassium-sparing diuretics are also used.
• Check the adequacy of potassium intake when potassium-wasting diuretics are used.
• Check the adequacy of iodine intake when salt is restricted.
• Watch for dilutional hyponatremia. Monitor serum levels of sodium.

Hypertension

PATHOPHYSIOLOGY

Hypertension is a symptom manifested by a sustained increase in the arterial diastolic or systolic pressure or both. A blood pressure measurement taken in the supine position is considered elevated in an adult if the readings are 160/95 mm Hg or higher. Because blood pressure increases with age, readings are compared to lower normal values for children and infants.

Hypertension may be secondary to kidney disorders. When no cause can be established, it is referred to as essential hypertension. Hypertension leads to death by contributing to coronary artery disease, cerebrovascular disease, and renal disease. Control of blood pressure reduces the incidence of stroke and congestive heart failure.

The blood pressure is determined by the muscle force exerted by the blood against the walls of the arteries as the heart contracts and relaxes and by the resistance to this force by other blood vessels in the body. This resistance is related to increased cardiac output when the pumped blood is in excess of the body's needs or when the heart pumps the required amount of blood through narrowed blood vessels.

TABLE 8-10

**FOODS USUALLY AVOIDED IN A MILDLY RESTRICTED SODIUM DIET,
2,400 to 4,000 MILLIGRAMS**[a]

Anchovies

Bacon/salt pork

Baking soda: as an antacid or in cooking vegetables

Barbeque sauce

Bouillon/bouillon cubes

Bread/rolls/crackers with salted tops

Catsup

Canned soups and stews

Caviar

Chili sauce

Chipped beef

Cheeses: regular, processed

  Camembert

  Gorgonzola

  Roquefort

Cold cuts

Corned beef

Codfish: salted or dried

Cooking wines

Frankfurters

Herring: salted or dried

Instant soups and instant cooked cereals

Kosher meats: if prepared kosher style by salting

Meat extracts/sauces/tenderizers

Mustard

Olives

Pickles

Popcorn: salted

Potato chips

Pretzels

Relishes

Salted nuts

Salted snacks

Sauerkraut

Sardines

Sausage

Sodium saccharin

Vegetables prepared in brine or heavy salted

Worcestershire sauce

[a]Reduce salt, monosodium glutamate, and soy sauce used in preparation of food and as seasoning as directed (usually about one-half normal intake). Celery, onion, or garlic salt may be used in place of the regular seasoning allowance.

TREATMENT

The treatment of secondary hypertension is directed toward eliminating the underlying cause. Essential hypertension is treated with antihypertensive drugs, sedatives, and relaxation.

DIET THERAPY

A low-sodium diet may be prescribed in conjunction with antihypertensive medications. The combination of drugs and diet may permit a lower drug dosage and a less rigid restriction of sodium. A low-Calorie diet may be prescribed for patients who are overweight. There is a 6.6 mm Hg rise in blood pressure in men for every 10% gain in weight (Mahan, 1979). Weight loss often results in a reduction of blood pressure. Weight reduction in women is only one-half as effective in reducing blood pressure.

Diet therapy for hypertension consists of a sodium-restricted, low-Calorie diet in which 50% of the Calories come from carbohydrates. Emphasis is on intake of complex carbohydrates rather than concentrated sugars. The protein content of the diet is normal, with high-biologic-value proteins recommended. The diet is moderately low in fats.

NURSING IMPLICATIONS

- Encourage the patient to have patience. It takes from 4 to 6 weeks for improvement in blood pressure to be noted when diet therapy is used as the sole treatment modality.
- Suggest that the patient remove the saltshaker from the table and develop the habit of tasting food before salting it.
- If added salt is permitted, suggest the substitution of a salt dish and salt spoon for a saltshaker. The amount of salt shaken on food tends to be grossly underestimated.
- Support patients in adhering to their diets. Assure them that in a month or so, they will adapt to the new level of sodium intake.
- Provide information on the use of alternative seasoning to replace sodium-rich additives.
- Fresh or powdered onion and garlic (not onion or garlic salt), lemon juice, table wine, and vinegar may be used to add flavor. Basil, rosemary, oregano, paprika, chili powder, and pepper are acceptable spices to use in low-sodium diets.
- Cooking without salt may permit the addition of a small amount of salt or seasoning at the table. It also eliminates the need for special cooking for the dieter.
- Because the American diet contains much more sodium on the average than is needed, families whose hypertension appears to be triggered by salt intake may wish to reduce their salt intake prophylactically.

References

Adams, C. *Nutritive value of American foods in common units* (Agriculture Handbook No. 456). Washington D.C.: U.S. Department of Agriculture, 1975.

American Heart Association. *Your 500 milligram sodium diet.* New York 1968a.

American Heart Association. *Your 1000 milligram sodium diet.* New York 1968b.

American Heart Association. *Your mild sodium-restricted diet.* New York 1969.

American Heart Association. *Diet and coronary heart disease.* New York 1978a.

American Heart Association. *Diet modification to control hyperlipidemia.* New York 1978b.

Brunner, L., & Suddarth, D. *Textbook of medical-surgical nursing* (4th ed.). Philadelphia: J. B. Lippincott Company, 1980.

Flynn, M. The cholesterol controversy. *Contemporary Nutrition,* March 1978, *3*(3).

Frederickson, D., Levy, R., & Lees, R. Fat transport in lipoproteins—An integrated approach to mechanisms and disorders. *New England Journal of Medicine,* January/February 1967, 276:34.

Gotto, A. M. Statement in diet-related killer diseases. Second Hearing Before Select Committee on Nutrition and Human Needs in United States Senate, Part I Cardiovascular Diseases. Washington, D.C.: United States Government Printing Office, 1977.

Hill, M. Helping the hypertensive patient control sodium intake. *American Journal of Nursing,* May 1979, *79,* 5.

Howe, P. *Basic nutrition in health and disease* (6th ed.). Philadelphia: W. B. Saunders Company, 1976.

Krause, M., & Mahan, L. K. *Food, nutrition and diet therapy* (6th ed.). Philadelphia: W. B. Saunders Company, 1979.

Luckmann, J., & Sorensen, K. *Medical-surgical nursing: A psychophysiologic approach* (2nd ed.). Philadelphia: W. B. Saunders Company, 1980.

Mahan, L. K. A sensible approach to the obese patient. *Nursing Clinics of North America,* June 1979, *14,* 2.

Mallison, M. Updating the cholesterol controversy: Verdict—Diet does count. *American Journal of Nursing,* October 1978, *78,* 10.

Mikkola, M. The cardiovascular system. In R. Howard & N. Herbold, *Nutrition in clinical care.* New York: McGraw-Hill Book Company, 1978.

Mitchell, H., Rynbergen, H., Anderson, L., et al: *Nutrition in health and disease* (16th ed.). Philadelphia: J. B. Lippincott Company, 1976.

National Heart, Lung, and Blood Institute. *The dietary management of hyperlipoproteinemia—A handbook for physicians and dietitians* (DHEW Publication No. [NIH] 78–110). Bethesda, Md.: National Institutes of Health, 1978.

North Dakota State Wheat Commission. *Sodium controlled diet.* Bismarck, 1978.

O'Malley, M., Scott, L., Foreyt, J., et al. Diet and heart disease: The basic concepts. *Health Values: Achieving High Level Wellness,* September/October 1978, *2,* 5.

Reiser, R. The three weak links in the diet-heart disease connection. *Nutrition Today,* August 1979, *14,* 4.

Robinson, C., & Lawler, M. *Normal and therapeutic nutrition* (15th ed.). New York: Macmillan Publishing Company, 1977.

Taylor, W., & Raizner, A. Prevention of cardiovascular disease: A research perspective. *Health Values: Achieving High Level Wellness,* September/October 1978, *2,* 5.

Williams, S. *Nutrition and diet therapy* (3rd ed.). St. Louis: C. V. Mosby Company, 1977.

World Health Organization. Heart and health—25 Facts about cardiovascular disease. *Nursing Mirror,* March 22, 1974, *138,* 1.

9

Diet Therapy in the Preoperative and Postoperative Periods

Pathophysiology of Surgical Intervention

Preoperatively, most patients are kept "nothing by mouth" for at least 8 hours before an operation. Depending on the patient and the nature of the surgical procedure, food intake may have been inadequate for an extended period before the operation. Apprehension, pain, and medications also induce anorexia. The surgical period is one of limited starvation.

Metabolism is the process by which the body uses the nutrients absorbed in the blood after digestion. The anabolic phase of metabolism is constructive: Ingested substances are converted into the constituents of protoplasm. The catabolic phase is destructive: Protoplasm is broken down into simpler compounds, and energy is released.

Carbohydrate is stored as glycogen in the liver and muscles, but glycogen is a relatively minor source of fuel and is usually reserved for emergency situations in which anaerobic metabolism occurs. The total amount of body protein is relatively fixed in a healthy person. Protein intake in excess of the body's need for growth and repair is converted to glucose for energy or stored as fat. Excessive burning of the body protein for energy may interfere with body function. Excessive protein catabolism also upsets nitrogen balance. Nitrogen balance is the difference between the amount of nitrogen ingested and the amount excreted. If intake is greater than output, a positive balance exists. Conversely, if output exceeds intake, a negative balance exists. Protein is an inefficient source of fuel, yielding only 1 to 2 kcal per gram. Except in extreme starvation, burning body fat for fuel does not affect body function.

138

During the first few days of starvation, fats and proteins are burned for energy, and the small carbohydrate reserve is spared for emergency situations. About 58% of muscle protein is capable of being converted to glucose; the nitrogen component is excreted in the urine. Oral intake is impossible during the surgical procedure and in the immediate postoperative period, so catabolism continues. Depending on the nature of the surgical procedure and the patient's response, oral feedings are gradually resumed postoperatively. However, it will be about 1 week, under the best conditions, before a patient who has undergone major surgery is able to ingest a diet sufficient to meet his or her body's need for nutrients.

When the body burns fat tissue for energy, metabolic acidosis develops. One result of metabolic acidosis is anorexia, which further complicates postoperative diet therapy. A standard procedure for most operative patients is intravenous feedings of glucose to forestall acidosis and spare body tissue. A solution of 5% glucose in water provides 170 Calories per liter. To attempt to supply the body's entire energy needs with intravenous glucose is impossible without causing fluid overload. Use of stronger solutions of glucose that are hypertonic is also limited by renal function, damage to the veins, and diuretic action. It has been estimated that the usual surgical patient loses 0.5 pound of body weight every day during the first few postoperative days. In addition to the medically imposed oral intake restrictions, the body responds to surgical intervention the same way it responds to any stress. The stress response is usually elicited by the operative procedure and anesthesia, but extreme apprehension can initiate the stress response in the preoperative period.

Characteristics of the stress response include retention of sodium and chloride and excretion of potassium. With these changes, body fluids are retained, and intracellular fluid is shifted into the extracellular areas. This action is viewed as protective against hypovolemia and hypotension. Further conservation of body fluids is achieved by increased secretion of antidiuretic hormone, which restricts urinary output. Increased secretion by the adrenal cortex promotes gluconeogenesis, which converts protein and fat to glucose to meet the body's need for energy.

Increased urinary losses of nitrogen, coupled with reduced intake of protein, leads the surgical patient into a negative nitrogen balance. Additional changes in body metabolism accompany specific surgical procedures, prolonged operations, and losses of body secretions and their electrolytes. All patients whose bodies are incised lose varying amounts of blood and tissue fluid in the course of surgical procedures.

Preoperative Treatment

A patient who is in good nutritional status can withstand the stress of surgical intervention better than can a patient who is in less than optimal condition. Except in cases of elective surgery, there is little opportunity to correct nutritional deficits before operations. The only absolute nutritional barrier to surgical intervention is dehydration, and even this condition can be quickly corrected by intravenous therapy.* In emergency situations, the relative danger of surgery in a patient with major deficiencies must be weighed against the danger of delay. The nutrients that have been identified as being important during the surgical experience are:

- Proteins to build new tissue during the healing process
- Carbohydrates and fats to supply the body's energy needs and spare proteins for repair
- Glucose to prevent postoperative ketosis and vomiting
- Vitamin K to aid in clotting of blood
- Vitamin C to aid in healing of wounds and in formation of collagen
- Vitamin B complex to form coenzymes necessary for metabolic reactions
- Thiamine to oxidize carbohydrate and to maintain gastrointestinal function.
- Zinc to aid in healing of wounds
- Iron for the synethesis of hemoglobin in the presence of blood loss

The two major nutritional problems in the preoperative period are undernutrition and obesity. An undernourished patient usually needs Calories, proteins, vitamins, and minerals. Hypoproteinemia predisposes the patient to shock, particularly when other surgical factors threaten maintenance of blood volume. Protein protects the liver from anesthesia toxicity and reduces edema at the incisional site. In the presence of long-standing protein deficiency, there is increased susceptibility to infection due to decreased ability to manufacture antibodies. Protein deficiency is also related to superficial atrophy of the mucous membrane of the respiratory and gastrointestinal tracts, which increases the risk for postoperative infections in these areas. Although it is possible to provide the needed nutrients intravenously to correct major deficiencies, it may not be possible to correct long-standing deficiencies before surgical intervention. Hyperalimentation offers an opportunity to provide optimal nutrition to counteract deficiencies if the surgical procedure can be postponed without increasing the risks for the patient.

The second major preoperative nutritional problem is obesity. An obese surgical patient is at greater risk than is one whose weight is normal. Excess adipose tissue places a greater strain on the heart. It has been estimated that there are 25 miles of blood vessels for every 30 pounds of

*Anemia can also be corrected by blood transfusions to ensure adequate hemoglobin for oxygen supply to the body cells.

excess weight. Fat tissue is less resistant to infection, placing the obese patient in increased danger of contracting postoperative infections. Fatty tissue is difficult to approximate and suture, so the obese patient is more prone to wound dehiscence. Some anesthetic substances are sequestered in fat and remain there for long periods after they have disappeared from the blood. Thus, these agents have a shorter duration of action and must be given in smaller doses if they need to be readministered within a few hours of the initial dose. Thiopental sodium (pentothal sodium), halothane (Fluothane) and trichloroethylene (Trilene) are examples of such anesthetic agents. The incidences of hypertension, congestive heart failure, and diabetes mellitus are also higher in obese persons, and these diseases further complicate surgical intervention.

DIET THERAPY

When possible, an undernourished patient should be prepared for a surgical procedure by receiving the required nutrients in amounts necessary to overcome deficiencies. Few people who are able to ingest food become seriously malnourished. Anorexia associated with malnutrition may be overcome by initial tube feedings, permitting the patient to progress to an enriched diet. Anorexia caused by the disease that has necessitated the operation may be alleviated by tube feedings. Supplemental liquid feedings may be the answer for patients who have limited appetites. Ideally, a poorly nourished patient should have a diet containing an adequate number of Calories to promote weight gain, protein to restore a positive nitrogen balance, and vitamins, minerals, and fluids to restore health.

An important consideration in the immediate preoperative period is the nutrients that cannot be stored by the body. Because no more than a 24-hour supply of glucose can be stored, the meals on the day before the operation should provide ample glucose. Vitamin C and vitamin B complex should also be provided in generous amounts. Fluids should be urged until the time that they are ordered withheld.

There is no quick way for an obese person to lose weight safely before an operation. The obese person who has time to prepare should be placed on a low-Calorie diet, but care must be taken to ensure that all essential nutrients are being provided in adequate amounts. Starvation diets have no place in preoperative preparation. When possible, increased activity may be suggested to augment the low-Calorie diet.

Preparation of a person who has no nutritional problems should also take into consideration the special nutritional implications of surgical intervention. A diet rich in carbohydrates, proteins, minerals, vitamins, and fluids may promote a more rapid recovery or at least a more comfortable convalescence in which incisions heal quickly, intravenous infusions are discontinued promptly, and postoperative complaints are fewer, permitting a fast return to a regular diet.

NURSING IMPLICATIONS

- Encourage preoperative patients to eat foods containing nutrients that provide protection during the surgical experience: proteins, carbohydrates, vitamins K, C, and B complex, thiamine, iron, zinc, and calcium.
- Provide and encourage fluid intake preoperatively.
- Unless contraindicated, provide a sweetened, vitamin C-rich beverage on the evening of the operation.
- Urge anesthetists to write realistic preoperative orders regarding the withholding of fluids.
- Lollipops may be a readily accepted source of preoperative glucose for pediatric patients.
- Popsicles provide both glucose and fluids.
- Remember that edema may mask undernutrition and gives an inaccurate indication of true body mass.

Postoperative Treatment

Most surgical patients have an intravenous infusion started preoperatively and are usually given 5% glucose in water to keep the intravenous line open in the event of need for special fluids, blood, or medications. One liter of 5% glucose in water provides 170 Calories; as little as 100 grams of carbohydrate daily (2 liters of 5% glucose) can reduce protein breakdown by one-half.

Ideally, postoperative nutrition is designed to satisfy the body's requirements, for fluids, electrolytes, energy, and replacement of any special losses until the patient is able to return to his or her regular diet and activities. The routine progression, once oral intake is permitted postoperatively, starts with sips of water or ice chips and progresses to clear liquids, then full liquids, to a soft diet, and finally to the patient's regular diet. The timing of this sequence is highly dependent on the patient's progress, the type of operation, complicating factors, and the surgeon's preference.

Many surgical procedures, because of their type or severity, preclude oral intake, and the patient's nutritional needs must be met intravenously or by tube feeding, gastrostomy, or hyperalimentation. The peristaltic and absorptive functions of the gastrointestinal tract are reduced after most operations, so that a gradual resumption of oral intake is the rule. The postoperative patient is in negative nitrogen balance until about the fifth to seventh postoperative days, so that the need for protein foods to replace lost nitrogen should be considered in selecting and offering foods and fluids.

Immobilization increases the loss of nutrients, especially proteins and calcium. Although the replacement of calcium in the immobilized patient is questionable due to the danger of renal calculi, the need for protein should be considered in meal planning for the bedfast patient.

NURSING IMPLICATIONS

- Intravenous infusions are only a stopgap measure, and nurses should do everything in their power to permit them to be discontinued as soon as possible.
- Because the body tends to retain sodium and fluids postoperatively, total fluid intake should be carefully assessed in light of total fluid losses to avoid circulatory overload.
- Patients tend to lose about 0.5 pound per day in the early postoperative period; weight gain during this period may be an indication of fluid excess.
- Encourage intake of foods and fluids to replace the most probable losses, that is, potassium after ileostomy, sodium (if not contraindicated) after cholecystectomy, and bile drainage.
- Ambulation not only prevents many postoperative complications but also increases appetite and prevents loss of proteins and calcium.
- Swallowed air contributes to the formation of gas in the postoperative period. Encourage patients to eat and drink slowly.
- Severe sepsis increases metabolic needs.
- Time dressing changes and other treatments that might cause anorexia as far away from mealtimes as possible.

Special Surgical Situations

Diabetes Mellitus

During the surgical experience, the diabetic faces increased threats to his or her already disturbed metabolism. The blood level of glucose must be controlled in the presence of the stress reaction, which elevates the blood level of glucose and increases the need for insulin. Protection must be provided from the ketoacidosis of starvation that accompanies surgical procedures as well as the ketoacidosis of diabetes.

Preoperative preparation for the diabetic patient includes increased caloric intake, with extra carbohydrate and proteins for several days before the operation. This increased intake must be combined with appropriate insulin coverage. The aim of this dietary expansion is to ensure an adequate glycogen store and to provide the extra protein needed during the surgical procedure.

The surgical experience includes other procedures that imply special concern for the diabetic patient. For example, both morphine and meperidine (Demerol), widely used preoperatively, may cause nausea and vomiting that decrease the blood level of glucose and reduce the need for insulin in the immediate postoperative period. Failure to equate the glucose and insulin needs of the patient during the operation could lead to hypoglycemia, which is more difficult to recognize in the unconscious patient.

The blood level of glucose in a diabetic patient should be monitored throughout the surgical experience. A blood sample should be drawn 1 hour before the operation for determination of the glucose level; if the level is below the patient's normal value, it should be increased by intravenous infusion of glucose. Many physicians believe that a slight degree of hyperglycemia is desirable during surgical procedures.

A diabetic surgical patient needs close observation in the postoperative period. The nurse must be prepared to assess the patient's condition and take steps to counter either ketoacidosis or hypoglycemia. An intravenous line is essential to provide glucose rapidly. Regular insulin is usually ordered by the subcutaneous route because of problems of control when it is added to intravenous solution. (Insulin tends to adhere to glass and plastic.) Various regimens exist for protecting the diabetic surgical patient from the twin dangers of ketoacidosis and hypoglycemia. The physician selects his or her plan on the basis of the severity of the diabetes and the magnitude and duration of the surgical procedure.

The use of nasogastric suction further complicates the problem of the surgical diabetic patient. The patient must be guarded against acidosis, electrolyte imbalance, and dehydration. The nurse must record all intake and output carefully. The intravenous infusion record is critical because glucose Calories as well as fluid intake are calculated on these notations. The dietary goal for the diabetic is to return to oral intake as soon as possible.

NURSING IMPLICATIONS

- Request specific written orders regarding insulin dosage on the day of the operation.
- Include specific written instructions for insulin in the preoperative nursing care plan. If the usual insulin dose is to be withheld, indicate this instruction. If alternative insulin coverage is being used, specify that it replaces the usual dosage.
- The usual intravenous replacement is 50 grams of glucose per missed meal. One liter of 5% glucose contains 50 grams.

In assessing diabetics postoperatively, evaluate all the factors that might contribute to ketoacidosis, namely, starvation, reduced insulin dosage, insulin added to intravenous solution, nausea and vomiting, lack of exercise, increased gluconeogenesis, and nasogastric suction. Evaluate all the factors that might contribute to hypoglycemia: too little glucose, slowing of the intravenous rate, or infiltration of the intravenous glucose solution without a comparable change in insulin coverage.

Neurosurgery

The type of surgical procedure influences the postoperative dietary regimen; however, some guidelines are usually followed. Some surgeons believe that it is not necessary to restrict fluids in the postoperative period to reduce cerebral edema. Other surgeons limit total fluid intake to 1,500 milliliters per day for several days after neurosurgery. If oral feedings are permitted, patients are usually fed for the first 48 hours postoperatively to ensure adequate intake and reduce exertion.

After supratentorial surgery, there is no contraindication to oral feedings as soon as the patient is able to swallow. Food may be allowed as early as the day of the operation. If vomiting occurs, feedings are withheld temporarily. Vomiting causes strain and could lead to intracranial bleeding.

After infratentorial surgery, the patient is usually not given food for at least 24 hours because of impaired gag and swallow reflexes. After 24 hours, water is given to test the reflexes, with suction equipment readily available. If the reflexes are impaired, feedings continue to be withheld. Tube feedings may be used if the swallowing muscles are involved more than 48 hours.

After spinal surgery, food and fluids are permitted as soon as nausea subsides. Diets are then expanded as tolerated.

Surgery of the Mouth and Throat

Unless the surgical procedure indicates another route of feeding, after patients have undergone surgical procedures on the mouth or throat, they are expected to take, chew, and swallow in the presence of incised, sutured, or manipulated tissue. This ingestion of food or fluid usually causes discomfort. Fluids are usually offered first. The use of a straw may be helpful, for example, in the case of a dental extraction, or it may be specifically contraindicated, as in the case of cleft palate repairs. Soft foods are sometimes less painful to swallow than are liquids. In selecting foods and fluids to offer the patient with mouth or throat surgery, avoid hot beverages, tart juices, and fiber. Milk, yogurt, sherbet, ice cream, ginger ale, and dilute fruit juices may be allowed. It is important to encourage swallowing, and any food that the patient will take within the limits of the prescribed diet is acceptable to accomplish this goal in the early postoperative period. Once the dysphagia subsides, concern for nutritional aspects should be considered in food selection.

Gastrectomy

When oral feedings are allowed after the complete or partial removal of the stomach, the loss or reduction of this food reservoir dictates the use of small feedings offered at frequent intervals. When gastric secretions, hydrochloric acid, and pepsin are absent, protein is digested in the small intestine. Gastrectomy causes other changes in digestion. These changes include reduced mixing of food, inadequate pancreatic and bile secretions, increased intestinal motility, deficiencies of vitamin B_{12} and folic acid, disordered calcium metabolism, and decreased absorption of calcium and vitamin D. These deficiencies are related to a decrease in the concentration of intrinsic factor or to inadequate absorption due to increased intestinal motility.

The usual diet progression after gastrectomy is a small amount of fluid every hour. The fluid in the initial feeding is water, and gradually the progression is to clear fluids and then to full fluids. Soft, low-fiber meals are then introduced. Five or six high-protein, high-fat, low-carbohydrate feedings are the next step. Fluids should not be given until about 1 hour after meals. Simple sugars should be avoided. Eventually, tissue expansion permits a return to a three-meal-a-day schedule.

Ileostomy

Ileostomy patients lose considerable amounts of fluid that contain sodium and potassium. Absorption of fat and vitamin B_{12} is reduced. Initial oral intake is fluids, and as these are tolerated, consideration should be given to the replacement of electrolyte losses by fluids rich in sodium and potassium.

Good Fluid Sources of Sodium

Milk
Bouillon
Broth

Good Fluid Sources of Potassium (all more 100 milliequivalents per deciliter)

Tomato juice
Grapefruit juice
Pineapple juice
Milk
Orange juice
Apricot nectar
Apple juice
Cocoa

The use of any of the sources of electrolytes just cited should also be evaluated in regard to their effect on the ileostomy drainage. Prune juice, the richest source of potassium among the fruit juices, has been omitted from the list because of its laxative effect. Other omissions may have to be made on the basis of individual response.

The addition of moderately low-fiber foods is made gradually. Only one food should be added at a time to allow evaluation of its effect. Eventually, a return to a regular diet is achieved, with elimination of foods that have been identified as producing problems. Excessive roughage is usually avoided because it may obstruct the stoma. Nuts, prunes, celery, corn, pineapples, turnips, beans, cabbage, and onions are examples of fibrous foods that are often troublesome to such patients. The highly fluid nature of the ileostomy drainage may prompt some patients to limit their fluid intake because of the misconception that this restriction thickens the ileostomy drainage or decreases the amount. Such patients must be cautioned against this practice, both because it is ineffective and because they have a high requirement for fluids.

Colostomy

The colostomy patient follows a dietary progression similar to that of the ileostomy patient once oral feedings are resumed. The location of the surgical opening permits an increase in fluid absorption and decreases the loss of electrolytes. The patient progresses from water to clear fluids to full fluids to a soft and, eventually, a regular diet. The person with a colostomy learns through experience which foods to omit because of their effect on the colostomy drainage. Like the ileostomy patient, the colostomy patient must be cautioned against intake of excessive roughage. Eating slowly and chewing food well is also helpful in preventing stomal obstruction.

Jejunoileostomy

A jejunoileostomy is a surgical procedure designed to allow food to bypass 90% of the small intestine. This surgical procedure is performed for extreme obesity. Weight loss occurs because food is in the small intestine for a much shorter period, thus reducing the absorption of nutrients. Nutritional problems associated with this operation include reduced absorption, diarrhea, and electrolyte imbalance. Electrolyte disturbances consist of substantial losses of potassium, magnesium, and calcium. Because lactose, fiber, and fat increase the occurrence of diarrhea and, therefore, electrolyte loss, the dietary plan should include:

- Restriction of fluids to between meals
- High-protein, low-fat, low-fiber, low-carbohydrate diet

- Six small feedings
- Replacement of electrolyte losses
- Supplementation of essential nutrients that are malabsorbed

Hemorrhoidectomy

After surgical removal of hemorrhoids, a low-residue diet is usually pre-scribed to delay defecation and to allow healing at the operative site. A slow progression from a clear fluid to a soft diet has the same effect be-cause such diets are low in residue. Once healing has occurred, return to a high-fiber diet is recommended to prevent constipation. If a high-fiber diet is too irritating for the patient, a low-fiber diet with plenty of stewed fruit, cooked vegetables, and fluids may be recommended.

References

Brand, J., & Tolins, S. *The nursing student's guide to surgery*. Boston: Little, Brown & Company, 1979.

Goldstein, S. Surgery, stress, burns and nutritional care. In R. Howard & N. Her-bold, *Nutrition in clinical care*. New York: McGraw-Hill Book Company, 1978.

Howe, P. *Basic nutrition in health and disease* (6th ed.). Philadelphia: W. B. Saunders Company, 1976.

Luckmann, J., & Sorensen, K. *Medical-surgical nursing: A Psychophysiologic approach* (2nd ed.). Philadelphia: W. B. Saunders Company, 1980.

Metheny, N., & Snively, W. *Nurses' handbook of fluid balance* (3rd ed.). Philadelphia: J. B. Lippincott Company, 1979.

Mitchell, H., Rynberger, H., Anderson, L., et al. *Nutrition in health and disease* (16th ed.). Philadelphia: J. B. Lippincott Company, 1976.

Robinson, C., & Lawler, M. *Normal and therapeutic nutrition* (15th ed.). New York: Macmillan Publishing Company, 1977.

Shils, M., & Randall, H. T. Diet and nutrition in the care of the surgical patient. In R. Goodhart, & M. Shils, (Eds.), *Modern nutrition in health and disease* (6th ed.). Philadelphia: Lea & Febiger, 1980.

Watson, J. *Medical-surgical nursing and related phsysiology* (2nd ed.). Philadelphia: W. B. Saunders Company, 1979.

10
Diet Therapy in Endocrine Disorders

Diabetes Mellitus

PATHOPHYSIOLOGY

Diabetes mellitus is characterized by disordered carbohydrate metabolism due to a deficiency of insulin. Eventually, the metabolism of proteins and fats is also affected, leading to ketosis and acidosis. Insulin deficiency may result from:

- Beta-cell damage in the islets of Langerhans
- Inactivation of insulin
- Increased requirements for insulin

Insulin deficiency initiates a series of reactions within the body because glucose cannot be transported from the extracellular fluid to the intracellular fluid. Without glucose, the cells have no source of energy. They are forced to use muscle protein and adipose tissue fat as alternative sources. Use of protein for energy leads to wasting of tissue and a negative nitrogen balance due to protein catabolism. Use of fat for energy leads to ketosis from rapid fat catabolism.

The glucose that is unable to leave the extracellular fluid accumulates, and the blood level of glucose rises, producing hyperglycemia. The increased glucose in the blood increases the osmotic pressure within the vessels and pulls fluid from the cells, leading to cellular dehydration. When the blood level of glucose exceeds the renal threshold, glucose spills over into the urine, producing glycosuria. Glycosuria increases the osmotic pressure of the urine and prevents tubular reabsorption of water, leading to extracellular dehydration. These physiologic changes produce the classic symptoms of diabetes mellitus: polyuria, polydipsia, and polyphagia. Weight loss is associated with the onset of juvenile diabetes, and obesity is a common finding in adult-onset diabetes.

Complications of diabetes mellitus include metabolic acidosis, which occurs in untreated and poorly controlled diabetes as a result of the excessive use of fat as an energy source. High levels of fat in the blood create a chronic hyperlipemia, which may be responsible for vascular lesions that can eventually lead to kidney damage and blindness. Neuropathic problems are related to increased blood levels of glucose. The increased glucose content of the blood leads to greater susceptibility to infections. Poor wound healing is associated with circulatory problems resulting from atherosclerosis.

TREATMENT

Diet therapy was the only treatment of diabetes mellitus before the discovery of insulin, and it remains the cornerstone of modern diabetic treatment. The management of diabetes mellitus is a balance of diet, insulin or hypoglycemic agents, and exercise. Insulin or oral hypoglycemic agents may be required to assure proper carbohydrate metabolism, although many people with adult-onset diabetes are able to control their disease with the proper diet alone. Exercise improves carbohydrate tolerance and reduces insulin requirements.

DIET THERAPY

The aim of diet therapy is to curtail excessive intake of carbohydrates, particularly in the form of concentrated sugars. Concentrated sugars produce a rapid rise in blood levels of glucose that cannot be handled in the presence of insulin deficiency. The avoidance or correction of obesity is another goal in diabetes mellitus. Weight loss alone may be sufficient therapy in situations where the disease has been precipitated by a demand for insulin beyond the body's ability to produce it.

There are two basic types of diets used in the treatment of diabetes mellitus, the qualitative and the quantitative. In the qualitative diet, the patient is advised not to add sugar to any foods, to avoid sweetened foods, and to limit foods with a high starch content. The quantitative diet uses exchange lists or a fixed-weight diet.

Exchange lists were devised by the American Diabetes Association and the American Dietetic Association to provide variety and control over diet for diabetics. Exchange lists include milk, vegetables, fruits, bread, meats, and fat. The serving sizes of foods in each group contain approximately the same number of Calories as well as approximately the same proportion of carbohydrate, protein, and fat. The patient is able to vary the diet by exchanging one food for another within the same exchange list. The exchange method allows the patient control within the limits of the diet. It provides a method that is easy to use and to understand. Diabetics are taught to use precise measuring devices until they are adept at gauging servings. They are also advised to measure foods at intervals to be sure they are using proper amounts. See Tables 10-1 through 10-8 for exchange lists. The fixed-weight diet requires that all food be weighed; this diet is rigidly prescribed, and amounts may not vary.

The physician orders the diet by prescribing the total Calories and percentages of carbohydrate, protein, and fat or the grams of carbohydrate, protein, and fat to be allowed. Caloric intake is calculated on the basis of ideal body weight for the patient, usually allowing 30 kcal for every kilogram of ideal body weight as a basic diet. If the patient is obese or elderly, 15 to 25 kcal per kilogram of body weight is used to calculate the total caloric intake. The person's level of activity affects caloric intake; 35 kcal per kilogram is used for light activity and 40 kcal per kilogram for strenuous activity.

There has been a trend toward increasing carbohydrate content of diabetic diets through the use of more starches. Starches are metabolized slowly into glucose and do not cause rapid rises in blood levels of glucose. Increased intake of complex carbohydrates increases glucose tolerance. The increased use of starches reduces the need for high fat intake in an

TABLE 10-1

MILK EXCHANGES

One exchange of milk contains 12 grams of carbohydrate, 8 grams of protein, a trace of fat, and 80 calories. Underlined exchanges are nonfat.

Nonfat fortified milk	
Skim or nonfat milk	1 cup
Powdered (nonfat dry, before adding liquid)	⅓ cup
Canned, evaporated skim milk	½ cup
Buttermilk made from skim milk	1 cup
Yogurt made from skim milk (plain, unflavored)	1 cup
Low-fat fortified milk	
1% fat fortified milk (omit ½ fat exchange)	1 cup
2% fat fortified milk (omit 1 fat exchange)	1 cup
Yogurt made from 2% fortified milk (plain, unflavored; omit 1 fat exchange)	1 cup
Whole milk (omit 2 fat exchanges)	
Whole milk	1 cup
Canned, evaporated whole milk	½ cup
Buttermilk made from whole milk	1 cup
Yogurt made from whole milk (plain, unflavored)	1 cup

Source: These exchange lists are based on material in Exchange lists for meal planning prepared by committees of the American Diabetes Association and the American Dietetic Association in cooperation with the National Institute of Arthritis, Metabolism, and Digestive Diseases and the National Heart and Lung Institute.

TABLE 10-2
VEGETABLE EXCHANGES

One exchange of vegetables contains about 5 grams of carbohydrate, 2 grams of protein, and 25 Calories. One exchange is ½ cup.

Asparagus	Greens
Bean sprouts	Mustard
Beets	Spinach
Broccoli	Turnip
Brussels sprouts	Mushrooms
Cabbage	Okra
Carrots	Onions
Cauliflower	Rhubarb
Celery	Rutabaga
Eggplant	Sauerkraut
Green pepper	String beans, green or yellow
Greens	Summer squash
Beet	Tomatoes
Chards	Tomato juice
Collards	Turnips
Dandelion	Vegetable juice cocktail
Kale	Zucchini

The following raw vegetables may be used as desired:

Chicory	Lettuce
Chinese cabbage	Parsley
Cucumbers	Pickles, dill
Endive	Radishes
Escarole	Watercress

Starchy vegetables are found in Table 10-4.

Source: These exchange lists are based on material in *Exchange lists for meal planning* prepared by committees of the American Diabetes Association and the American Dietetic Association in cooperation with the National Institute of Arthritis, Metabolism, and Digestive Diseases and the National Heart and Lung Institute.

attempt to meet caloric needs. The older diabetic diets were usually proportioned as 40% carbohydrates and fats and 20% proteins. The modern diabetic diet is proportioned as 50 to 60% carbohydrates, 30 to 35% fats, and 15% proteins.

Once the total intake has been determined, the food is divided into meals and snacks on the basis of eating habits and the time of administration and duration of action of the hypoglycemic agents used. Table 10-9 shows the calculation of a diabetic diet.

Juvenile Diabetes Mellitus

When diabetes mellitus develops during childhood, it is usually characterized by an abrupt onset in an underweight or normal-weight child. Juvenile diabetes increases in severity during the growth period. All diabetic

TABLE 10-3

FRUIT EXCHANGES

One exchange of fruit contains 10 grams of carbohydrate and 40 Calories.

Apple	1 small	Mango	½ small
Apple juice	⅓ cup	Melon	
Applesauce (unsweetened)	½ cup	Cantaloupe	¼ small
Apricots, fresh	2 medium	Honeydew	⅛ medium
Apricots, dried	4 halves	Watermelon	1 cup
Banana	½ small	Nectarine	1 small
Berries		Orange	1 small
Blackberries	½ cup	Orange juice	½ cup
Blueberries	½ cup	Papaya	¾ cup
Raspberries	½ cup	Peach	1 medium
Strawberries	¾ cup	Pear	1 small
Cherries	10 large	Persimmon, native	1 medium
Cider	⅓ cup	Pineapple	½ cup
Dates	2	Pineapple juice	⅓ cup
Fig, fresh	1	Plums	2 medium
Fig, dried	1	Prunes	2 medium
Grapefruit	½	Prune juice	¼ cup
Grapefruit juice	½ cup	Raisins	2 tablespoons
Grapes	12	Tangerine	1 medium
Grape juice	¼ cup		

Cranberries may be used as desired if no sugar is added.

Source: These exchange lists are based on material in *Exchange lists for meal planning* prepared by committees of the American Diabetes Association and the American Dietetic Association in cooperation with the National Institute of Arthritis, Metabolism, and Digestive Diseases and the National Heart and Lung Institute.

children require insulin because the beta-cells of the islets of Langerhans are nonfunctional. Insulin dosage usually increases with the age of the child.

The goal of treatment for children with diabetes mellitus is to provide a diet that permits normal growth and activity and that controls the disease. The diet should also allow children self-expression and independence by recognizing their food preferences and aversions. Children need to be as much like their peers as possible, and the diet should include suggestions for eating with friends. Insulin dosage is calculated to cover the prescribed diet. Food restriction is never used for diabetic control for a child with diabetes because the child needs food for growth and development of body systems in addition to energy requirements.

The diet is planned to allow 75 to 90 kcal per kilogram of ideal body weight for the child's age. Protein requirements are 3.3 grams per kilogram for younger children and taper to 2.2 grams per kilogram for older children. The protein allowance is usually about 20% of the total caloric allotment. About 50% of the total Calories come from complex carbohydrates; the remaining 30% come from fats. Another method used to cal-

TABLE 10-4

BREAD EXCHANGES (INCLUDES BREADS, CEREALS, AND STARCHY VEGETABLES)

One exchange of bread contains 15 grams of carbohydrate, 2 grams of protein, and 70 Calories. Starchy vegetables are included in this list because they contain the same amounts of carbohydrate and protein as 1 slice of bread. Underlined exchanges are low fat.

Breads

White (including French and Italian)	1 slice
Whole wheat	1 slice
Rye or pumpernickel	1 slice
Raisin	1 slice
Bagel, small	½
English muffin, small	½
Plain roll, bread	1
Frankfurter roll	½
Hamburger bun	½
Dried bread crumbs	3 tablespoons
Tortilla, 6 inch	1

Cereals

Bran flakes	½ cup
Other ready-to-eat, unsweetened cereal	¾ cup
Puffed cereal (unfrosted)	1 cup
Cereal (cooked)	½ cup
Grits (cooked)	½ cup
Rice or barley (cooked)	½ cup
Pasta (cooked)	½ cup
Spaghetti, noodles, macaroni	
Popcorn (popped, no fat added, large kernel)	3 cups
Cornmeal (dry)	2 tablespoons
Flour	2½ tablespoons
Wheat germ	¼ cup

Crackers

Arrowroot	3
Graham 2½-inch square	2
Matzo 4 × 6 inch	½
Oyster	20
Pretzels 3⅛ inch long × ⅛ inch diameter	25
Rye, wafer 2 × 3½ inch	3
Saltines	6
Soda 2½ inch square	4

Dried beans, peas, and lentils

Beans, peas, lentils (dried and cooked)	½ cup
Baked beans, no pork (canned)	¼ cup

TABLE 10-4 (Continued)

Starchy vegetables	
Corn	⅓ cup
Corn on cob	1 small
Lima beans	½ cup
Parsnips	⅔ cup
Peas, green (canned or frozen)	½ cup
Potato, white	1 small
Potato (mashed)	½ cup
Pumpkin	¾ cup
Yam or sweet potato	¼ cup
Winter squash, acorn or butternut	½ cup
Prepared foods	
Biscuit 2 inch diameter (omit 1 fat exchange)	1
Corn bread 2 × 2 × 1 inch (omit 1 fat exchange)	1
Corn muffin 2 inch diameter (omit 1 fat exchange)	1
Crackers, round butter type (omit 1 fat exchange)	5
Muffin, plain small (omit 1 fat exchange)	1
Potatoes, french fried, length 2 to 3½ inch (omit 1 fat exchange)	8
Potato or corn chips (omit 2 fat exchanges)	15
Pancake 5 × ½ inch (omit 1 fat exchange)	1
Waffles 5 × ½ inch (omit 1 fat exchange)	1

Source: These exchange lists are based on material in *Exchange lists for meal planning* prepared by committees of the American Diabetes Association and the American Dietetic Association in cooperation with the National Institute of Arthritis, Metabolism, and Digestive Diseases and the National Heart and Lung Institute.

culate the diet for a diabetic child is to allow 1,000 kcal for 1 year of age and add 100 kcal for every additional year of age. In this method, a 3 -year-old child with diabetes would receive 1,300 kcal and a 12-year-old child 2,200 kcal. A third method allows 100 kcal per kilogram between the ages of 1 and 4 years, 75 kcal per kilogram between the ages of 5 and 9 years, 50 kcal per kilogram between the ages of 10 and 14 years, and 40 kcal per kilogram at 15 years. Protein accounts for 20% of the total caloric intake.

The total food intake is usually divided into three meals and three snacks but can be arranged in other ways to meet particular needs imposed by the type of insulin(s) used, the dosage, and the life-style of the child. Total Calories are divided into eighteenths and usually allotted as follows:

Breakfast 4/18
Morning snack 2/18
Lunch 5/18
Afternoon snack 1/18

Dinner   5/18

Bedtime snack   1/18

Snacks can be rearranged and eaten before activities. The use of concentrated glucose may be needed during sustained activity. The importance of providing a diet that the child will accept and that will permit full participation in peer activities is one of the best assurances against noncompliance.

The child should be taught how to use the exchange lists and should be permitted to manage the diet as soon as competence is demonstrated. Exchange lists for fast foods are available from the American Diabetes Association. These lists permit the adolescent to join peer groups and still adhere to the prescribed allowances.

TABLE 10-5

MEAT EXCHANGES, LEAN MEATS

One exchange of lean meat (1 ounce) contains 7 grams of protein, 3 grams of fat, and 55 Calories. Trim off all visible fat. To plan a diet low in saturated fat and cholesterol, choose only exchanges that are underlined.

Beef	
Baby beef (very lean), chipped beef, chuck, flank steak, tenderloin, plate ribs, plate skirt steak, round (bottom, top), all cuts rump, spare ribs, tripe	1 ounce
Lamb	
Leg, rib, sirloin, loin (roast and chops), shank, shoulder	1 ounce
Pork	
Leg (whole rump, center shank), ham, smoked (center slices)	1 ounce
Veal	
Leg, loin, rib, shank, cutlets	1 ounce
Poultry	
Meat without skin of chicken, turkey, Cornish hen, Guinea hen, pheasant	1 ounce
Fish	
Any fresh or frozen	1 ounce
Canned salmon, tuna, mackerel, crab, lobster	¼ cup
Clams, oysters, scallops, shrimp	5, or 1 ounce
Sardines, drained	3
Cheeses containing less than 5% butterfat	1 ounce
Cottage cheese, dry and 2% butterfat	¼ cup
Dried beans and peas (omit 1 bread exchange)	½ cup

Source: These exchange lists are based on material in *Exchange lists for meal planning* prepared by committees of the American Diabetes Association and the American Dietetic Association in cooperation with the National Institute of Arthritis, Metabolism, and Digestive Diseases and the National Heart and Lung Institute.

TABLE 10-6

MEAT EXCHANGES, MEDIUM-FAT MEATS

One exchange of medium-fat meat (1 ounce) contains 7 grams of protein, 5 grams of fat, and 75 Calories. Trim off all visible fat.

Beef	
Ground (15%), corned beef (canned), rib eye, round (ground commercial)	1 ounce
Pork	
Loin (all cuts tenderloin), shoulder arm (picnic), shoulder blade, Boston butt, Canadian bacon, boiled ham	1 ounce
Liver, heart, kidney, sweetbreads	1 ounce
Cottage cheese, creamed	¼ cup
Cheese	
Mozzarella, ricotta, farmer cheese, Neufchâtel, Parmesan	1 ounce
Egg	1
Peanut butter (omit 2 fat exchanges)	2 tablespoons

Source: These exchange lists are based on material in *Exchange lists for meal planning* prepared by committees of the American Diabetes Association and the American Dietetic Association in cooperation with the National Institute of Arthritis, Metabolism, and Digestive Diseases and the National Heart and Lung Institute.

TABLE 10-7

MEAT EXCHANGES, HIGH-FAT MEATS

One exchange of high-fat meat (1 ounce) contains 7 grams of protein, 8 grams of fat, and 100 Calories. Trim off all visible fat.

Beef	
Brisket, corned beef (brisket), ground beef (more than 20% fat), hamburger (commercial), chuck (ground commercial), roasts (rib), steaks (club and rib)	1 ounce
Lamb	
Breast	1 ounce
Pork	
Spare ribs, loin (back ribs), pork (ground), country-style ham, deviled ham	1 ounce
Veal	
Breast	1 ounce
Poultry	
Capon, duck (domestic), goose	1 ounce
Cheese	
Cheddar types	1 ounce
Cold cuts	4½ × ⅛-inch slice
Frankfurter	1 small

Source: These exchange lists are based on material in *Exchange lists for meal planning* prepared by committees of the American Diabetes Association and the American Dietetic Association in cooperation with the National Institute of Arthritis, Metabolism, and Digestive Diseases and the National Heart and Lung Institute.

TABLE 10-8
FAT EXCHANGES

One exchange of fat contains 5 grams of fat and 45 Calories. Underlined exchanges are polyunsaturated.

Margarine, soft, tub or stick[a]	1 teaspoon
Avocado (4 inch diameter)	1/8
Oil, corn, cottonseed, safflower, soy, sunflower	1 teaspoon
Oil, olive[b]	1 teaspoon
Oil, peanut[b]	1 teaspoon
Olives[b]	5 small
Almonds[b]	10 whole
Pecans[b]	2 large whole
Peanuts[b]	
Spanish	20 whole
Virginia	10 whole
Walnuts	6 small
Nuts, other[b]	6 small
Margarine, regular stick	1 teaspoon
Butter	1 teaspoon
Bacon fat	1 teaspoon
Bacon, crisp	1 strip
Cream, light	2 tablespoons
Cream, sour	2 tablespoons
Cream, heavy	1 tablespoon
Cream cheese	1 tablespoon
French dressing[c]	1 tablespoon
Italian dressing[c]	1 tablespoon
Lard	1 teaspoon
Mayonnaise[c]	1 teaspoon
Salad dressing, mayonnaise type[c]	2 teaspoons
Salt pork	3/4-inch cube

To plan a diet low in saturated fat, select only exchanges that are underlined. They are polyunsaturated.

Source: These exchange lists are based on material in *Exchange lists for meal planning* prepared by committees of the American Diabetes Association and the American Dietetic Association in cooperation with the National Institute of Arthritis, Metabolism, and Digestive Diseases and the National Heart and Lung Institute.

[a]Made with corn, cottonseed, safflower, soy, or sunflower oil only.

[b]Fat content is primarily monounsaturated.

[c]If made with corn, cottonseed, safflower, soy, or sunflower oil, can be used on a fat-modified diet.

Diabetes Mellitus During Pregnancy

The goal of care for the diabetic is to provide frequent evaluation to prevent the diabetes from adversely affecting the pregnancy and the pregnancy from adversely affecting the diabetes. In the early stages of pregnancy, food intake is usually reduced due to nausea and vomiting. Maternal glucose is also transferred to the fetus. Consequently, insulin requirements are reduced because there is less glucose circulating in the mother's blood. Insulin requirements are usually lower than prepregnancy requirements throughout the first half of pregnancy.

Fetal insulin is secreted at about 12 weeks of gestation, and the fetus is no longer dependent on maternal insulin after the first 3 months. In the second half of pregnancy, placental hormones act as insulin antagonists and offset the transfer of glucose to the fetus; consquently, insulin requirements increase. An increased tendency toward diabetic ketoacidosis is present in the second half of pregnancy that should be minimized to protect the fetus. Ketosis can result in fetal brain damage. Postpartum hormonal changes usually cause insulin requirements to fall below prepregnant levels.

The diet for a pregnant diabetic is based on about 30 kcal per kilogram of ideal body weight but should not fall below a total caloric intake of 1,400 kcal. Protein intake should be based on 1.5 to 2 grams per kilogram of ideal body weight, or approximately 20% of the total Calories. Carbohydrate intake is usually increased to about 45% of the total Calories, but a minimal carbohydrate intake of at least 200 grams per day is mandatory. Carbohydrate intake is supplied by starches, fruits, and vegetables.

Weight gain is not as rigidly controlled as in the past; this approach follows the trend for nondiabetic pregnant women. Weight reduction during pregnancy of a diabetic woman should be avoided.

Food intake is divided into three meals and two or three snacks to provide a continuous release of glucose and to prevent insulin reactions.

Diabetes Mellitus During Illness

A diabetic may become ill with a nonrelated complaint that interferes with food intake. If the illness is of a short-term nature, the diabetic is advised not to stop taking insulin. Oral hypoglycemic agents may be discontinued if the patient is anorexic. The diabetic should take liquids every hour and record the type and amount taken. If vomiting and diarrhea occur, salty liquids, such as broth, should be included.

When the diabetic is unable to eat the usual diet, carbohydrate foods should be replaced by carbohydrate liquids and semiliquids. This type of replacement should not continue more than 36 hours without consultation with a physician. Any illness that persists more than 72 hours or that interferes with liquid intake should be reported to a physician promptly.

TABLE 10-9

CALCULATION OF A DIABETIC DIET

Ideal body weight for a 65-inch middle-aged woman weighing 125 pounds, or 57 kilograms:

57 kg × 35 Calories (moderate activity) = 2,000 Calories

50% carbohydrate = 1,000 Calories, or 250 grams

30% fat = 600 Calories, or 66 grams

20% protein = 400 Calories, or 100 grams

Exchanges	Calories	Carbohydrates	Proteins	Fats
Breakfast				
1 fruit exchange				
½ small grapefruit	40	10		
2 bread exchanges				
¾ cup of dry cereal	70	15	2	
1 slice of toast	70	15	2	
1 fat exchange				
1 teaspoon of margarine	45			5
1 milk exchange				
1 cup of skim milk	80	12	8	
1 cup of black coffee				
	305	52	12	5
Midmorning				
2 vegetable exchanges				
1 cup of tomato juice	50	10	4	
2 meat exchanges				
2 ounces of cheddar cheese	200		14	16
2 bread exchanges				
12 saltines	140	30	4	
	390	40	22	16
Lunch				
3 meat exchanges				
¾ cup of tuna fish	165		21	9
3 bread exchanges				
2 slices of bread	140	30	4	
3 arrowroot crackers	70	15	2	
Allowed vegetables				
Lettuce and parsley				
1 fruit exchange				
1 small apple	40	10		
1 fat exchange				
1 teaspoon of margarine	45			5
	460	55	27	14
Dinner				
3 meat exchanges				
3 ounces of chicken	165		21	9
3 bread exchanges				

TABLE 10-9 (Continued)

1 baked potato	70	15	2	
1 slice of bread	70	15	2	
1 1½-inch cube of angel food cake	70	15	2	
1 vegetable exchange				
½ cup of broccoli	25	5	2	
List 2 vegetables				
½ cup of endive				
1 fruit exchange				
¼ cantaloupe	40	10		
3 fat exchanges				
2 teaspoons of margarine	90			10
2½ tablespoons of dressing	112			12
1 cup of black coffee				
	642	60	29	31
Bedtime				
1 milk exchange				
1 cup of skim milk	80	12	8	
2 bread exchanges				
4 graham crackers	140	30	4	
	220	42	12	0
Daily total	2,017	249	102	66

NURSING IMPLICATIONS

- A normal potassium level is necessary for production of insulin.
- Diabetic diets are expensive, but special diabetic foods are neither necessary nor desirable.
- Assist patients to differentiate between "dietetic" and "diabetic" foods. Dietetic foods are those that are produced for special restrictive diets (without sugar, salt, or sodium). Diabetic foods are those that are designed specifically for diabetic diets (sugar free).
- Increased intake of fiber may improve diabetic control by reducing blood levels of glucose (Anderson & Chen, 1979).
- Large doses of vitamin C affect some of the dip and tape tests for urinary levels of glucose, resulting in false-positive and false-negative results. Question all patients about prescription and nonprescription drug usage.
- Caution clients about claims regarding the use of fructose for diabetics. Although it is true that fructose is metabolized without insulin, it is still stored as glycogen and released as glucose. At the time of

release, insulin is needed to prevent an abnormal rise in blood levels of glucose.

- Sorbitol and mannitol are sugar alcohols used in some diabetic foods. These substances are carbohydrate in nature and are absorbed slowly from the intestine and converted to glucose. Diabetics tolerate small amounts of sugar alcohols better than they tolerate sucrose, but they should use sugar alcohols with discretion. Large amounts of sorbitol or mannitol eventually affect blood levels of glucose and may also cause diarrhea.

- All diabetic diets should provide at least 80 grams of carbohydrates daily to prevent ketosis.

- Diabetics may have other disorders that require diet therapy. One of the most common lipid abnormalities that occurs in diabetics is Type IV hyperlipoproteinemia, the carbohydrate-induced disorder related to excessive carbohydrate intake and elevated blood levels of triglycerides. The treatment of Type IV hyperlipoproteinemia is weight reduction, diet therapy, or both. Another frequent finding in diabetics is Type II hyperlipoproteinemia, which is treated by a diet that restricts fats to 30% of the total intake and limits saturated fats to 10% of the total intake (see Chapter 8).

- Low-sodium diet plans for diabetics are available from Eli Lilly Company.

- Encourage patients to adhere to regular mealtimes and snack times. The timing of food intake is as important as the total intake of Calories. Caution clients not to substitute exchanges between meals but to make substitutions only within the same meal or snack.

Functional Hypoglycemia (Hyperinsulinism)

PATHOPHYSIOLOGY

Functional, or reactive, hypoglycemia occurs when excessive amounts of insulin are secreted in response to the intake of carbohydrate-rich foods. The increased level of insulin in the blood causes symptoms that resemble the hypoglycemic reaction of diabetes mellitus or the dumping syndrome. Two to 4 hours after a meal, the patient feels weak, hungry, agitated, and becomes diaphoretic and sometimes unconscious. These symptoms are the result of the body's attempt to compensate for low blood levels of glucose by increasing the secretion of epinephrine. Epinephrine stimulates the liver to convert glycogen to glucose to increase the blood levels of glucose.

TREATMENT

Treatment focuses on reducing carbohydrate intake to a level that does not overstimulate the pancreas to secrete inappropriately large amounts of insulin.

DIET THERAPY

Carbohydrate intake is limited to 75 to 100 grams per day. Dietary carbohydrates should come mainly from low-carbohydrate fruits and vegetables. Milk is usually limited to 1 pint daily to reduce the insulin-triggering effect of lactose.

Protein intake is increased to 100 to 150 grams per day to provide energy as well as nutrients for growth and repair. Protein is metabolized into energy at a slow rate and does not stimulate excessive secretion of insulin. Fat provides the remainder of the caloric requirements. Food is divided into equal amounts at each meal to provide steady stimulation of the pancreas. A pattern of three small meals and three snacks is usual.

NURSING IMPLICATIONS

- Check the need for calcium and riboflavin supplementation in the adult diet. Children may need calcium supplementation due to their limited intake of milk.
- Alcohol intake can potentiate hypoglycemia by blocking gluconeogenesis. The use of alcohol by the patient should be discussed with a physician.
- Caffeine increases blood levels of glucose and is omitted from the diet. This restriction removes coffee, tea, chocolate, and cola beverages from the diet.
- Concentrated carbohydrates are avoided. Saccharine is allowed.
- Large amounts of carbohydrate should not be eaten at one time. Refined carbohydrates should be completely eliminated from the diet.
- The patient is taught to always have available a high-protein snack, such as cheese and crackers, to avoid hypoglycemic attacks.
- Dividing the daily food intake into five to eight feedings per day is usually preferable to larger, less frequent meals.
- The patient should be cautioned about skipping meals or excessive delays in usual mealtimes.
- Fresh, canned, or frozen fruits without added sugar may be used. Dried fruits should be avoided due to the concentrating of sugar that occurs in the drying process.

Chronic Primary Adrenocortical Insufficiency (Addison's Disease)

PATHOPHYSIOLOGY

In chronic primary adrenocortical insufficiency, the adrenal gland becomes shrunken and contracted. Medullary function continues, but cortical cells atrophy, with the resulting loss of the hormones aldosterone, cortisol, and androgens.

Aldosterone functions to conserve sodium and excrete potassium. When aldosterone is no longer secreted in adequate amounts, the following chain of events occurs:

- Excretion of sodium increases
- Loss of sodium causes a concurrent loss of body water, leading to dehydration, hypotension, and decreased cardiac output
- The heart becomes smaller due to a reduced work load
- Increased serum levels of potassium lead to cardiac arrhythmias and, possibly, arrest
- Death may occur from circulatory collapse due to hypotension and decreased cardiac action

Glucocorticoid deficiencies result in reduced conversion of fats and proteins to glucose. This decreased gluconeogenesis leads to hypoglycemia. The patient also has a reduced stress tolerance.

Cortisol deficiency causes increased secretion of ACTH and melanocyte-stimulating hormone, resulting in the skin color changes associated with the disease. Reduced secretion of androgens leads to sparse development of pubic and axillary hair in women.

TREATMENT

The treatment of chronic primary adrenocortical insufficiency is replacement of the secretions of the adrenal cortex with synthetic hormones. Various preparations are available to permit individualization of treatment on the basis of specific symptoms.

DIET THERAPY

Diet therapy is used in conjunction with drug therapy to permit smaller doses of drugs to be used. The aim of diet therapy is prevention of hyponatremia, hypoglycemia, and dehydration.

A high-protein, moderate-carbohydrate diet is usually prescribed. A high sodium intake is used to compensate for the increased loss of sodium. If a sodium-retaining hormone (fludrocortisone) is part of the drug therapy, salt intake is not increased.

Intake of simple sugars is restricted, and the total intake of carbohydrates is reduced to avoid stimulation of insulin secretion and to prevent hypoglycemic attacks. A high-protein food should be included with each feeding to provide a steady source of glucose.

Sodium and potassium levels are usually controlled through medication rather than dietary modification.

NURSING IMPLICATIONS

- Patients should be instructed to take corticosteroid medications with milk or antacids to minimize gastric irritation.
- Periodic weight checks are important in assessing the patient's progress. An increase in weight may indicate retention of fluids related to medication. Weight loss may be indicative of poor control of disease.
- Patients should be advised to state that they have adrenal insufficiency when any procedure requiring fasting is contemplated. The practice of skipping meals should be avoided.
- The importance of keeping appointments for blood chemistry measurements should be stressed. The potential for both hypokalemia and hyperkalemia exists.
- Foods that are extremely high in potassium or combinations of foods that would result in a high intake of potassium should be avoided, unless the potassium level is well controlled by medication. (See Chapter 2 for a list of potassium-rich foods.)
- A cheese-and-cracker snack should be carried at all times and ingested when necessary to prevent hypoglycemic attacks.
- A bedtime feeding is usually part of the diet plan to prevent hypoglycemia in the early morning.
- Supplements of vitamins B and C may be needed to support the increased metabolism associated with the disease management.

Hyperthyroidism

PATHOPHYSIOLOGY

Oversecretion of thyroxine, triiodothyronine, or both hormones results in an increase in the body's metabolic rate. The accelerated metabolism affects production of heat and energy; the circulatory, muscular, and nervous systems; and the function of other endocrine glands. All body processes are speeded up. An increased metabolic rate leads to the rapid loss of glycogen from the liver and is usually associated with some tissue wasting.

TREATMENT

The aim of treatment is to reduce the secretion of the thyroid hormones and to prevent or treat the complications associated with the accelerated metabolism. This goal may be accomplished by the use of antithyroid drugs, surgical removal of a portion of the thyroid gland, or radioactive iodine therapy.

DIET THERAPY

A well-balanced, high-Calorie, high-carbohydrate, high-protein diet divided into six feedings is usually prescribed. The caloric intake should be sufficient to offset weight loss. The high carbohydrate intake is needed to replenish glycogen stores. Protein intake of 1 to 2 grams per kilogram of ideal body weight is recommended to correct a negative nitrogen balance. Fluid intake should average from 3,000 to 4,000 milliliters per day, unless cardiac or renal problems contraindicate increased fluid intake. A generous fluid allowance is needed to replace water losses in diarrhea, diaphoresis, and increased respirations.

Highly seasoned and fibrous foods are usually eliminated from the diet because they tend to increase peristalsis, which has already been speeded up by the disease. Use of stimulants, such as coffee, tea, and cola beverages, is also discouraged because they tend to increase nervousness, which is a symptom of the disease.

Vitamin supplements may be needed, with particular concern for adequate intake of B complex and vitamins A and C. At least 1 quart of milk daily is needed to supply the calcium, phosphorus, and vitamin D required by patients with hyperthyroidism. If these mineral and vitamin needs are not met by milk intake, supplementation is indicated. The increased secretion of thyroid hormones causes bone demineralization, with loss of large amounts of calcium and phosphorus in the urine. Vitamin D is needed to increase absorption of calcium.

NURSING IMPLICATIONS

• The patient's environment should be quiet and pleasant, particularly at mealtime, to encourage an adequate intake of food.

- Highly seasoned foods, coffee, and alcohol may produce reflex diarrhea.
- Decaffeinated coffee should replace regular coffee to prevent reflex diarrhea and nervousness.
- Alcohol taken without food may produce hypoglycemia in a susceptible patient.
- Increased secretion of thyroid hormone causes increased absorption of carbohydrates and a rise in blood levels of glucose after carbohydrate-rich meals.
- In the presence of exophthalmus, salt and fluid intake may be limited. Exophthalmus is thought to be due to increased accumulation of extracellular fluid.
- Increased intake of carbohydrates necessitates an increase in the intake of thiamine to metabolize the carbohydrates.
- If Lugol's solution is prescribed preoperatively, it should be administered in fruit juice or milk to disguise the unpleasant taste and to reduce irritation of the mucous membrane.
- Appetite increases with hyperthyroidism but does not decrease as the disease is controlled. Obesity could become a problem if the diet is not altered appropriately.
- The patient should be involved in all aspects of the diet plan to ensure understanding of its rationale and to improve compliance.

Hypothyroidism

PATHOPHYSIOLOGY

In hypothyroidism, the pituitary gland fails to secrete thyroid-stimulating hormone or the thyroid gland is unable to secrete adequate amounts of thyroid hormones. In either situation, there is a deficiency of thyroxine and triiodothyronine that leads to a reduced metabolic rate and slowing of body processes. A decrease in thyroxine activity is reflected in low thyroxine test results. Reduced thyroxine activity may be due to inadequate intake of iodine, increased intake of goitrogens (fruits and vegetables that contain an antithyroid substance), or congenital absence, malformation, or malfunction of the thyroid gland.

When hypothyroidism is present at birth or occurs in early infancy, it affects brain development and is referred to as cretinism. Hypothyroidism in adults is called myxedema, a term used to describe the puffiness of the face and eyelids. The puffiness is due to edema resulting from a negative nitrogen balance and from the deposition of mucoproteins in the subcutaneous and extracellular spaces that pull fluid into these spaces.

TREATMENT

The aim of treatment is to restore normal metabolism by means of administration of thyroid hormone preparations.

DIET THERAPY

A patient with hypothyroidism is usually given a low-Calorie, high-protein diet with adequate content of fiber and laxative foods. Fluid intake is usually increased to aid in the treatment of constipation but must be monitored because excessive intake of fluids could lead to fluid retention.

Cholesterol intake may be limited because the rate of cholesterol breakdown is slowed, and patients with hypothyroidism tend to have elevated serum levels of cholesterol.

Intake of goitrogens may be restricted in patients who suffer from goiter as a result of excessive intake of these foods coupled with an inadequate intake of iodine. Goitrogens contain progoitrin, an antithyroid agent. Goitrin is usually destroyed by heat, so that thorough cooking may render these foods acceptable in the diet. The following foods contain substantial amounts of goitrin:

Cabbage
Rutabagas
Turnips
Brussels sprouts
Soybeans
Peanuts
Peaches
Peas
Strawberries
Spinach
Radishes

NURSING IMPLICATIONS

- Encourage the use of iodized salt. Salt used in processing is noniodized. Noniodized salt is less expensive and accounts for 50% of the salt sold.
- Adequate intake of iodine is 40 to 150 micrograms per day; 2½ teaspoons of iodized salt (6.2 grams) is equivalent to 474 micrograms. Iodine is necessary for the production of thyroid hormones.
- Check the adequacy of a pregnant woman's intake of iodine, particularly when a salt restriction is imposed.

- Encourage the use of iodized salt, and urge thorough cooking of vegetables that contain goitrin for patients who have "cabbage" goiter.
- Measure weight frequently to evaluate weight loss and to check for retention of fluid.
- Encourage the use of fibrous and laxative foods to correct constipation.

Diabetes Insipidus

PATHOPHYSIOLOGY

Diabetes insipidus results from a deficiency of vasopressin, the antidiuretic hormone (ADH) secreted by the posterior lobe of the pituitary gland. A patient with a deficiency of ADH excretes a large volume of very dilute urine. The functions of ADH include promotion of the reabsorption of water by the kidney tubules and regulation of the osmotic pressure of extracellular fluid. When ADH is deficient, excessive fluid is lost through the kidneys, and the body becomes dehydrated. Uncontrolled diabetes insipidus leads to hypovolemic shock.

TREATMENT

Diabetes insipidus can be controlled in most patients by the administration of vasopressin (Pitressin) tannate intramuscularly or by inhalation. Some patients with mild deficiencies have found benzothiadiazine diuretics effective. These drugs are capable of reducing urine volume by 50%; however, the rationale for this paradoxical use of diuretics has not been established. Other patients with diabetes insipidus elect simply to replace the fluid lost by increasing their intake of fluids.

DIET THERAPY

Special diets are not indicated in the treatment of diabetes insipidus. Potassium supplementation may be indicated, especially for patients who are taking benzothiadiazine diuretics.

NURSING IMPLICATIONS

- Caution patients not to limit fluid intake in an attempt to reduce urinary output.
- Weights should be recorded three times per week to check for retention of fluid and to evaluate the effectiveness of drug therapy.
- Patients who increase their intake of fluids to offset urinary output

should be assisted in the selection of low-Calorie beverages. The caloric content of the increased volume of fluids could lead to obesity.

Nephrogenic Diabetes Insipidus

PATHOPHYSIOLOGY

Nephrogenic diabetes insipidus is an inherited disorder in which the renal tubules are unable to reabsorb water and thus produce an excessive volume of urine and fluid loss.

TREATMENT

Nephrogenic diabetes insipidus does not respond to vasopressin (Pitressin) tannate; however, thiazide diuretics are effective in nephrogenic diabetes insipidus as well as in the pituitary form.

DIET THERAPY

The diet used in nephrogenic diabetes insipidus is designed to reduce obligate water loss by decreasing the solute load of the food intake. This type of diet is helpful in infants and young children. Initially, protein intake is limited to 1 to 2 grams per kilogram of body weight. The diet includes unlimited amounts of cooked and fresh fruits and vegetables. Water is allowed in generous amounts to prevent dehydration. Salt is permitted only in cooking. The following foods are allowed in limited amounts:

Salt-free white bread
Puffed wheat
Noodles
Cauliflower
Orange juice
Salt-free butter

The following foods are not permitted:

Meats
Eggs
Milk
Milk products, except salt-free butter
Fish
Soups

This diet is strictly followed for the first year of life and becomes more liberal as the child learns to satisfy fluid needs.

Gout

PATHOPHYSIOLOGY

Gout results from abnormal metabolism of purine. Purines are components of protein that patients with gout are unable to metabolize; the result is accumulation of uric acid in the serum (hyperuricemia). Uric acid is the end product of the metabolism of purine compounds, such as nucleic acids and xanthines.

Hyperuricemia leads to deposition of urate crystals throughout the body, which causes local inflammation and the formation of tophi (nodular deposits of sodium urate crystals that act as foreign bodies).

TREATMENT

Bed rest and analgesics are recommended for acute attacks of gout. Colchicine or other uricosuric medications are used to prevent acute attacks. Uricosuric drugs, such as probenecid (Benemid), sulfinpyrazone (Anturane), or salicylates block reabsorption of urates by the kidneys. Allopurinol (Zyloprim), a xanthine oxidase inhibitor, is used in ongoing therapy to block the formation of uric acid. Phenylbutazone (Butazolidin), indomethacin (Indocin), or corticotropin (ACTH) is used to reduce fever and inflammation.

DIET THERAPY

A high-carbohydrate, low-fat diet is usually recommended. Carbohydrates increase excretion of uric acid, whereas fats are believed to block excretion of this metabolite. Purine restriction is used temporarily to reduce serum levels of urate. A diet that produces an alkaline ash or high urinary pH has been replaced for the most part by antacid medications. Ample intake of fluids is important, particularly in patients taking uricosuric drugs.

Weight control is important, but weight loss should occur slowly; fasting should be avoided. Fasting results in acidosis and dehydration, both of which should be avoided by the patient with gout.

The following foods are high in purine and should be avoided during the purine-restricted phase of diet therapy:

Shellfish
Anchovies

Smoked meats
Sardines
Meat extracts

Limited amounts of the following foods are permitted in a purine-restricted diet:

Meats
Squab
Fowl
Beans
Mushrooms
Peas
Spinach
Asparagus
Cauliflower

The foods usually permitted on a low-purine diet include:

Eggs
Fat-free milk
Cottage cheese
Cereals
Fruits
Vegetables, except those previously noted

NURSING IMPLICATIONS

- Caution the patient that alcohol or fatty foods may precipitate an acute attack.
- Potassium supplements may be needed when sodium bicarbonate or acetazolamide is used in drug therapy.
- Uricosuric drug therapy may stimulate the formation of uric acid stones, particularly in a patient with a history of renal calculi. Stress the importance of intake of fluids and alkalies to reduce the risk for stone formation.
- Fluids and alkalies should also be ingested with allopurinol.
- A liberal intake of fruits and vegetables results in an alkaline urine.
- Patients with gout should avoid fasting and alcoholic binges; discontinuation of food intake leads to cellular breakdown and increased serum levels of uric acid.

- If the patient is unable to eat solid foods, urge intake of high-carbohydrate fluids so that adipose tissue is not burned excessively for energy.
- Colchicine may reduce the absorption of fats, carotene, sodium, potassium, vitamin B_{12}, lactose, and folic acid (Roe, 1976).
- Coffee, tea, and chocolate contain methylxanthine but are allowed in the diet because they do not lead to deposits in the tissues.
- If colchicine causes diarrhea, constipating foods may be added to the diet from the list of permitted foods. Boiled skim milk usually has a constipating effect. Antacids that contain calcium or aluminum have a constipating effect and could be helpful.
- Phenylbutazone should be taken with meals or with at least 1 glass of milk to reduce gastric irritation.
- Stress may precipitate an acute attack of gout. A diet that is too restrictive is a form of stress. Allow the patient adequate input into the diet plan.

References

Anderson, J., & Chen, W. Plant Fiber, Carbohydrate and Lipid Metabolism. *American Journal of Clinical Nutrition* 32:346, 1979.

American Diabetes Association and American Dietetic Association. *Exchange lists for meal planning*. New York, 1976.

Bierman, E. Diabetes mellitus. *Contemporary Nutrition*, December 1977, *2*, 12.

Boykin, L. Controlling gout through diet. *Nursing Care*, October 1977, *10*, 10.

Brazeau, P. Agents affecting the renal concentration of water. In L. Goodman, & A. Gilman, (Eds.), *The pharmacologic basic of therapeutics* (5th ed.). New York: Macmillan Publishing Company, 1975.

Danowski, T. S. Sugar and disease. *Contemporary Nutrition*, December 1978, *3*, 12.

Garofano, C. Pregnant diabetics: Dispelling myths. In *Managing diabetics properly*. Horsham, Pa.: Nursing 77 Books, 1977.

Guthrie, D. Diabetic children: Preparing them to live. In *Managing diabetics properly*. Horsham, Pa.: Nursing 77 Books, 1977.

Hunt, S., Groff, J., & Holbrook, J. *Nutrition: Principles and clinical practice*. New York: John Wiley & Sons, 1980.

Kaufmann, S. Diet: Enforcing the sine qua non. In *Managing diabetics properly*. Horsham, Pa.: Nursing 77 Books, 1977.

Kozak, G. *Diabetic teaching guide*. Boston: Joslin Diabetic Foundation, 1977.

Krall, L. (Ed.). *Joslin diabetes manual* (11th ed.). Philadelphia: Lea & Febiger, 1978.

Lavine, R. How to recognize—And what to do about hypoglycemia. *Nursing 79*, April 1979, *9*, 4.

Lilly Research Laboratories. *Diabetes mellitus* (8th ed.). Indianapolis, Ind.: Eli Lilly Company, 1979.

Mayer, J. *Human nutrition.* Springfield, Ill.: Charles C Thomas, Publisher, 1972.

Nursing 77. Giving gout the clout. *Nursing 77,* August 1977.

Petrokas, D. Explaining axioms for sick days. In *Managing diabetics properly.* Horsham, Pa.: Nursing 77 Books, 1977.

Roe, D. A. *Drug-induced nutritional deficiencies.* Westport, Conn.: AVI Publishing Company, 1976.

Suitor, C., & Hunter, M. *Nutrition: Principles and application in health promotion.* Philadelphia: J. B. Lippincott Company, 1980.

White, P. Prudent diet in diabetes. *Consultant,* June 1976, *16,* 6.

Williams, S. *Nutrition and diet therapy* (3rd ed.) St. Louis: C. V. Mosby Company, 1977.

11
Diet Therapy
in Renal Disorders

Acute Glomerular Nephritis

PATHOPHYSIOLOGY

Acute glomerular nephritis develops as the result of an antigen-antibody reaction in which complexes form and circulate throughout the body. Some of the complexes become trapped in the glomeruli of the kidney and set up an inflammatory response. Acute inflammation is characterized by edema, hyperemia, and white blood cell aggregation, leading to scarring and loss of filtering surface within the glomeruli. Because of these processes, blood and albumin are lost in the urine, urinary output is reduced, blood pressure rises, and renal function is impaired, as evidenced by a rising blood urea nitrogen level.

TREATMENT

Acute glomerular nephritis is usually a self-limiting disease. Treatment consists of bed rest, antibiotic therapy for residual Group A beta-streptococcal infection, and recognition and treatment of complications. Antihypertensive drugs are used in hypertensive encephalopathy, and diuretics are employed for edema. Dialysis may be necessary if other measures fail to promote adequate urinary clearance of metabolic wastes.

DIET THERAPY

The dietary treatment of acute glomerular nephritis usually includes the provisions of nutritional support until the disease is limited. However, dietary modifications are used when serum chemistry values indicate that metabolic wastes are accumulating in the blood.

Protein intake may be restricted in patients with oliguria. Sodium restriction is indicated in the event of edema or oliguria and in the prevention of hypertensive encephalopathy, congestive heart failure, and pulmonary edema. Potassium restriction may also be necessary when urinary output is greatly reduced.

After the oliguric phase has ended, protein intake is usually increased to compensate for urinary loss of proteins. Emphasis is placed on providing high-biologic-value proteins (milk, eggs) in controlled amounts and reducing intake of low-biologic-value proteins. Fluids are restricted during the oliguric phase and limited to the amount of the previous day's output. When the oliguric phase is over, an additional 500 to 1,000 milliliters is allowed above the previous day's output.

NURSING IMPLICATIONS

- A high caloric intake is important but difficult to achieve when low-biologic-value proteins (grains, vegetables) are limited. A concentrated high-biologic-value protein diet is unpalatable, and nausea, vomiting, and anorexia may accompany the disease.
- Fluid intake should be adjusted for additional losses when diarrhea or diaphoresis occurs.
- Cream and concentrated sweets may be used to increase caloric intake.
- The patient with edema should be positioned carefully for food intake. Ascites may make the normal upright position uncomfortable and lead to anorexia.
- Apportion the limited fluid intake equally throughout the waking hours.
- Keep the patient's mouth clean and moist when fluids are restricted.

Chronic Glomerular Nephritis

PATHOPHYSIOLOGY

Repeated episodes of nephritis lead to loss of renal tissue and kidney function; in particular, the glomeruli disappear, and normal filtering capabilities are lost. The kidneys lose their ability to concentrate urine, and increased amounts of urine are voided in an attempt to rid the body of waste products. Protein and blood are lost in the urine. Blood pressure rises, causing vascular changes.

TREATMENT

The aims of treatment in chronic glomerular nephritis are to control hypertension, to correct metabolic abnormalities, and to reduce edema.

DIET THERAPY

The diet used in chronic glomerular nephritis is modified according to the progression of the disease. Protein intake is maintained at a high level as long as the kidneys are able to eliminate the waste products of protein metabolism. The usual practice is to calculate the normal protein requirement for the patient and to increase this requirement by the amount of protein that was lost in the urine in the previous 24-hour period. As the blood urea nitrogen level rises, protein intake becomes restricted to 40 grams or less per day.

Intake of carbohydrates and fats makes up the remainder of the body's energy requirements, which range between 2,000 and 3,000 kcal. Sufficient carbohydrate and fat must be consumed to prevent the catabolism of body protein for energy. Catabolism of body protein would contribute to the production of urea and other protein waste products.

Sodium is restricted in patients with edema and sometimes prophylactically in an attempt to forestall the retention of fluid. Careful assessment of blood sodium levels is critical because sodium depletion can occur during the diuretic phase of chronic glomerular nephritis.

NURSING IMPLICATIONS

- Potassium may also be lost during the diuretic phase, so that careful monitoring of serum levels of electrolytes is important.
- Nocturia is a common and troublesome symptom that is related to deranged kidney function and not to the timing of fluid intake. Patients should be cautioned not to deprive themselves of allotted fluids in a vain attempt to prevent nocturia.
- Edematous patients are often thirsty despite water retention. Edema fluid is trapped fluid that is not available for the body's use.
- Fluid retention is more apt to be managed successfully by means of sodium restriction than by fluid restriction. Fluids are needed to replace the increased urinary losses.
- Position the edematous patient for optimal comfort at mealtimes.

Nephrotic Syndrome

PATHOPHYSIOLOGY

The nephrotic syndrome is a complex of biochemical and clinical symptoms that develop from a variety of diseases. The end result in these diseases is glomerular injury that permits plasma proteins, which normally cannot permeate the glomerular filter, to pass into the urine, leading to massive proteinuria and hypoalbuminemia. An elevated serum level of cholesterol is also typical of this syndrome.

TREATMENT

The aim of treatment in nephrotic syndrome is to preserve remaining kidney function as long as possible. Bed rest and diuretics are used. Corticosterioids are administered to reduce urinary losses of proteins. Intravenous albumin has been given to raise serum levels of albumin and to reverse edema.

DIET THERAPY

A high-protein, high-Calorie diet is usually prescribed. At least 1.5 grams of protein per kilogram of body weight is used as a baseline, with more protein added to replace the amounts lost in the urine. Some authorities recommend a very high intake of proteins (120 grams per day) and Calories to replace losses of albumin and other proteins and to maintain a positive nitrogen balance. Such a diet may have to be given as a tube feeding because of its unpalatability and the patient's lack of appetite.

Sodium is usually restricted, and low-sodium milk and bread may need to be used to keep within the allotted limits, yet still provide variety and taste appeal.

The practice of limiting cholesterol intake to reduce the serum level of cholesterol is debatable in the nephrotic syndrome, as well as is in other clinical situations.

NURSING IMPLICATIONS

- Position the patient for maximal comfort before meals. Extensive edema may make positioning difficult.
- Use all appropriate nursing strategies to promote food intake. Nephrotic children present a particular challenge in this area. Games and devices that prove successful at one time may fail when repeated, taxing the nurse's patience and inventiveness.

- Twenty-four-hour urine collections may be needed to measure urinary losses of proteins.
- Daily weights are essential to evaluate the status of edema and the effectiveness of diuretic therapy.

Chronic Pyelonephritis

PATHOPHYSIOLOGY

Chronic bacterial infection of the kidneys leads to fibrosis, scarring, and dilatation of the tubules, which results in impaired renal function. Hypertension and some degree of renal failure is usually present.

TREATMENT

The aims of treatment are to preserve kidney function and to control blood pressure.

DIET THERAPY

Sodium restriction is usually prescribed to control blood pressure. However, some patients with chronic pyelonephritis lose excessive amounts of sodium in the urine and must be monitored for sodium depletion rather than having their intake limited. Protein intake may be restricted if the blood urea nitrogen level indicates inability to handle protein wastes. Potassium intake is restricted when the serum level of potassium is elevated.

NURSING IMPLICATIONS

- When protein intake is restricted, the protein allowance should be satisfied primarily by high-biologic-value proteins, such as eggs and milk, with limited contributions from vegetable proteins.
- See Chapter 10 for additional nursing implications related to the dietary control of hypertension.

Renal Calculi (Nephrolithiasis)

PATHOPHYSIOLOGY

In patients with infection, urinary stasis, or prolonged immobilization, some of the crystalline substances normally present in the urine may precipitate out as gravel or stones. These crystalline substances are primarily calcium, phosphorus, calcium oxalate, and uric acid. An excessive level of calcium or uric acid in the blood favors precipitation of stones composed mainly of these substances. Calculi may lodge at any point in the urinary tract, causing obstruction, infection, and pain.

TREATMENT

The aims of treatment are to remove the stone, to identify its composition, and to preserve renal function. Relief of pain is of immediate concern. Surgical crushing or stone removal is indicated if spontaneous passage does not occur. Thiazide diuretics are sometimes used in an attempt to flush out the stone by increasing urinary output.

DIET THERAPY

A sustained fluid intake over a 24-hour period is critical to reduce the concentration of the crystals in the urine and encourage a large urinary output. Three to 4 liters of fluid per day, spread out over the 24 hours, is recommended.

Dietary modification in relation to the composition of the stone is most effective when there is an increased level of stone components in the urine. Most renal calculi are composed of calcium phosphate, or calcium oxalate. A low-calcium (250 to 400 milligrams) diet is sometimes used to reduce the urinary excretion of calcium. The avoidance of dairy products usually leads to a substantial decrease in calcium intake. See Table 11-1 for an example of a low-calcium diet.

When excessive levels of oxalates are found in the urine, a diet limited in oxalates may be prescribed. The following foods have high oxalate contents and would be eliminated from such a diet:

Rhubarb

Spinach

Asparagus

Dandelion greens

Cranberries

Almonds

Cashews

Chocolate

Cocoa

Tea

Uric acid stones may be treated by a low-purine diet (see Chapter 10), although allopurinol (Zyloprim) is more effective.

TABLE 11-1
LOW-CALCIUM DIET

	Milligrams of Calcium
Breakfast	
½ cup of fresh orange juice	14
1 cup of corn flakes	4
½ cup of whole milk	144
2 slices of Italian bread, toasted	7
1 tablespoon of margarine	3
Coffee	
Lunch	
Tuna sandwich	
2 slices of Italian bread	7
3 ounces of tuna	7
1 tablespoon of mayonnaise	3
1 apple	8
½ cup of whole milk	144
Dinner	
3 ounces of broiled chicken	8
1 baked potato	9
½ cup of green peas	18
½ cup of carrots	24
2 slices of French bread	7
1 tablespoon of margarine	3
1 4-inch sector of apple pie	11
½ ounce of cheddar cheese	112
Tea	
Total daily intake	533

The acidity or alkalinity of urine influences the solubility of the crystals that form stones. Altering the pH of urine is an adjunctive therapy for urinary stones and is most commonly accomplished by drug administration. It is possible to raise or lower the urinary pH by dietary intervention. An acid urine favors the excretion of calcium. The following foods would be emphasized in the diet to produce an acid urine:

Large amounts of protein
Cereals
Meats
Fish
Eggs
Bread

Sodium may be restricted in the acid-ash diet because it buffers acid. Salt and baking powder would be eliminated, as would their common substitutes. Cranberry juice is a favorite beverage used to produce an acid urine.

An alkaline-ash diet is sometimes helpful in the treatment of uric acid stones and cystine stones. The foods that produce an alkaline urine include:

Fruits (except plums, prunes, cranberries)

Vegetables (except corn)

Milk (limited to 1 pint per day because of calcium content)

NURSING IMPLICATIONS

- The importance of a generous intake of fluids spaced out over the entire 24 hours should be emphasized to the patient and the family.
- Milk must be used with caution in patients with renal calculi. Although milk produces an alkaline ash, it is high in calcium, so it may have to be avoided if calcium is a component of the stones.
- The calcium content of the patient's drinking water should be ascertained. Some water supplies have a high concentration of calcium. The use of distilled water as a beverage and in cooking may be desirable.
- A low-calcium diet should include foods fortified with vitamin D, which promotes absorption of calcium.
- Vitamin B_6 reduces production of oxalates by 50% and may be an effective form of therapy for oxalate stones.
- The patient should be cautioned to avoid becoming dehydrated. Excessive perspiration or other fluid losses indicates the need for increased intake of fluids.
- Scheduling of tests that require withholding of fluids should be questioned because of dehydration.

Nephrosclerosis

PATHOPHYSIOLOGY

Nephrosclerosis is hardening of the renal arteries, usually as a result of renal hypertension and generalized arteriosclerosis. In nephrosclerosis, albumin is lost in the urine, nitrogenous wastes are retained, and retinal changes occur. Death is usually due to circulatory failure or the sequelae of hypertension.

TREATMENT

Treatment is directed toward preservation of renal function and control of hypertension.

DIET THERAPY

The diet is maintained at normal intake as long as possible. Low-Calorie diets may be prescribed for obese patients because weight loss reduces the circulatory load on the kidney. Protein intake is guided by the blood urea nitrogen level and is usually normal in the early stages and reduced as kidney function fails.

Intake of fluids is usually encouraged to enable the patient to maintain an adequate urinary output for the elimination of wastes. In patients with fluid retention, fluids may be restricted. Sodium restriction is prescribed to reduce edema and to control blood pressure. (See Chapter 8 for low-sodium diets in hypertension.)

Acute Renal Failure

PATHOPHYSIOLOGY

The failure of the kidneys to function because of circulatory, glomerular, or tubular insufficiency is called renal failure. When renal failure occurs abruptly, it is labeled acute. Acute renal failure often occurs after burns, severe crushing injuries, nephrotoxicity, shock, or sepsis. The kidneys excrete less then 500 milliliters per day in acute renal failure. At least 600 milliliters per day must be excreted to eliminate solute metabolic wastes. In renal failure, these wastes accumulate in the blood, eventually reaching toxic levels.

There are three phases of acute renal failure, classified on the basis of volume of urinary output. The first phase is the oliguric phase, which lasts about 10 days; urinary output is less than 500 milliliters per day. The second phase, the diuretic phase, is characterized by gradually increasing urinary output. Output may be normal during this phase, although kidney function remains deranged. The final phase is the period of recovery and is characterized by improved renal function, although some permanent loss of filtration, concentration, or acidification may be present. The recovery period may last from 3 months to 1 year.

TREATMENT

The aims of treatment are to correct the underlying abnormality when possible and to maintain the body in a homeostatic state until the kidneys

resume adequate functioning. Supportive treatment includes maintenance of fluid and electrolyte, acid-base, and mineral balances. Maintenance of adequate nutritional status is essential in view of the variety of
devastating conditions that precipitate acute renal failure. The prevention of uremia may be handled by enhancing existing renal function with
diuretics or, in patients with severe oliguria or anuria, the use of dialysis.

DIET THERAPY

The energy needs of patients in acute renal failure are increased, and
they must receive sufficient Calories to prevent catabolism of body protein. The daily caloric intake may range from 2,000 to 5,000 kcal and
should include at least 100 grams of carbohydrate. This high caloric intake is frequently combined with fluid restriction. Intravenous solutions
of 25 to 50% glucose or total parenteral nutrition may be necessary to
meet the combined requirements.

If food can be taken by mouth, a concentrated carbohydrate and fat,
low-protein diet is selected initially. Protein is initially limited to 1.5 grams
per kilogram of body weight but should be increased as kidney function
improves because the body needs the protein to repair damaged tissues
and to cope with the stress of catastrophic illness. High-biologic-value
protein is selected for the major portion of the protein allowance.

Fluids are restricted in the oliguric phase to the basal insensitive fluid
loss (approximately 600 milliliters) plus an amount of fluid equal to the
previous day's output. During the diuretic phase, fluid intake is increased
to offset fluid losses. Daily weight measurements are essential for monitoring fluid status.

Potassium intake is restricted during the anuric phase, and potassium
levels must be monitored closely. Many causes of acute renal failure are
characterized by destruction of tissues, which causes potassium to be released from the damaged cells. The major pathway of potassium excretion is the kidneys. In patients with anuria, it may be necessary to use exchange resins to rid the body of potassium via the bowel. Intravenous
glucose and insulin, or calcium gluconate, can be used to drive potassium
into the cells to reduce the serum levels of patients who are not undergoing dialysis. During the diuretic phase, potassium levels are assessed to
watch for excessive loss. Excessive loss of sodium may also occur during
the diuretic phase. When exchange resins are used in the treatment of
hyperkalemia excessive retention of sodium may occur.

NURSING IMPLICATIONS

- Exchange resins given by enema must be retained for 30 to 45 minutes to be effective.

- Sorbitol is sometimes taken by mouth or by rectum to increase fluid loss via the gastrointestinal tract.
- Failure to lose 0.5 pound per day during the oliguric phase indicates retention of fluids.
- A rising blood pressure is also an indication of retention of fluids.
- Metabolic acidosis accompanies acute renal failure because the body is unable to eliminate the hydrogen ions produced by metabolic processes. Hydrogen ions in the form of fixed acids are normally excreted by the kidneys.
- Assess the patient for anemia, which frequently accompanies acute renal failure as a result of blood loss, interference with production of erythropoietin, and reduced life span of red blood cells. The kidneys secrete a substance that acts on plasma proteins to produce erythropoietin.

Chronic Renal Failure

PATHOPHYSIOLOGY

Failure of kidney function to return after acute renal failure, or progressive loss of kidney function due to renal disease, results in chronic renal failure. The kidneys are no longer able to fulfill their role in removing metabolic wastes from the blood, and the body's homeostatic mechanism is irreversibly upset. When 60 to 75% of the nephrons are not functioning, loss of kidney function is severe enough to interfere with homeostasis. The kidneys normally excrete 70% of the body's protein wastes. When the kidneys fail to function, they cannot excrete urea and other nitrogenous products, and the blood urea nitrogen level rises. The serum levels of creatinine and phosphate also rise.

Chronic renal failure is usually divided into four stages. The first stage is characterized by reduced renal reserves, a loss of one-half to two-thirds of the functioning nephrons. In the second stage, destruction of nephrons has progressed to the degree that the kidneys can no longer maintain homeostasis, and a mild degree of azotemia (excess levels of urea and nitrogenous wastes in the blood) develops. The third stage in renal failure is characterized by moderate to severe azotemia. The fourth stage is uremia, in which 90% of kidney function has been lost.

A major complication of chronic renal failure is renal osteodystrophy. As a result of kidney dysfunction, phosphorus is retained in the blood. Because calcium and phosphorus have a reciprocal relationship, the elevated serum level of phosphorus causes the serum level of calcium to fall. Normally, hypocalcemia stimulates the parathyroid glands to secrete parathyroid hormone and stimulates the kidneys to increase their output of vitamin D_3, which, in turn, causes reabsorption of the calcium from the bones and intestines to increase the serum level of calcium. In renal failure, the activity of vitamin D_3 is reduced, and the increased secretion of parathyroid hormone leads to bone demineralization, osteitis, and metastatic calcification.

TREATMENT

The aim of treatment is to help the failing kidneys maintain homeostasis as long as possible. Dialysis or transplantation is the only treatment when conservative therapy is no longer adequate. Drug therapy is used to control hypertension.

DIET THERAPY

When the kidneys can no longer adequately excrete metabolic wastes, dietary modification is instituted to regulate the intake of proteins, fluids, sodium, potassium, and phosphate to maintain homeostasis. In the first stage of chronic renal failure, dietary restriction is usually not indicated, unless weight reduction is desirable to lower blood pressure from hypertensive levels. An adequate caloric intake is essential to prevent the use of body protein for energy needs, which would also increase the load of protein waste for the failing kidneys to handle.

In the second stage of chronic renal failure, sodium restriction is frequently prescribed. The degree of restriction depends on the degree of hydration and hypertension. Intake of potassium and phosphate is also restricted when urinary output is reduced.

In the third and fourth stages of chronic renal failure, intake of protein is restricted to 0.6 to 1.0 gram per kilogram of ideal body weight. Three-fourths of the protein should come from high-biologic-value proteins, such as eggs and milk. The rationale for restricting protein intake is the need to control protein metabolism so that the amount of nitrogenous waste products is minimized. Ideally, all protein and nitrogen provided by the diet would be used by the body to manufacture hormones and enzymes and for repair and maintenance.

The Giordano-Giovannetti diet and its many modifications have been used successfully in chronic renal failure. These diets are high-Calorie diets that include approximately 24 grams of protein. Seventy percent of this protein allowance comes from high-biologic-value proteins. These diets contain enough essential amino acids to maintain a positive nitrogen balance. Limiting the intake of low-biologic-value proteins keeps the nonessential amino acids in the diet at a minimal level, forcing the body to manufacture them by using up some of the urea that the kidneys are unable to excrete. The diet must also contain sufficient Calories to prevent catabolism of body protein for energy needs. This catabolism produces an increase in the amount of nitrogenous waste products, which the kidney cannot excrete. Sodium restriction is determined by hydration and blood pressure. Some patients with chronic renal failure are salt-losers and should not be subjected to sodium restriction because their kidneys are unable to retain sodium to the degree required by their bodies. Intake of potassium and phosphorous is restricted in relation to the serum levels of these minerals, although intake of phosphorus is usually restricted to 1 to 1.5 grams or less.

Fluid intake is usually limited to the amount of insensible losses plus an amount equal to the previous day's urinary output. In some facilities, the amount of fluid intake is determined by the patient's weight. Fluid intake is restricted to the amount necessary to keep the body weight at a stable level.

Amino acid analogues are being used to increase the palatability of low-protein diets and to maintain a positive nitrogen balance while still reducing blood urea levels. Amino acid analogues are also referred to as carbohydrate skeletons or ketoacids. They are synthetic compounds that are used as protein substitutes; they possess the carbohydrate skeleton of essential amino acids but lack the amino group. In the body, these skeletons pick up the necessary amino groups from urea, reducing the accumulation of urea as a result of protein anabolism. The diet that includes amino acid analogues contains 15 to 20 grams of protein and is supplemented by four essential amino acids: tryptophan, lysine, threonine, and histidine (considered an essential amino acid in renal failure), and the analogues of five other essential amino acids: valine, leucine, isoleucine, methionine, and phenylalanine. Amino acid analogues have an unpleasant taste and may have to be administered by tube feeding or total parenteral nutrition.

NURSING IMPLICATIONS

- Low-protein diets, particularly those that stress high-biologic-value proteins, tend to be unpalatable. Compliance can be improved by combining allowed high- and low-biologic-value proteins in a varied diet.
- Histidine is considered an essential amino acid for patients in renal failure. Histidine supplementation increases hemoglobin levels and promotes maintenance of a positive nitrogen balance.
- Essential amino acids can be given in liquid or tablet form, so that the vegetable, cereal, and bread contents of the diet can be increased to improve palatability.
- The absolute minimal daily protein intake that will maintain a positive nitrogen balance is 0.23 gram per kilogram of ideal body weight.
- Meat is a high-biologic-value protein, but it contains more nitrogen

than do eggs or milk, which reduces its usefulness in renal failure diets.

- Most high-calcium foods are also high in phosphorus, so that intake of calcium may have to be increased by the use of such drugs as calcium gluconate, calcium carbonate, or calcium lactate rather than by the use of calcium-containing foods.
- Phosphorous-binding gels that contain aluminum, for example, Amphojel or Basogel, may be used to reduce the absorption of phosphorus. Magnesium products should be avoided because of their risk for triggering hypermagnesemia.
- Iron supplementation may be needed to treat anemia.
- Children in renal failure need enough protein and Calories for growth and cannot be kept on rigid protein or Calorie restrictions for protracted periods without interfering with growth.
- Taste changes occur in uremia. Sharp, distinct flavors may be preferred.
- Glucose intolerance may accompany renal failure; however, fructose, galactose, and sorbitol are well tolerated.
- Abnormal carbohydrate metabolism occurs in uremia and is only partially corrected by dialysis.
- High-carbohydrate, protein-free supplements are available to increase caloric intake without increasing protein intake. Controlyte produces 1,000 kcal per 7 ounces of powder. Cal-Powder contains 675 kcal per 240 milliliters and Hycal Liquid contains 425 kcal per 175 milliliters.
- Other protein-free sources of concentrated carbohydrate include gumdrops, hard candies, jelly, popsicles, sugar, and honey.
- Low-protein wheat starch can be used to make bread and similar products to provide variety in protein-restricted diets.
- Foods high in phosphorus include milk, organ meats, nuts, cocoa, chocolate, and whole-wheat grains.
- The potassium content of foods can be reduced by cutting foods into small pieces, soaking them in water, cooking them in large amounts of water, and then discarding the soaking or cooking fluid. Meats can be cooked in large amounts of water, which should be discarded. Canned fruits can be used if the juices are discarded and only the solid pieces are served. The bran layer of wheat has a high potassium content, so that white bread is preferable in potassium-restricted diets.
- Wheat starch, cornstarch, arrowroot, and tapioca are low in potassium and can be used in potassium-restricted diets.
- The patient with uremia tends to have a better appetite in the morning. Serving a large breakfast may be a way of increasing intake.

Diet Therapy During Peritoneal Dialysis

Peritoneal dialysis removes metabolic wastes and excess fluid from the body of a patient in renal failure, but it does not make diet therapy unnecessary. Considerable losses of proteins and amino acids occur in the dialysate fluid, so that protein intake must be liberalized to compensate for these losses. One gram of protein per kilogram of ideal body weight is recommended; high-biologic-value protein is preferred. Intravenous protein can be used, if necessary.

At least 35 to 45 kcal per kilogram of body weight per day is recommended, with one-third of the Calories coming from carbohydrates. Sodium intake is usually liberal, but assessment of hydration, blood pressure, and losses in the dialysate fluid is essential in determining individual needs.

Intake of potassium and phosphorus is directly related to serum levels of these minerals. Fluid intake is determined by the state of hydration and may be encouraged or restricted. The diet should be supplemented with multivitamins, particularly vitamin B complex, folic acid, pyridoxine, and vitamin C.

Between peritoneal dialysis treatments, the patient returns to the third-stage diet for chronic renal failure.

Diet Therapy During Hemodialysis

There is less protein loss in hemodialysis than in peritoneal dialysis; however, losses still occur, especially of amino acids. Usually, 1 to 1.5 grams per kilogram of ideal body weight of protein is prescribed, with 60 to 70% contributed by high-biologic-value proteins. Sodium intake is usually limited, unless there are large urinary losses of this mineral. Intake of potassium and phosphorus is usually determined on the basis of predialysis serum chemistry values and frequently must be limited. Daily fluid intake is usually 500 to 1,000 milliliters plus an amount equal to the previous day's output or sufficient fluid to permit a gain of 1 to 1.5 kilograms between treatments. Energy requirements are usually calculated on the basis of 30 to 35 kcal per kilogram of body weight. Vitamin supplementation is important because vitamins, particularly water-soluble vitamins, are removed by hemodialysis.

Children undergoing hemodialysis need protein for growth; 3 to 4 grams per kilogram of ideal body weight is usually permitted. If potassium and phosphorus are restricted, intake of protein may be reduced because the potassium and phosphorus contents of protein foods are high. Intake of sodium is determined on the basis of blood pressure and hydration status. Intake of potassium is based on predialysis serum levels and is usually limited. Intake of phosphorus is kept as low as possible, and milk is usually limited to 4 ounces per day. Children's diets usually contain 100 to 150 kcal per kilogram of body weight to encourage growth. Fluid intake is 20 milliliters per kilogram of body weight plus an amount equal to the previous day's output. Multivitamin and folic acid supplements are necessary.

Diet Therapy After Renal Transplantation

After renal transplant, the patient has a functioning donor kidney and is receiving high doses of glucocorticoid drugs to prevent rejection. Diet therapy may be used to reduce the side effects of the immunosuppressant drug therapy. The usual side effects of corticosteroids include:

- Increased catabolism of proteins
- Negative nitrogen balance
- Decreased glucose tolerance
- Retention of sodium
- Retention of fluid
- Impaired absorption of calcium

The posttransplant diet includes a generous allowance for protein, 2 grams per kilogram of ideal body weight. Sodium is limited to 2,000 to 4,000 milligrams per day. Calcium intake is increased to 800 to 1,200 milligrams per day to offset the poor absorption. Intake of phosphorus is also increased to 800 to 1,200 milligrams per day. Intake of carbohydrates is restricted to 1 to 1.5 grams per kilogram of ideal body weight. The restriction of carbohydrate is designed to prevent hyperglycemia associated with decreased glucose tolerance; however, sufficient carbohydrate must be provided to prevent excessive catabolism of body protein. Calcium, vitamin D, thiamine, and magnesium supplements may be necessary.

Adequate intake of calcium is of particular importance in children to prevent suppression of growth as a result of impairment of epiphyseal growth.

The diet may be discontinued when the drug dosage is reduced to maintenance levels.

References

Anderson, C., Nelson, R., Margie, J., et al. Nutritional therapy for adults with renal diseases. In *Nutrition reviews' present knowledge of nutrition*. Washington, D.C., The Nutrition Foundation 1976.

Greenburg, J. Why your hospitalized patient won't eat. *Consultant,* September 1979, *19,* 9.

Henry, R. The kidney and urinary tract. In R. Howard & N. Herbold, *Nutrition in clinical care.* New York: McGraw-Hill Book Company, 1978.

Hetrick, A., Frauman, A., & Gilman, C. Nutrition in renal disease: When the patient is a child. *American Journal of Nursing,* December 1979, *79,* 12.

Kark, R., & Oyama, J. Nutrition, hypertension and kidney disease. In R. Goodhart & M. Shils (Eds.), *Modern nutrition in health and disease* (6th ed.). Philadelphia: Lea & Febiger, 1980.

Krause, M., & Mahan, L. *Food nutrition and diet therapy* (6th ed.). Philadelphia: W. B. Saunders Company, 1979.

Lancaster L. (Ed.). *The patient with end stage renal disease.* New York: John Wiley & Sons, 1979.

Luckmann, J., & Sorensen, K. *Medical-surgical nursing: A psychophysiologic approach* (2nd ed.). Philadelphia: W. B. Saunders Company, 1980.

Luke, B. Nutrition in renal disease: The adult on dialysis. *American Journal of Nursing,* December 1979, *79,* 12.

Massachusetts General Hospital Dietary Department. *Diet manual.* Boston: Little, Brown & Company, 1979.

Mitchell, H., Rynberger, H., Anderson, L., et al. *Nutrition in health and disease* (16th ed.). Philadelphia: J. B. Lippincott Company, 1976.

Robinson, C., & Lawler, M. *Normal and therapeutic nutrition* (15th ed.). New York: Macmillan Publishing Company, 1977.

Suitor, C., & Hunter, M. *Nutrition Principles and applications in health promotion.* Philadelphia: J. B. Lippincott Company, 1980.

Thiele, V. *Clinical nutrition.* St. Louis: C. V. Mosby Company, 1976.

Vaamonde, C. Diet does make a difference for patients with chronic uremia. *Consultant,* April 1979, *19,* 4.

Williams, S. *Nutrition and diet therapy* (3rd ed.). St. Louis: C. V. Mosby Company, 1977.

12

Diet Therapy in Burns

Immediate Postburn Period

PATHOPHYSIOLOGY

Burns destroy skin that protects against infection. The severity of the burn depends on the depth of the burn and on the amount of body surface involved. Burn depth is usually classified as first, second, or third degree. A first-degree burn is characterized by redness due to vasodilatation. A second-degree burn is characterized by formation of vesicles and damage to capillaries. Third-degree burns involve destruction of the full thickness of the skin, formation of capillary thrombosis, and a crust of dead tissue (eschar). The proportion of body surface area involved is estimated by the "rule of nines" (a method of estimating percentages of body surface area in which the head and both arms each represent 9%; the truck, front, and back each 18%; each leg 18%; and the perineum 1%) or by a more precise division of body surface area based on the person's age. The severity of a burn is based on the person's age, the depth, extent, and type of burn, and the area involved. Burns in the very young and very old tend to be more serious. Burns that involve the face and respiratory tract are more serious. Chemical and electrical burns are more difficult to treat than are thermal injuries.

Fluid loss is a major, immediate concern after a serious burn. A burn exudate, consisting of interstitial fluid and plasma, is lost at the denuded areas. Additional fluid is trapped in the intravascular spaces around the burned area. The damaged capillaries leak blood into the surrounding tissue. The metabolic needs of the body are greatly increased due to stress and the energy expended in evaporation of the fluid exudate.

Serious burns are characterized by a major increase in protein catabolism that leads to increased glucocorticoid activity and the mobilization of amino acids to meet energy needs. There is loss of albumin and plasma proteins at the site of the burn injury; in addition urinary losses of nitrogen and potassium are increased. The fluid and electrolyte losses are greater than the protein losses, resulting in increased concentrations of plasma proteins and a drawing of fluid from nonburn areas. At the same time, a plasma-to-interstitial fluid shift occurs in the burn area.

A sodium deficit develops as a result of extracellular fluid losses and intracellular fluid entrapment around the burn. Potassium excess develops during the first 48 hours after a serious burn as a result of the escape of potassium from traumatized cells. After 48 hours, a potassium deficit develops as potassium shifts back into undamaged cells. Metabolic acidosis occurs within a few hours of burns as a result of liberation of fixed acids from damaged tissues.

After 2 days, the edema fluid shifts back into the blood, renal circulation is increased, and diuresis occurs. Increased urinary output is accompanied by increased sodium losses. Paralytic ileus may also accompany burns.

TREATMENT

The initial aims of treatment are support of the circulatory and respiratory systems, relief of pain, and prevention of infection. Replacement of fluid and electrolyte losses is of major concern to forestall hypovolemic shock. There are several formulas commonly used to calculate intravenous fluid and electrolyte replacement requirements. These formulas consider the patient's age, body surface area involved, and depth of the burn. They usually take into account needs for colloids, glucose, water, and electrolytes, primarily sodium. The principal colloid used is plasma, dextran, or blood. Electrolytes are supplied in the form of lactated Ringer's solution or isotonic saline. Glucose and lactated Ringer's solutions aid in the correction of metabolic acidosis and also supply fluid. The volume of replacement fluid required is guided by central venous pressure readings and urinary output. The urinary output should be at least 15 milliliters per hour for an infant, 25 milliliters for a child, and 30 milliliters for an adult.

Antibiotics are usually prescribed prophylactically against infection, and tetanus toxoid or antitoxin is usually given. Various methods of dressing burns are used to prevent infection and to aid in healing or in the establishment of healthy granulation tissue as a base for skin grafts.

DIET THERAPY

Most patients with serious burns are administered nothing by mouth for at least 48 hours. Oral electrolyte solutions may be used in situations where immediate medical treatment is unavailable, and such solutions are occasionally used in conjunction with intravenous therapy. The emergency oral solution used consists of 1 teaspoon of sodium chloride, and ½ teaspoon of sodium bicarbonate dissolved in 1 liter of water.

Once oral feedings are permitted, clear fluids are given first and, if well tolerated, are advanced to high-Calorie, high-protein liquids and, later, to a high-Calorie, high-protein diet.

Long-Term Postburn Period

PATHOPHYSIOLOGY

Burn patients face long periods of convalescence with increased metabolism and a negative nitrogen balance. Increased secretion of catecholamines results in increased secretion of glucagon and increased metabolism for 6 to 8 weeks after the burn injury. The action of insulin is reduced, and glucose intolerance is common.

Protein is needed for replacement and repair and for reestablishment of a positive nitrogen balance. Inadequate protein intake is associated with delayed healing of burns, rejection of skin grafts, increased susceptibility to infection, and poor healing of donor sites. A calcium deficit may occur in the convalescence period because the calcium that rushed to the trauma site in the immediate postburn period was lost in the sloughing of tissue. Prolonged immobilization also increases excretion of calcium. Sodium and potassium deficits may continue into the convalescence period.

TREATMENT

The aim of treatment in the convalescence period is to prevent infection, promote healing, and support the body's increased needs for nutrients and fluids. Topical burn care continues, and grafting may be performed to reestablish the skin barrier.

DIET THERAPY

The aim of diet therapy is to sustain the patient until an intact skin cover is achieved and until the metabolic rate returns to normal. The use of tube feedings, parenteral nutrition, and elemental diets has greatly increased the medical team's ability to provide the 3,000 to 6,000 kcal and the 150 to 200 grams of protein that may be required each day. All routes may be used to ensure an adequate intake for the patient, who may be in pain, depressed, anorexic, and subjected to frequent upsetting changes of dressings and surgical procedures.

In addition to the high-Calorie, high-protein diet, supplementation with vitamin B complex is usually prescribed to aid in the metabolism of proteins and carbohydrates, and additional vitamin C is given to aid in wound healing. Fat-soluble vitamins may also be administered in increased amounts.

Frequent, small feedings are used to promote the patient's acceptance of the high-Calorie, high-protein intake. An accurate record of feedings is essential to ensure that the actual intake is as has been prescribed.

Constipation and fecal impaction are common and should be avoided by dietary measures (increased fluid, fiber, fruit, and vegetable intake) when possible. Milk and antacids are frequently used to prevent Curling's ulcer.

Oral feedings are preferred. Tube feedings are unpleasant, although effective, particularly when used with high-nitrogen elemental diets. Total parenteral nutrition has been lifesaving in patients with severe burns, despite the danger of sepsis.

Anemia is a frequent complication that results from blood losses during changes of dressings and depression of bone marrow function. This anemia appears to be treated more effectively by transfusion than by diet or drug therapy, particularly in patients with infection.

NURSING IMPLICATIONS

- Nutrient intake is essential to the burn patient's survival. A loss of more than 10% of preburn body weight places the patient at risk for sepsis and, possibly, death.
- The increase in metabolism is related to the depth and extent of the burn injury. Peak metabolic needs occur 6 to 10 days after the injury. Grafting procedures and healing result in a gradual return to a normal metabolic rate.
- Fats are high in Calories and low in bulk and help increase caloric intake. Intake of fats may also lessen the tendency toward constipation.
- Eating with other persons may improve oral intake, especially for children and adolescents.
- Thirst is a problem in the early postburn period. Despite the patient's edematous appearance, the unburned areas are dehydrated. Oral hygiene may relieve discomfort for the patient who receives nothing by mouth. Oral electrolyte fluids provide fluid, although they tend to be unpalatable. If water is permitted, monitor intake carefully to prevent water intoxication.
- Oral electrolyte solutions are more acceptable if served well chilled and flavored with lemon or frozen into ice chips.
- The incidence of Curling's ulcer increases with the severity of the

burn and the presence of sepsis. Be alert for gastric distention, which is an early sign of developing ulcer.

- When 0.5% silver nitrate is used in the topical treatment of burns, monitor serum chemistry values with care. Silver nitrate tends to draw electrolytes from the body in the early phases of its use, and intravenous replacement may be indicated. Adding salt to the diet may help replace sodium. Potassium and calcium supplements may also be indicated.
- Metabolic acidosis may occur during the period when topical mafenide acetate (Sulfamylon) is being used. If this acidosis arises, it must be corrected, and treatment with mafenide acetate may have to be discontinued.
- Be alert for potassium deficits during periods of diuresis.
- Burn patients may fight against their dependence by seeking to control aspects of their care. Allow patients some control in planning their diets, but do not permit them to manipulate food intake.
- Patients should be educated about the importance of diet to their recovery and well-being. Tube feedings should be described as auxiliary treatment to increase intake and not as punishment for failure to eat.
- Consider the effects on gastrointestinal function and appetite of drugs used to control pain.
- Schedule dressing changes away from mealtime, and do not permit meals to be interrupted by other aspects of care.
- Tube feedings, total parenteral nutrition, and high-Calorie liquid feedings may lead to the dumping syndrome and osmotic diarrhea.
- Stress-induced hyperglycemia may necessitate institution of insulin therapy.
- Watch serum levels of chloride when intravenous sodium chloride is used and during periods of diuresis. Excessive chloride may lead to or aggravate existing metabolic acidosis.
- Intake of zinc appears to be associated with more rapid wound healing. Meats, liver, eggs, and seafood are good dietary sources of zinc.
- Encourage the family to prepare favorite dishes as occasional treats. An occasional requested fast-food item may provide variety and aid in increasing intake of Calories.
- Children may eat larger amounts of vegetables if they are served raw as finger foods.
- Early ambulation improves appetite, reduces losses of calcium and protein due to immobilization, helps prevent contractures, and improves morale.
- Be alert for renal calculi when intake of high protein foods is combined with prolonged immobilization. Encourage generous intake of fluids.

References

Campbell, L. Special behavior problems of the burned child. *American Journal of Nursing*, February 1976, *76*, 2.

Goldstein, S. Surgery, stress, burns and nutritional care. In R. Howard & N. Herbold, *Nutrition and clinical care*. New York: McGraw-Hill Book Company, 1978.

Holli, B., & Oakes, J. Feeding the burned child. *Journal of the American Dietetic Association*, September 1975, *67*, 9.

Hunt, S., Groff, J., & Holbrook, J. *Nutrition: Principles and clinical practice*. New York: John Wiley & Sons, 1980.

Krause, M., & Mahan, L. *Food, nutrition and diet therapy* (6th ed.). Philadelphia: W. B. Saunders Company, 1979.

Luckmann, J., & Sorensen, K. *Medical-surgical nursing: A psychophysiologic approach* (3rd ed.). Philadelphia: W. B. Saunders Company, 1980.

Metheny, N., & Snively, W. *Nurses' handbook of fluid balance* (3rd ed.). Philadelphia, J. B. Lippincott Company, 1979.

Phipps, W., Long, B., & Woods, N. *Schafer's medical-surgical nursing* (7th ed.). St. Louis: C. V. Mosby Company, 1980.

Stephenson, C. Stress in critically ill patients. *American Journal of Nursing*, November 1977, *77*, 11.

Suitor, C., & Hunter, M. *Nutrition: Principles and application in health promotion*. Philadelphia: J. B. Lippincott Company, 1980.

Watson, J. *Medical-surgical nursing and related physiology* (2nd ed.). Philadelphia: W. B. Saunders Company, 1979.

Whaley, L., & Wong, D. *Nursing care of infants and children*. St. Louis: C. V. Mosby Company, 1979.

13
Diet Therapy in Respiratory Disorders

Cystic Fibrosis

PATHOPHYSIOLOGY

Cystic fibrosis is an inherited disease that is manifested by a generalized dysfunction of the mucous-producing (exocrine) glands. The following physiologic changes occur in cystic fibrosis:

- Increased viscosity of mucous gland secretions in the pancreas, bronchi, bile ducts, and small intestine
- Increased concentrations of electrolytes in the sweat
- Increased concentrations of sodium and chloride in the saliva and tears

The thickened mucus accumulates within pancreatic ducts, causing them to dilate. Small passageways become obstructed. Back pressure from obstruction causes atrophy and fibrosis of the pancreatic cells. Pancreatic enzymes are unable to reach the duodenum, at first because of obstruction and, eventually, because of lack of production. Digestion and absorption of proteins, fats and, to a lesser degree, carbohydrates are impaired due to lack of pancreatic secretions. The decrease in these bicarbonate-rich secretions reduces buffering and further reduces digestion and absorption. Proteins and fats are lost in the characteristic bulky stools. Absorption of fat-soluble vitamins is impaired.

In the bronchi and bronchiolar structures, thickened mucus causes obstruction, back pressure and, eventually, loss of pulmonary function. The pulmonary abnormalities are the most serious threat to life. The thickened mucus and obstructed air passages increase the incidence of infection and reduce gaseous exchange. Progressive lung dysfunction leads to pulmonary hypertension and cor pulmonale.

Excessive sweating leads to excessive loss of sodium and chloride and to heat prostration. The presence of increased levels of sodium and chloride in the tears and saliva is useful in detecting cases but results in few physiologic problems.

TREATMENT

The major goals of treatment in cystic fibrosis are to prevent or control pulmonary infections, to preserve pulmonary function, and to provide adequate nutrition despite the excessive loss of nutrients due to malabsorption and fecal losses. Pancreatic enzymes (pancreatic granules, Viokase, or Cotazym) improve digestion and absorption. Antibiotics, expectorants, and iodides are drugs used to combat infection and to liquefy and remove the obstructing mucus. Mist tents, aerosol therapy, and chest physiotherapy are also used to preserve pulmonary function by liquefying and removing mucus.

DIET THERAPY

The diet prescribed for a patient with cystic fibrosis usually contains one and one-half to two times the usual number of calories for age and activity to compensate for losses. Protein intake is doubled to provide for growth and repair in the face of poor digestion and absorption of proteins. Fat intake is reduced in the presence of steatorrhea but can be increased if tolerated. Medium-chain triglycerides can be used to provide a more absorbable source of fat. Fat intake is reduced if fatty stools recur.

Pancreatic enzymes must be taken at the beginning of all meals and with all snacks. They are discontinued when oral feedings are withheld. Food should be salted generously during hot weather or whenever production of sweat increases substantially. Iron supplements and water-miscible forms of fat-soluble vitamins are indicated. Supplementary water-soluble vitamins may also be needed. Riboflavin may be given to prevent cheilosis (fissuring of the lips and at the corners of the mouth), which is frequently seen in patients with cystic fibrosis.

Infants with cystic fibrosis are usually given high-protein formulas with low curd tension. Probana and Nutramigen are formulas that contain protein hydrolysates that are better tolerated than evaporated or whole milk formulas and that promote weight gain. Soybean milks do not contain sufficient protein and should not be used unless other sources of protein compensate for the inadequacy.

A child with untreated cystic fibrosis has an appetite that is often described as ravenous; however, once treatment with pancreatic enzymes is instituted, appetite decreases. During acute episodes of infection or gastrointestinal upset, anorexia can become a problem, and strategies to encourage the child to eat should be employed.

NURSING IMPLICATIONS

- Provide snacks as a means of increasing caloric intake as well as to conform to typical childhood eating patterns.
- Encourage eating at a table to improve posture and lung expansion.
- Provide mouth care after postural drainage, which is usually scheduled before meals.
- Encourage good dental hygiene. Children with cystic fibrosis may have unhealthy teeth as a result of nutritional inadequacies.
- Skim or low-fat milk may be used to reduce stool bulk.
- Medium-chain triglycerides are not usually palatable, unless they are flavored. Medium-chain triglycerides may also cause diarrhea.
- Encourage fluid intake as a means of liquefying secretions.
- When iodines are used as liquefiers, watch for iodine sensitivity and goiter.
- Iodine medications are least objectionable when administered in grape juice.
- Powdered pancreatic enzymes can be mixed with small amounts of pureed fruits. Do not add enzymes to infant formulas; if all the formula is not taken, the dose of enzymes is unknown.
- Enteric-coated pancreatic enzymes should not be crushed.
- Do not add pancreatic enzymes to warm or hot foods.
- The return of a voracious appetite and increased bulk in the stools suggest inadequate enzyme dosage.
- Excessive enzyme dosage may result in constipation and anorexia.
- Allergy to pork protein in commercial pancreatic enzymes may necessitate the use of beef enzymes.
- Rectal prolapse, a common complication of cystic fibrosis, tends to abate as the nutritional status improves.
- Pancreatic enzyme therapy interferes with oral iron therapy.

Emphysema

PATHOPHYSIOLOGY

Repeated or chronic respiratory infections, smoking, and pulmonary irritants lead to mucous plugs, obstruction and, eventually, alveolar destruction, enlargement of airspaces, and loss of airway support. Loss of elasticity allows the bronchi to collapse during expiration, so that the lungs remain chronically hyperexpanded. Secretions are increased and retained due to ineffectual coughing. Failure of the lungs to empty during expiration results in poor gaseous exchange, with retention of carbon dioxide, leading to respiratory acidosis. The walls of the alveoli may rupture. The size of the pulmonary capillary bed is decreased, whereas the pulmonary blood flow rate increases in an attempt to compensate. Eventually, the increased pressure within the right ventricle caused by the pumping of blood against pulmonary resistance leads to cor pulmonale.

TREATMENT

The aims of treatment for a patient with emphysema are to slow the progression of the disease, to relieve hypoxia, and to prevent or treat pulmonary infections. Drugs are used to liquefy secretions, dilate the bronchi, and treat infections. Pulmonary therapy is used to maintain remaining lung function. Intermittent positive-pressure breathing and aerosol treatments may supplement physiotherapy and breathing exercises. Oxygen at low concentrations may be used with extreme caution for short periods.

DIET THERAPY

A soft, high-Calorie diet is usually recommended for patients with emphysema. Concentrated foods in small amounts are used to ensure adequate intake in the face of anorexia. Small, frequent feedings are less apt to cause fatigue. Liquid supplements may need to be added to increase caloric intake.

An adequate fluid intake is important for hydration and liquefaction of secretions. Gas-producing foods are avoided because they cause upward pressure on the diaphragm and limit thoracic expansion. Large meals cause distention of the abdomen and also make breathing more difficult.

Patients who experience dyspnea tend to have poor appetites. They lack the strength to eat or fear that eating may bring on coughing spells or increase their breathing difficulties. Small, attractive, appealing meals are most likely to be eaten if they are scheduled after periods of rest. Pulmonary therapy should be scheduled to take into consideration the patient's fatigue level and mealtimes and should be combined with other approaches to encourage food intake.

NURSING IMPLICATIONS

• Plan rest periods before and after meals for patients who experience dyspnea as a result of eating.

- Avoid excessively hot or cold liquids that may trigger coughing spells.
- Make sure that patients who wear dentures have them in place for all feedings.
- Many patients have difficulty eating breakfast. A light breakfast, followed by a more substantial food intake at coffee break time, may increase food intake.
- A warm beverage as soon as the patient awakens may be helpful. Have the patient inhale the steam and then hold the warm liquid in the mouth before swallowing to aid in loosening mucus.
- Obese patients should be given support to adhere to a weight reduction regimen. Obesity complicates emphysema by increasing respiratory demands.
- Underweight patients should be given support in their attempts to gain weight. Patients who are underweight have flattened diaphragms and impaired respirations.
- Patients should be instructed to eat slowly and to refrain from talking while eating to avoid swallowing air, which can lead to discomfort and reduced intake.
- Fibrous fruits and vegetables and tough meats should be avoided to reduce excessive chewing, which could contribute to fatigue.

Laryngotracheobronchitis

PATHOPHYSIOLOGY

Viral and bacterial diseases that affect the small passages of the larynx, trachea, and bronchi in infants and young children are characterized by dyspnea, fever, prostration, and inspiratory distress. The already small airways are further narrowed by mucus and edema.

TREATMENT

The treatment of laryngotracheobronchitis includes oxygen, humidity, antibiotics, intravenous fluids and, possibly, tracheostomy.

DIET THERAPY

Intravenous feedings provide fluid and Calories without taxing the infant's limited energy reserve. When oral feedings are permitted, they should be high in Calories. Some authorities believe that milk tends to thicken mucus and do not permit its use until the infant's condition improves substantially. A careful record of intake and output is essential to ensure adequate intake of fluids and Calories.

NURSING IMPLICATIONS

- An infant with respiratory difficulty may become a mouth-breather. It is impossible for the infant to breath through his or her mouth and suck at the same time. A medicine cup may be effective in administering fluids.
- The infant's nose and mouth should be cleared of mucus and crusts before feedings.
- Feedings should be given slowly, providing ample rest periods.
- When infants must remain in mist tents during feeding, they should be supported in a comfortable position with their heads and shoulders elevated. An infant seat may be helpful in relieving dyspnea as well as in providing support during feedings.
- Adequate hydration is one of the best ways to liquefy secretions.

Tuberculosis

PATHOPHYSIOLOGY

Invasion of the lungs by the tubercle bacillus sets up an inflammatory process. White blood cells are mobilized and wall off the primary infection. If not successfully contained, the infection may spread throughout the body (miliary tuberculosis). The walled off infection may become reactivated. In untreated or reactivated cases, caseation occurs; the cheesy formation later dissolves, leaving an open cavity. Healing occurs with calcification of the caseation.

TREATMENT

The treatment of tuberculosis is chemotherapy. Three major drugs are used, isoniazid, streptomycin, and ethambol, alone or in combination. Rifampin is used in isoniazid-resistant cases.

DIET THERAPY

A well-balanced diet that contains liberal amounts of proteins, minerals, and vitamins is recommended. Protein is needed for healing, a positive nitrogen balance, and raising serum levels of albumin. Calcium is needed for calcification of the tubercular lesion. At least 1 quart of milk per day is advised to meet calcium requirements. Other sources of calcium include cheese and yogurt. If fortified milk is used, vitamin D is also provided to aid in absorption of the calcium. Extra protein and calcium can be included by adding nonfat dry milk to beverages, casseroles, soups, and desserts.

Iron may be needed for replacement of hemoglobin in instances of hemorrhage. Vitamin C is needed to aid in healing of wounds, and vitamin D is needed to assist in absorption of calcium. Vitamin B complex may stimulate appetite and aid in increasing food intake. Vitamin B_6 has proved helpful in counteracting the peripheral neuritis associated with isoniazid therapy. Carotene appears to be converted poorly to vitamin A in tubercular patients, so that adequate amounts of performed vitamin A should be provided by diet or supplementation.

NURSING IMPLICATIONS

- Failure to meet the protein requirements of adolescent patients is thought to be related to reduced resistance to tuberculosis and other infections.
- Aminosalicylic acid, which is sometimes used in the treatment of tuberculosis, may interfere with the absorption of vitamin B_{12}.
- *P*-Aminosalicylic acid may cause gastrointestinal upset, which may necessitate its discontinuation.
- Isoniazid is the drug of choice in pediatric patients. It can be crushed and administered in small amounts of pureed fruit or jam to disguise its taste.
- There is a high incidence of alcoholism in tubercular patients, which places them at greater risk. Alcohol should not be allowed to replace essential nutrients in the diet.

References

Barber, J., Stokes, L., & Billings, D. *Adult and child care* (2nd ed.). St. Louis: C. V. Mosby Company, 1977.

Brunner, L., & Suddarth, D. *Textbook of medical-surgical nursing* (4th ed.). Philadelphia: J. B. Lippincott Company, 1980.

Fletcher, M. Intensive care of asthma, cystic fibrosis, and other pediatric respiratory diseases. In G. Burton, G. Gee, & J. Hodgkin, (Eds.), *Respiratory care.* Philadelphia: J. B. Lippincott Company, 1977.

Krause, M., & Mahan, L. *Food, nutrition and diet therapy* (6th ed.). Philadelphia: W. B. Saunders Company, 1979.

Luckmann, J., & Sorensen, K. *Medical-surgical nursing: A psychophysiologic approach* (2nd ed.). Philadelphia: W. B. Saunders Company, 1980.

Pillitteri, A. *Nursing care of the growing family—A child health text.* Boston: Little, Brown & Company, 1977.

Robinson, C., & Lawler, M. *Normal and therapeutic nutrition* (15th ed.). New York: Macmillan Publishing Company, 1977.

Whaley, L., & Wong, D. *Nursing care of infants and children.* St. Louis: C. V. Mosby Company, 1979.

14

Diet Therapy in Allergic Disorders

Food Allergy

PATHOPHYSIOLOGY

Food allergy follows the typical hypersensitivity response associated with all allergies. The antigen is a food that stimulates the production of antibodies, which provoke a reaction when the food is subsequently ingested. Manifestations of allergic responses are due to the release of histamine and serotonin, which cause smooth muscle contraction and increase capillary permeability. The major tissues affected are located in the nose, bronchi, gastrointestinal tract, skin, and brain, although any area can be affected. The most common responses to food antigens are vomiting, diarrhea, cramping, nausea, abdominal distention, and abdominal pain. If large quantities of food allergens are ingested, eczema, urticaria, rhinitis, and asthma may occur. Food allergies may also cause behavioral changes.

Many food antigens are rendered inactive by the digestive process. Children are more likely than are adults to have food allergies because the decreased efficiency of the gastrointestinal tract allows incompletely digested food to be absorbed and thus become a potential antigen.

Food allergy reactions may be immediate or delayed. The immediate, or obvious, reaction occurs within 1 hour of ingestion of the antigen. Immediate food allergy responses are less common and are potentially life threatening. The amount of food allergen ingested is not related to the response. The response is a predictable, shocklike reaction that usually occurs in only one organ. Delayed allergic reactions, or occult responses, can occur up to 5 days after ingestion of an offending food. Delayed reactions account for about 95% of all food allergies. Delayed responses may be related to faulty digestive or absorptive mechanisms. They are not life threatening but are a chronic source of morbidity. Immediate responses can develop from prolonged delayed sensitivity. The food antigen is easy to identify in the immediate type and difficult to pinpoint in the delayed type.

TREATMENT

The treatment of food allergy is avoidance of the food that provokes the response. The food antigen must be identified for it to be eliminated from the diet. Antihistamine drugs are helpful in immediate reactions but are of no use in delayed responses. Disodium cromoglycate (Nalcrom) in oral doses of 100 milligrams has been used with some success. This drug is 99% unabsorbed in the gastrointestinal tract and appears to prevent degranulation of the mast cells, which release serotonin and histamine.

DIET THERAPY

Diet therapy is used both in the identification of the food allergen and in the avoidance of reactions. Skin testing for the identification of food antigens has not been reliable in most instances. Identification of the food responsible for an immediate response is usually simpler than it is in the delayed type. A complete history is a necessary starting point. A family history of allergy is important, as are past allergies of the patient. Any allergy or possible allergic response should be completely investigated to identify the antigen.

A food history can be kept: The patient records all the foods eaten and symptoms noted in an attempt to uncover relationships. If a food is implicated, it can be eliminated from the diet for 6 weeks. If symptoms disappear during that period, the food is reintroduced as a challenge to see if symptoms reappear. This type of elimination diet is useful only when a single food is the offender. Many patients have less obvious and, frequently, more than one food allergy. For such patients, a more stringent elimination diet is required. The test diets devised by Rowe consist of three different diets that contain foods that are most likely to be nonallergenic. One diet is selected on the basis of the patient's diet history. This diet is followed for 3 weeks, unless it initiates severe reactions. If the diet does not alleviate symptoms in 3 weeks, a second diet is tried for 3 weeks and, if necessary, the third diet is tried. When a diet relieves symptoms, the trial period is extended for another week, and foods are added to the diet one at a time at intervals of 10 days. The most common food antigens (wheat, eggs, milk) are added last. Any food that causes a return of symptoms is eliminated from the diet permanently. If milk is eliminated from the diet, meat is given twice daily to provide adequate protein, and calcium supplements are used. Supplemental vitamins and minerals may be necessary during the test period. See Tables 14-1, 14-2, and 14-3 for the Rowe diets.

Another dietary approach to the identification of food antigens is the use of diets that eliminate the most common food allergens, wheat, eggs, and milk. The wheat-free diet provides a list of foods that can be substituted so that all sources of wheat are avoided. This diet is deficient in iron, thiamine, and riboflavin and requires supplementation. Meat, fish, and poultry serve as protein sources in an egg-free diet. Although it is

TABLE 14-1
FOODS ALLOWED IN THE CEREAL-FREE ELIMINATION DIET[a] (ROWE)

Tapioca	Apricots[f]
White potatoes	Grapefruit[b]
Sweet potatoes or yams	Lemons
Soybean-potato bread[g]	Peaches[f]
Lima bean-potato bread[g]	Pineapples
Soy milk (Mull-Soy)[cd]	Prunes
Lamb	Pears[f]
Chicken, fryers, roosters, and capon (no hens)	Cane or beet sugar
	Salt
Bacon	Sesame oil (not Chinese)
Liver (lamb)	Soybean oil
Peas	Willow Run oleomargarine[e]
Spinach	Gelatin (Knox's) with flavoring of allowed
Squash	fruits and juices
String beans	White vinegar
Tomatoes	Vanilla extract
Artichokes	Lemon extract
Asparagus	Cornstarch-free baking powder[e]
Carrots	Baking soda
Lettuce	Cream of tartar
Lima beams	Maple syrup or syrup made with cane sugar flavored with maple

[a]This diet was revised in 1970.

[b]The canned fruits should be preserved with cane sugar and not corn sugar. Water-packed fruits may be used and sweetened with cane sugar syrup.

[c]Mull-Soy (free of corn glucose) may be used. It may cause indigestion.

[d]Other soy milks contain corn sugar. Neo-Mull-Soy contains sucrose. Neo-Mull-Soy is more palatable than Mull-Soy.

[e]A baking powder that contains tapioca or potato starch instead of cornstarch and no tartaric acid and also Willow Run oleomargarine can be obtained from Bray's, 3764 Piedmont Avenue, Oakland, California.

[f]Fruit may be peeled and be fresh or cooked with water or with cane or beet sugar (not with corn sugar, glucose).

[g]If a baker trusted and supervised by the physician is not available, it is best to make these bakery products at home by our recipes. Bray's, 3764 Piedmont Avenue, Oakland, California, has cooperated with us for over 35 years.

Source: From Rowe, A. H., & Rowe, A., Jr. *Food allergy: Its manifestations and control and the elimination diets.* Springfield, Ill.: Charles C Thomas, Publisher, 1972, by permission of the publisher.

TABLE 14-2

FOODS ALLOWED IN THE FRUIT-FREE, CEREAL-FREE ELIMINATION DIET (ROWE)

Tapioca (pearl)[a]	Lamb
White potatoes	Bacon
Potato starch	Chicken (no hens)
Sweet potatoes or yams	Cane or beet sugar
Soybean-potato bread	Willow Run oleomargarine[b]
Lima bean-potato bread	Soybean oil
Neo-Mull-Soy (Borden's)	Gelatin (Knox's)
Cooked carrots	Salt
Squash	Syrup made with cane sugar
Artichokes	(no maple syrup)
Peas	Corn-free tartaric acid-[c] free baking powder[d]
Lima beans	
String beans	

[a]Minute tapioca contains citric acid (not allowed in this diet).

[b]Kosher margarine is allowed if it contains no cow's milk or its products or if allergy to its vegetable oil is not present.

[c]Tartaric acid is made from grapes (not allowed in this diet).

[d]For corn-free baking powder, see Table 14-1.

Source: From Rowe, A. H., & Rowe, A., Jr., *Food allergy: Its manifestations and control and the elimination diets.* Springfield, Ill.: Charles C Thomas, Publisher, 1972, by permission of the publisher.

usually possible to provide an adequate diet without eggs, there is concern for the provision of an adequate number of Calories when egg-containing baked goods are eliminated. Egg-free bakery products can be made with substitute thickeners or leavening agents. The milk-free diet is of particular concern when the patient is an infant or young child. Soybean, meat-based, or hypoallergenic formulas can be used. When goat's milk is used as a milk substitute, supplementary vitamin B_{12}, folic acid, and vitamin D are required.

Elimination diets are simpler to manage in infants because the formula is the mainstay of the diet. A milk-free formula can be used as the only food during the trial period, with other foods added one at a time at spaced intervals as the infant grows.

Appropriate substitution or supplementation of essential nutrients is important in any elimination diet. Foods that cause allergic responses may be reintroduced after a period of abstinence because many people, particularly children, tend to outgrow food allergies.

NURSING IMPLICATIONS

- Hereditary transmission of an allergic potential is a common occurrence. Newborn infants of parents with allergies should be protected

TABLE 14-3
FOODS ALLOWED IN THE MINIMAL ELIMINATION DIETS (ROWE)

1. Lamb, white potatoes, pearl tapioca, carrots, peas, cottonseed or sesame oil,[a] salt, sugar, water, and Neo-Mull-Soy[b] may be tried. This diet eliminates beef, all cereals and fruits, soybeans and lima beans, and most vegetables, which are in the diet shown in Table 14-1 or Table 14-2 or both of those diets.

2. Chicken, turkey, rice, pearl tapioca, cottonseed or sesame oil, salt, sugar, water, and Neo-Mull-Soy,[b] which eliminates all cereals, legumes, meats, vegetables, and fruits, or a similar diet may be used.

3. Fin fish, crab, eggs, pearl tapioca, soy tapioca bread, cake and cookies, Willow Run oleomargarine, sugar, salt, water, and Neo-Mull-Soy.[b]

[a]Chinese sesame oil is made from roasted sesame seeds and is not acceptable.

[b]Neo-Mull-Soy (Borden's) or other soy products, if tolerated, can be used in any of these minimal diets. Neo-Mull-Soy can be diluted with one-third water with cane sugar and salt added to taste and taken three times per day to increase caloric intake if allergy to soy is absent.

Source: From Rowe, A. H., & Rowe, A., Jr. *Food allergy: Its manifestations and control and the elimination diets.* Springfield, Ill.: Charles C Thomas, Publisher, 1972, by permission of the publisher.

from the highly sensitizing antigens (milk, fish, eggs, wheat, nuts), both those ingested directly and those in breast milk.

• Breast milk is the best food for a potentially allergic infant.

• Some children have a history of refusing foods to which they are allergic. It is also possible to be addicted to a food that causes an allergic response.

• Solid foods should be introduced into an infant's diet one at a time and evaluated for several days to aid in the identification of potential allergens.

• Delayed introduction of solids into the infant's diet permits maturation of the gastrointestinal tract and reduces the absorption of undigested, potential antigens.

• Pregnant women with histories of allergy should not ingest large amounts of any highly sensitizing food to reduce the risk of in utero sensitization of their unborn children. Milk ingested by such women should be boiled to reduce its antigenic potential.

• The foods that most frequently cause immediate allergic reactions are eggs, fish, seafood, berries, and nuts.

• The foods that are most frequently responsible for delayed allergic reactions are wheat, corn, milk, chocolate, pork, legumes, white potatoes, beef, and oranges.

• Patients who are allergic to a specific food are also likely to react adversely to other foods in the same category.

• Hidden sources of wheat include packaged soup mixes and sauces.

• Hidden sources of corn include cornstarch, corn syrup, corn oil, baking powder, confectioner's sugar, and frozen yogurt.

- A component of milk (sodium caseinate) is used in the manufacture of margarine.
- Egg albumin is used in the preparation of marshmallows and frozen dinners.
- The diet must be carefully evaluated, and substitutes should be provided to fill the gaps created by elimination of foods.
- People with food allergies should wear a Medic-Alert tag.
- People who are allergic to eggs should not be immunized with vaccines prepared from egg components (chick embryos).
- Diabetics who are allergic to pork may be unable to use insulin prepared from hog pancreas.
- Careful reading of labels is critical in adhering to any elimination diet.
- Children with food allergies should be provided with allowable substitutes to permit full participation in peer group activities.
- The use of decals to label special foods fosters independence in a child with a food allergy.
- Patients who manifest the immediate-type response must be careful when dining out. They should inform the person who is cooking that they are allergic to a food and should stress that even a minute amount of the food could cause a severe reaction.
- Foods are more likely to be allergenic when raw than when cooked.
- Allergens are usually proteins, and cooking or digestion may eliminate their allergenic properties.
- Some foods generally considered nonallergenic can cause severe reactions. Allergies to soybean milk, rice, and lamb do occur, although the incidence is rare.

Atopic Dermatitis (Infantile Eczema)

PATHOPHYSIOLOGY

Although its exact cause is unknown, atopic dermatitis has been related to physical, emotional, and hypersensitivity factors. The skin of the infant is typically thin and fragile, with a high water content. It reacts to irritation with weeping lesions, severe itching, dryness, and crusting. The emotional factor is felt to be a response to "smother love." The allergic factor is commonly hypersensitivity to milk, egg albumin, or wheat. A familial incidence has been noted.

In atopic dermatitis, there is capillary dilatation, erythema, and edema. Papules develop into vesicles that break as weeping lesions. The weeping lesions eventually dry and crust. The intense pruritus leads to scratching and secondary infection.

TREATMENT

The treatment of atopic dermatitis involves removal of the allergen and provision of supportive care. Local treatment of the skin and measurements to prevent scratching and infection are critical.

DIET THERAPY

Infants with atopic dermatitis are often fat, well-nourished babies whose eczema improves with weight loss. A controlled-Calorie diet may be used for the obese infant. The usual diet is a hypoallergenic diet that restricts intake of the foods that are most frequently identified as allergens in infants.

An approach similar to the one used in food allergy is instituted. The infant is given a soybean, meat-based, or hypoallergenic formula for 10 days. New foods are added, one at a time, at weekly intervals. The least allergenic foods are added first. Wheat, eggs, and milk are often not introduced into the diet until the child is more than 2 years old, the age at which infantile eczema usually clears.

NURSING IMPLICATIONS

- Synthetic vitamins may be needed to supplement the restricted diet.
- Calcium intake should be carefully evaluated in the absence of milk intake.
- Read baby food labels carefully; some preparations of bananas contain orange juice. Citrus fruits are common allergens.
- When the child is ready for table foods, read labels carefully for hidden sources of allergens.
- Use care in scheduling immunizations, especially those prepared from egg or chick embryo components (measles, mumps).
- Do not force foods or permit ingestion of restricted foods to improve food intake.

Chinese Restaurant Syndrome

PATHOPHYSIOLOGY

Chinese restaurant syndrome is an allergic response to monosodium glutamate (MSG) that causes a temporary burning sensation in the neck and forearms, tightness in the chest, and headache. Because of the frequency of use of MSG, a flavor enhancer, in the preparation of Chinese food, this allergic response has been called Chinese restaurant syndrome.

TREATMENT

The symptoms usually subside without treatment.

DIET THERAPY

People who are allergic to MSG usually avoid Chinese food and attempt to eliminate all sources of MSG from their diets.

NURSING IMPLICATIONS

- MSG is a flavor enhancer, not a preservative or tenderizer, and can easily be eliminated from foods prepared at home.
- Any commercially processed product, except mayonnaise, salad dressings, and French dressing, must list MSG on its label. Consumers can easily check for this ingredient when selecting products.
- MSG is 14% sodium, which is a consideration in low-sodium diets.

References

Breneman, J. Food allergy. *Contemporary Nutrition,* March 1979, *4,* 3.

Fontana, V., Morena-Pagan, F. Allergy and diet. In R. Goodhart & M. Shils (Eds.), *Modern nutrition in health and disease* (6th ed.). Philadelphia: Lea & Febiger, 1980.

Greene, G. Food allergies. *American Baby,* May 1979, *41,* 5.

Lambert, M. Drug and food interactions. *American Journal of Nursing,* March 1975, *75,* 3.

Krause, M., & Mahan, L. *Food, nutrition and diet therapy* (6th ed.). Philadelphia: W. B. Saunders Company, 1979.

Marino, M. Food allergy. In R. Howard & N. Herbold, *Nutrition in clinical care.* New York: McGraw-Hill Book Company, 1978.

Marlow, D. *Textbook of pediatric nursing* (5th ed.). Philadelphia: W. B. Saunders Company, 1977.

Parker, C. Food allergies. *American Journal of Nursing,* February 1980, *60,* 2.

Pilliteri, A. *Nursing care of the growing family. A child health text.* Boston: Little, Brown & Company, 1977.

Stordy, B., & Hubbard, R. Allergy: When the body takes a stand. *Nursing Mirror,* March 6, 1980 (Supplement), *150,* 10.

15

Diet Therapy in Neurologic, Neurosurgical, and Psychiatric Disorders

The cells of the nervous system have a special relationship to nutritional intake. Glucose and ketones are the only fuel substances that can pass the blood-brain barrier. The central nervous system is particularly vulnerable to variations in glucose and oxygen levels. Thiamine and niacin are needed for the utilization of glucose by nervous system cells and other body cells. Vitamin B_6 is involved in the formation of neurotransmitters and neurohormones. The neurotransmitters acetylcholine, γ-aminobutyric acid, norepinephrine, dopamine, and serotonin are either amino acids or amino acid derivatives. Adequate neurotransmission is dependent on diet.

Neurologic Trauma

The pathophysiology and treatment of nervous system injuries vary with the nature and extent of the trauma; however, some general dietary guidelines do exist.

DIET THERAPY

Patients who experience severe head injuries are usually maintained on intravenous feedings for several days. Control of acid-base and electrolyte balances is essential; intravenous solutions are selected on the basis of blood gas and chemistry values.

213

Tube feedings may be used when peristalsis returns, usually 48 hours after injury. Tube feedings are omitted when distention or gastric retention is present. Oral feedings are avoided if vomiting is present because of the danger of aspiration. Vomiting also increases intracranial pressure.

Paraplegics initially require a high protein intake (150 to 300 grams) combined with a high-vitamin, high-Calorie diet. Caloric intake is restricted in the ongoing care of the paraplegic patient to prevent weight gain, which complicates rehabilitation. Calcium is restricted in the first few months after spinal cord injury to reduce the incidence of urinary calculi.

Cerebral Palsy

PATHOPHYSIOLOGY

Cerebral palsy is the result of damage to the motor centers of the brain before, during, or shortly after birth. This motor damage causes varying degrees of physical disability and mental impairment. Sensory involvement is also common, with sight, hearing, or speech impaired. Cerebral palsy is generally classified as spastic paralysis, in which there is hyperactivity of the stretch muscle reflexes; as chorioathetosis, in which involuntary movements occur; as ataxia, in which coordination and balance are impaired; or as flaccidity, in which muscle tone is decreased.

TREATMENT

There is no cure for cerebral palsy. Rehabilitation programs that help patients use their abilities to the greatest advantage are the recommended treatment. Surgical procedures may aid in the correction of orthopedic deformities.

DIET THERAPY

A patient with cerebral palsy may suffer from nutritional deficiencies because of an inability to close the lips, suck, bite, chew, or swallow. Sucking and swallowing problems may prevent adequate nutritional intake in affected infants. Fluids may be lost because of drooling and dribbling, so that actual intake should be carefully assessed. Chewing problems necessitate the elimination of coarse and stringy foods from the diet. Vomiting may be a problem and may increase the loss of nutrients. When the total food intake is limited, the quality of the intake becomes especially important.

A spastic patient who moves with difficulty may require fewer Calories; an athetoid patient may need additional Calories to cover the involuntary movements. Any patient whose disability makes ambulation impossible may become obese; excess body weight is a special problem during adolescence.

NURSING IMPLICATIONS

- Food may be fortified with dry skim milk, evaporated milk, wheat germ, or bran when the quantity of intake is limited.
- Fluids may be thickened with cereal or yogurt to reduce dribbling.
- To aid patients who have difficulty drinking from a cup, stand behind them and cup their jaws firmly in one hand while holding the cup in the other hand.
- When feeding a patient with cerebral palsy put the food to one side of the patient's mouth, and direct the patient to use his or her tongue to move the food around in the mouth.
- Remind patients to keep their lips closed to avoid pushing food out of their mouths or allowing food to fall out of their mouths.
- Allow patients to bite off pieces of toast and crackers rather than breaking off pieces for them.
- Place patients in a good anatomic position for feeding. Spastic patients tend to hyperextend their heads, which throws the swallowing mechanism out of line.
- Provide special eating devices to promote independence as much as possible.
- Avoid rushing the patient at mealtime; provide a quiet, unhurried environment.
- Constipation may become a problem due to atonic muscles and reduced fiber intake. Laxative foods may be helpful; unprocessed bran can be added to foods.

Seizure Disorders (Epilepsy)

PATHOPHYSIOLOGY

Seizure disorders are paroxysmal disturbances of the nervous system that result in recurrent attacks of loss of consciousness, convulsions, motor activity, or behavioral abnormalities. The seizures are a result of excessive neuronal discharges in various parts of the brain.

TREATMENT

Seizure disorders are treated by means of anticonvulsant drug therapy, surgery, or electrical stimulation. It is important to eliminate any precipitating factor. The promotion of physical and mental health is an essential part of the treatment plan.

DIET THERAPY

The drugs that are used to control seizures have side effects related to diet. In general, such drugs interfere with vitamin D metabolism and lead to calcium imbalance and, possibly, rickets or osteomalacia. Vitamin D supplementation, usually with the active form (25-hydroxy vitamin D), is usually prescribed in conjunction with anticonvulsant drug therapy.

Ethosuximide (Zarontin), trimethadione (Tridione), and primidone (Mysoline) may cause gastrointestinal disturbances and weight loss. Primidone, phenobarbital, and phenytoin decrease vitamin B levels, so that supplementation may be indicated. Phenytoin (Dilantin) also causes gum hyperplasia and carbohydrate intolerance. All these drugs are usually taken with meals to reduce gastric irritation.

The diet usually recommended for patients with seizure disorders is one that is well balanced and that avoids excesses of food or fluid. When anticonvulsant drugs are ineffective, ketogenic diets may be tried. Ketogenic diets are most effective in controlling intractable myoclonic or akinetic seizures in infancy. Ketogenic diets are designed to produce high plasma levels of ketones, which tend to decrease restlessness and irritability. These diets have severe restrictions for carbohydrate intake; fats are the major energy source. A ratio of 3:1 or 4:1 fat to carbohydrate and protein is used. Sufficient protein to meet basal requirements (1 gram per kilogram of body weight per day) is provided. The diet is rigidly monitored, and all food is weighed.

Medium-chain triglycerides have been used in ketogenic diets; they produce a high degree of ketosis because of their rapid metabolism and absorption. When medium-chain triglycerides are included in a ketogenic diet, they account for 60% of the Calories; 10% of the Calories are provided by fats, 10% by proteins, and 20% by carbohydrates.

NURSING IMPLICATIONS

- Patients with seizure disorders are usually advised to avoid stimulants, such as tea, coffee, and cola beverages.
- Alcoholic beverages are usually eliminated completely because they tend to induce seizures.
- Ketogenic diets are more effective in younger patients; the young brain has a greater capacity for oxidizing ketone bodies.
- Ketogenic diets are unpalatable and are easier to administer to very young or severely retarded patients.
- Daily urine collections are obtained for monitoring the degree of ketosis when ketogenic diets are used.
- Serum levels of cholesterol are not elevated when medium-chain triglycerides are used as the major source of fats.
- Ketogenic diets may cause nausea and vomiting. Orange juice usually relieves these symptoms.

- Ketogenic diets tend to lose some of their effectiveness with time.
- A combination of dietary intervention and drug therapy may prove effective.
- Ketogenic diets may be deficient in calcium, iron, vitamin B complex, vitamin C, and vitamin D.

Multiple Sclerosis

PATHOPHYSIOLOGY

Multiple sclerosis is a condition in which multifocal areas of demyelination are found scattered throughout the central nervous system. As a result of the loss of the myelin sheath, a progressive neurologic disability occurs and affects the myelinated nerve fibers and the muscles innervated by them. Although the precise cause of multiple sclerosis is unknown, there is thought to be a relationship between abnormal metabolism of fatty oils and the development of multiple sclerosis. Patients with multiple sclerosis have reduced serum levels of linoleic acid, the essential fatty acid. The condition is characterized by remissions and exacerbations.

TREATMENT

Treatment is symptomatic and varies with the individual patient. During remissions, the patient is advised to be as active as possible and to avoid coming in contact with infections. Corticosteroids are used for exacerbations. Treatment in the chronic phase centers around the management of bladder and bowel problems, muscle spasticity, and the prevention of decubiti and contractures.

DIET THERAPY

There is no evidence that special diets are helpful in the treatment of multiple sclerosis; however, if the diets are nutritionally sound, there is no reason not to try them. The advocates of low-fat diet claim that it retards the disease process and reduces the risk for exacerbations. This diet consists of 40 to 50 grams of polyunsaturated fatty acids, 10 grams of saturated fatty acids, normal protein intake, and carbohydrates in amounts that satisfy caloric requirements. A teaspoon of cod liver oil daily is recommended. The diet is based on the theory that multiple sclerosis is related to abnormal metabolism of fatty oils.

Other patients with multiple sclerosis select a well-balanced diet that can be easily assimilated. As muscle atrophy increases and coordination decreases, food may be liquefied for ease in swallowing. Weight control may become important with decreased activity; caloric intake must be adjusted to activity levels.

Constipation and fecal impaction are common in the chronic phase; laxative foods and adequate fluids may be helpful in the management of these problems.

NURSING IMPLICATIONS

- Feeding aids maintain independence in eating.
- If meat intake is less than 2 ounces per day (as it would be in a diet containing 10 grams of saturated fats), intake of proteins, iron, and vitamin B complex should be investigated.
- Linoleic acid is found in plant oils.
- The presence of bladder stones may indicate the need for a high-protein, acid-ash diet (see Chapter 11) as well as increased intake of fluids.

Myasthenia Gravis

PATHOPHYSIOLOGY

In myasthenia gravis, there is fluctuating weakness of some voluntary muscles. The weakness appears to be related to a defect in the transmission of nerve impulses at the neuromuscular junction. The muscles most commonly affected are those innervated by cranial nerves originating in the brain stem (ocular, facial, lingual, and muscles of mastication and deglutition). The defect in transmission is thought to be inadequate synthesis or release of acetylcholine. Myasthenia gravis may have an autoimmune basis.

TREATMENT

Myasthenia gravis is treated medically by use of short-acting anticholinesterase compounds (neostigmine [Prostigmin] or pyridostigmine bromide [Mestinon]) or corticosteroids. Surgical treatment involves removal of the thymus.

DIET THERAPY

Special diets are not used in the treatment of myasthenia gravis. However, the weakened condition of the muscles used in chewing and swallowing increases the difficulty of ensuring adequate nutrition. Easily swallowed foods are included in the diet; other foods can be minced or altered in consistency for ease in chewing and swallowing.

Patients sometimes can handle food intake in the early part of the meal but then encounter difficulty. Small, frequent feedings may circumvent this problem. When chewing and swallowing difficulties become too severe, tube feedings may be used.

NURSING IMPLICATIONS

- Do not rush the patient at mealtime. Allow adequate time for completion of meals.
- Meals may be served on a warming tray to keep the food hot during the time it takes the patient to consume it.
- Anticholinesterase medications should be administered 30 to 60 minutes before meals for maximal effect at mealtime.
- Potassium supplementation may be needed in conjunction with anticholinesterase drug therapy.
- Suction equipment should be available unobtrusively during feeding in the event of regurgitation.

Parkinsonism

PATHOPHYSIOLOGY

Parkinson's disease is a progressive neuromuscular disorder characterized by a low concentration of the neurotransmitter dopamine at the basal ganglia of the brain. The cause of the dopamine deficiency is unknown. Lack of dopamine results in tremor, rigidity, and akinesis.

TREATMENT

The treatment of parkinsonism includes the use of levodopa, which is a precursor of dopamine, or a combination of levodopa and carbidopa (Sinemet). Sinemet is used to reduce the dosage of levodopa. If levodopa cannot be used, anticholinergic drugs are prescribed to reduce tremor or rigidity. Other aspects of treatment are directed toward maintaining optimal physical and emotional health so that the patient can cope with this chronic and progressively disabling disease.

DIET THERAPY

Diet therapy in parkinsonism is related to drug therapy. When levodopa is used, appropriate dietary measures help make the drug optimally effective. A high protein intake reduces the effectiveness of levodopa. Intake of protein is restricted in patients receiving levodopa; emphasis is placed on the inclusion of high-biologic-value proteins and the restriction of low-biologic-value proteins. Food intake is usually divided into four to six small, low-protein meals. Protein intake should be consistent as well as restricted. High intake of protein results in loss of control over symptoms; too little protein causes an increase in involuntary movements (dyskinesia) in patients taking levodopa.

When given alone, levodopa is transformed into dopamine before reaching the brain. Vitamin B_6 increases this transformation. Foods fortified with vitamin B_6 (cereals) and vitamin supplements that contain vitamin B_6 should be avoided by patient who are taking levodopa as their sole medication.

Patients with parkinsonism may lose weight because of difficulty in ingesting sufficient food. Obesity also is a problem, not only because mobility is reduced but also because obesity interferes with the dosage regulation of levodopa.

Constipation may develop as a side effect of drug therapy and diminished activity; generous amounts of laxative foods and fluids may aid in preventing this problem.

NURSING IMPLICATIONS

- High-biologic-value proteins include eggs, milk, and meats. Low-biologic-value proteins include cereals, vegetables, and fruits.
- Eating may be complicated by an inability to close the lips, suck, chew, bite, or swallow. Semisolid foods may be easier to swallow than fluids.
- Dysphagia may occur in advanced cases. Foods can be cut, minced, or softened in a blender to reduce chewing difficulties.
- Foods should be served on a warming tray to keep them warm during the time it may take to consume them.
- Fluids may be consumed best with a straw if sucking ability is not impaired.
- Alcohol can antagonize levodopa and is best avoided.
- Sinemet, a combination drug (levodopa and carbidopa), reduces by about three-fourths the amount of levodopa taken. Sinemet is not affected by protein intake, vitamin B_6, or alcohol.

Anorexia Nervosa

PATHOPHYSIOLOGY

Anorexia nervosa is thought to be a biopsychosocial disorder that results in self-imposed starvation as a means of establishing identity and control. There may be a metabolic and, possibly, hereditary predisposition to this condition. Early feeding patterns and attitudes toward food may be involved. Society's emphasis on the desirability of slenderness has also been implicated. The patient (usually a teenage girl) denies being excessively thin despite extreme emaciation, denies hunger despite prolonged malnutrition, and denies fatigue despite frantic exercise. There is usually a problem in family dynamics.

Extreme malnutrition leads to secondary endocrine disorders, such as amenorrhea. In addition to refusal to eat adequate amounts of food, patients with anorexia nervosa sometimes go on food binges. Such binges are followed by self-induced vomiting or the use of enemas or cathartics.

TREATMENT

Various team approaches have been tried to restore normal nutrition and improve family interactions. Psychotherapy or behavior modification is frequently used. A period of hospitalization may be needed for the initial nutritional therapy or to separate the patient from the family.

DIET THERAPY

The aim of diet therapy is to return the patient to a normal diet and appropriate weight. Such patients resist measures designed to increase food intake. Punishment has no place in the therapy; gentle persuasion or a matter-of-fact approach is used. Elimination of privileges, followed by their gradual return in exchange for compliance to the treatment regimen, may be a viable approach. Tube feedings or hyperalimentation can be tried.

The initial dietary intake is designed to meet the basal caloric needs. These needs are diminished because of the patient's emaciated and hypometabolic condition. A liquid diet may be more acceptable to the patient because fluids appear to contain fewer nutrients. Through the use of elemental diets or liquid dietary supplements, fluids can be made nutritionally complete, except for fiber content.

NURSING IMPLICATIONS

- The team approach is essential, and all members of the team must be consistent in their handling of feeding behavior.
- Patients may be manipulative; they should not be allowed to dictate food intake.
- Feeding periods should be closely supervised; patients with anorexia nervosa are ingenious in making intake appear adequate.
- Patients may also hide food for later binges or to avoid eating.
- A prolonged mealtime is required to ensure intake.

- All conversation related to food or weight should be avoided. Nutritional education should be postponed until the patient is discharged from the hospital.
- Bathroom privileges should be denied for 30 minutes after meals to prevent self-induced vomiting.
- Patients with anorexia nervosa show major sleep disturbances that abate as they gain weight.

Hyperkinesia

PATHOPHYSIOLOGY

Hyperkinetic is a term used to describe children who, according to their parents and teachers, are persistently hyperactive, distractible, impulsive, and excitable. The reasons for this behavioral pattern have not been established.

TREATMENT

Treatment modalities include drug therapy, dietary intervention, and behavior modification. The drugs used are cerebral stimulants that, paradoxically, have a calming effect on such hyperactive children.

DIET THERAPY

In the early 1970s, Dr. Ben Feingold suggested that hyperkinesia might be caused by the ingestion of low-molecular-weight chemicals found in certain foods, artificial colorings, and artificial flavorings. He devised the Feingold diet, which eliminates foods that contain the salicylate radical, artificial colorings, and artificial flavorings (Feingold, 1975). Dr. Feingold's claims of dramatic improvement in hyperactive children have not been supported by subsequent research; however, some children appear to improve on the diet, and groups of enthusiastic parents have organized to support Dr. Feingold's claims. Other physicians use elimination diets that restrict intake of wheat, sugar, dyes, eggs, chocolate, and corn (Rapp, 1977). It would appear reasonable to try diet therapy for hyperkinesia for at least 1 week and evaluate the results on an individual basis.

The Feingold diet is based on the elimination of two groups of foods. Group I consists of all natural foods that contain the salicylate radical. Group I foods include:

Fruits

 Almonds
 Apples

Apricots

Blackberries

Boysenberries

Gooseberries

Raspberries

Strawberries

Cherries

Currants

Grapes and raisins (including all products made from grapes: wine, wine vinegar, jellies)

Oranges

Peaches

Plums

Prunes

Vegetables

Tomatoes

Cucumbers

Group II foods include all foods that include any of the seven synthetic colorings and flavorings that contain the salicylate radical. Identification of Group II foods is difficult, and labels must be studied carefully. Any food that contains "artificial color" or "artificial flavor" according to its labeling cannot be used. Homemade products, fresh meats, fresh milk, and fresh vegetables are recommended. The diet is continued for 4 to 6 weeks without any deviation. Then, one at a time, foods from Group II are added and evaluated. Parents are encouraged to keep diaries of the child's intake and behavior.

NURSING IMPLICATIONS

- The Feingold diet may not be adequate for meeting long-term nutritional needs.
- Exclusion of oranges from the Feingold diet may result in inadequate intake of vitamin C. Grapefruits, lemons, and limes are permitted on the diet.
- Many pediatric medications contain artificial colorings and flavorings. Vitamin supplements should be carefully selected for this reason.
- Toothpastes, mouthwashes, cough drops, and antacids are also artificially colored and flavored and must be eliminated when the Feingold diet is followed.

- Younger children appear to respond better to diet therapy than do older children.
- All children who are following elimination diets should be carefully monitored by medical personnel to assure that they are receiving a nutritionally adequate intake.
- Children who respond to diet therapy may also need drug therapy, psychologic counseling, or educational counseling.

Mental Illness

There are many forms of mental illness and various treatment modalities. Mentally ill people have the same basic needs for nutrition as do mentally well people. Good physical health, fostered by sound nutritional intake, should be an adjunct to psychiatric treatment. In the past, theories that related individual psychiatric disorders to the lack of some substance found in food enjoyed some popularity. Lithium is used in the treatment of manic-depressive states, dopamine percursors are used in parkinsonism, and a biochemical basis for schizophrenia has been suggested for years (Davis, 1978).

Food has emotional connotations that may become more pronounced in mentally ill patients. Food provides a sense of security and pleasurable feelings. Some people ease their anxiety with compulsive eating, whereas others lose their appetites when anxious. Depressed patients lose interest in food. Guilt-ridden patients may deny themselves food as a form of self-punishment. Hyperactive patients cannot sit still long enough to eat a proper meal. Deluded patients may have fears and suspicions related to food.

Just as the emotional component of care is essential in nursing physically ill patients, the physical needs of mentally ill patients must also be given adequate consideration.

NURSING IMPLICATIONS

- Shock therapy increases caloric needs.
- Patients who are taking monoamine oxidase inhibitors should avoid foods with high tyramine content (cheese, wine, fish, beer, yogurt). See Chapter 25 for a more complete discussion of food-drug interactions.
- Many tranquilizers and antipsychotic drugs cause dry mouth, which could discourage food intake.
- The fact that a mentally ill person's tray is empty does not necessarily mean that he or she has eaten the food. Food may have been hidden or consumed by others.

- Nutritional assessment should be included as part of the periodic evaluation of mentally ill patients. Weekly weight measurements might suggest nutritional problems and provide the basis for further investigation.

References

Beecham Foods Nutrition Information Center. How diet affects your sleep. *Nursing Mirror,* November 16, 1978, *147,* 20.

Boykin, L. Nutrition and hyperkinesis: Is there an association? *Journal of Psychiatric Nursing and Mental Health Services,* December 1978, *16,* 12.

Ciseaux, A. Anorexia nervosa: A view from the mirror. *American Journal of Nursing,* August 1980, *80,* 8.

Claggett, M. Anorexia nervosa: A behavioral approach. *American Journal of Nursing,* August 1980, *80,* 8.

Conway, B., Carini, E., Owens, G. *Neurological and neurosurgical nursing* (7th ed.). St. Louis: C. V. Mosby Company, 1978.

Davis, C. Dietary pathogenesis of schizophrenia. *Nursing Times,* December 7, 1978, *74,* 49.

Feingold, B. *Why your child is hyperactive.* New York: Random House, 1975.

Gresh, C. Parkinson's disease. *Nursing 80,* January 1,980, *10,* 1.

Growdon, J., & Wurtman, R. Nutrients and neurotransmitters. *Contemporary Nutrition,* December 1979, *4,* 12.

Hartley, J., & Matthews, C. The Feingold hypothesis: Current studies. *Contemporary Nutrition,* April 1978, *3,* 4.

Howard, R., Fetters, L., & MacDonald, D. The nervous system and handicapping conditions. In R. Howard & N. Herbold, *Nutrition in clinical care.* New York: McGraw-Hill Book Company, 1978.

Howe, P. *Basic nutrition in health and disease* (6th ed.). Philadelphia: W. B. Saunders Company, 1976.

Krause, M., & Mahon, L. *Food, nutrition and diet therapy* (6th ed.). Philadelphia: W. B. Saunders Company, 1979.

Lucas, A. Anorexia nervosa. *Contemporary Nutrition,* August 1978, *3,* 8.

Luckman, J., & Sorensen, K. *Medical-surgical nursing: A psychophysiologic approach* (2nd ed.). Philadelphia: W. B. Saunders Company, 1980.

Marlow, D. *Textbook of pediatric nursing* (5th ed.). Philadelphia: W. B. Saunders Company, 1977.

Rapp, D. A diet that could help the hyperactive child. *Consultant,* May 1977, *17,* 5.

Richardson, T. Anorexia nervosa: An overview. *American Journal of Nursing,* August 1980, *80,* 8.

Sheridan, M. Diet and hyperactivity: Is there a relationship? *American Baby,* August 1979, *41,* 15.

Suitor, C., & Hunter, M. *Nutrition: Principles and application in health promotion.* Philadelphia: J. B. Lippincott Company, 1980.

Watts, C. Nutrition and mental health. *Psychiatric Nursing,* September/October 1978, *19,* 5.

Wilson, H., & Kneish, C. *Psychiatric nursing.* Menlo Park, Calif.: Addison-Wesley Publishing Company, 1979.

16
Diet Therapy in Musculoskeletal Disorders

Fractures

PATHOPHYSIOLOGY

A fracture is a disruption in the normal continuity of a bone. Fractures heal by the formation of new bone tissue to unite the fragments at the fracture site. At the time of injury, bleeding occurs at the fracture site. A hematoma forms, surrounding the bone injury and filling the gap between bone fragments. A fibrin mesh forms around the fracture. Within a few days, the hematoma is replaced by granulation tissue. Fibroblasts invade the granulation tissue to form a soft callus. Six to 10 days after the injury, newly formed cartilage and bone matrix invade the callus. Calcium salts are deposited in the callus to form a permanent callus of rigid bone.

TREATMENT

The treatment of fractures involves reduction of the fracture and immobilization to permit the development of callus and healing. Immobilization may be accomplished by means of casts, splints, bandages, internal fixation devices, or traction. When the fracture heals, physiotherapy may be used to offset the effects of disuse.

DIET THERAPY

After fractures of the long bones and the immobilization required for healing, the body loses protein, nitrogen, potassium, phosphorus, sulfur, and calcium. A diet that is liberal in protein content is desirable to foster formation of bone matrix and calcium deposits in the callus. Adequate calcium and phosphorus are necessary for the building of new bone cells. Vitamin D encourages the effective use of calcium; vitamin C is needed to manufacture the intercellular cement that is required for healing.

Increased caloric intake is usually desirable in the early healing phase to compensate for the increased requirements imposed by stress. Caloric restriction may be indicated in the recovery phase if lack of activity leads to weight gain. Physical therapy usually increases the caloric requirements.

NURSING IMPLICATIONS

- The combination of immobilization and excess calcium may lead to renal or bladder calculi. Excessive intake of calcium should be avoided, and a generous fluid intake should be provided to prevent urinary stasis.
- Early mobilization is the best therapy for the bone demineralization that is associated with immobilization. Range-of-motion exercises for uninjured limbs should be encouraged if the activity does not jeopardize the fracture therapy.
- Patients in hip spica, jacket, or body casts should avoid gas-producing foods that could cause excessive tightness of the cast.

Rheumatoid Arthritis

PATHOPHYSIOLOGY

Rheumatoid arthritis is a chronic, progressive, inflammatory tissue disorder of unknown origin that results in stiff joints, ankylosis, and deformity. An autoimmune response centered in the synovial joints is suspected as the cause of the disease. Inflammatory changes occur in the synovial tissue, with swelling and thickening of the synovial lining of the involved joints. Eventually, granulation tissue covers the articular cartilage and is subsequently replaced by fibrous connective tissue. As the articular cartilage is eroded, bone is exposed, leading to ankylosis and deformity. During the course of the disease, negative nitrogen and calcium balances develop. Bone decalcification and muscle atrophy result from lack of use of the involved limb. Hemolytic anemia accompanies the disease.

TREATMENT

The treatment of rheumatoid arthritis is drug therapy with antiinflammatory and antirheumatic agents. Anaglesic drugs and comfort measures for the relief of pain are an important aspect of therapy. The patient is encouraged to remain as active as possible. Total joint replacements are being used to mobilize patients with ankylosed joints. Blood transfusions are used to treat anemia.

DIET THERAPY

There is no special diet that cures rheumatoid arthritis or alleviates its symptoms, despite many claims for certain vitamins and minerals. A well-balanced, nutritious diet with an adequate amount of vitamins and minerals is recommended. Some alteration of food intake may be associated with drug therapy. Many drugs used in rheumatoid arthritis cause gastric irritation and may be less disturbing if taken with bland meals or antacids. Small, frequent feedings tend to decrease gastric irritation when large doses of aspirin are taken at frequent intervals.

Rheumatoid arthritis is a chronic, painful disease; in any chronic condition, optimal nutritional support is essential. The recommendation of a nutritious, well-balanced diet appropriate for the patient's ideal weight and activity should be actively promoted. Patients with rheumatoid arthritis are often the victims of quackery related to diet or nutritional supplements. They should be encouraged, instead, with sound nutritional education. A specific diet plan to meet the individual needs of the patient should be an important aspect of therapy. Deformities that interfere with eating indicate the need for careful planning to ensure optimal intake.

NURSING IMPLICATIONS

- Drug therapy with corticosteroids may necessitate restriction of sodium intake.
- Iron, folic acid, and vitamin B_{12} are usually not effective in treating the anemia associated with rheumatoid arthritis. Blood transfusions are usually necessary.
- Anorexia is a symptom of anemia; red blood cell counts should be monitored.
- Discourage quackery and substitute sound health practices.
- Explain the untoward effects of massive doses of vitamin D.
- Adapt feeding methods to the patient's abilities. Provide for independence in eating as much as possible.
- During the active stage of the disease, carbohydrate tolerance is reduced because of chronic inflammation; adapt carbohydrate intake to carbohydrate tolerance.

Osteoarthritis

PATHOPHYSIOLOGY

Osteoarthritis is characterized by degenerative changes in the articular cartilage of weight-bearing joints, particularly the hips, knees, and spine. As part of the aging process, the elasticity of the joint capsules, articular cartilage, and ligaments is reduced. Cartilage atrophies, bones harden at the articular surfaces, and ligaments calcify.

TREATMENT

The aims of treatment are to relieve pain, to preserve joint function, and to protect the joints from trauma. These goals are usually accomplished by use of alternate periods of rest and activity, analgesics, and corrective surgical procedures.

DIET THERAPY

Osteoarthritis is aggravated by obesity, so that weight reduction diets are recommended for overweight patients. The diet should be high in proteins and moderately low in fats and carbohydrates.

Osteoarthritis is associated with aging. Older people frequently do not eat nutritious, well-balanced meals for a variety of reasons. The diet of the patient should be evaluated, and suggestions should be made for improvement. Older people should be encouraged to consume adequate amounts of proteins, calcium, iron, and vitamins.

NURSING IMPLICATIONS

- When aspirin is used as an analgesic, it may cause gastric distress. Taking aspirin with meals may reduce gastric irritation. Nonaspirin analgesics may be tried.
- Suggest the use of dry skim milk as a less expensive, lower-Calorie source of calcium and proteins than whole milk.

Osteomalacia

PATHOPHYSIOLOGY

Osteomalacia is the deossification of bone as a result of deficiency of vitamin D, calcium, or phosphorus. The bones become softened and deformed.

TREATMENT

Osteomalacia is treated by providing the deficient calcium, phosphorus, or vitamin D.

DIET THERAPY

Osteomalacia can be prevented by an adequate intake of calcium, phosphorus, and vitamin D. Milk is a good source of calcium and phosphorus; fortified milk has vitamin D added to it.

NURSING IMPLICATIONS

- Patients with milk intolerance should have their diets evaluated to ensure that they obtain adequate amounts of calcium and phosphorus from other sources. If the diet cannot be made adequate, supplementation should be provided.
- Exposure to sunlight provides vitamin D. Fortified margarine and milk are good sources of vitamin D. Vitamin supplementation can also be used.
- It is important to monitor serum levels of calcium during treatment with calcium salts to prevent hypercalcemia.

Osteoporosis

PATHOPHYSIOLOGY

Osteoporosis is increased porosity of the bone as a result of demineralization. There is reduced bone mass, which may lead to spontaneous fractures. The development of osteoporosis is related to age, and the condition tends to arise when secretion of sex and pituitary hormones is reduced, namely, postmenopausally. A reciprocal relationship exists between parathyroid hormone and the thyroid hormone calcitonin. In normal calcium metabolism, parathyroid hormone affects bone resorption, whereas calcitonin influences bone formation. Prolonged inadequate intake of calcium in adult life has been suggested as a cause of osteoporosis. Reduced physical activity causes calcium loss from bone. Some forms of periodontal disease characterized by bone resorption are believed to be forerunners of osteoporosis. It is known that the efficiency of calcium absorption decreases with age.

TREATMENT

Osteoporosis has been treated by estrogen therapy in postmenopausal women; however, the safety of this treatment is questionable in light of the carcinogenicity of estrogen. Recently, the modified male hormone stanozolol has been used to halt the loss of bone density. Increased activity in later life is recommended to prevent or slow the development of osteoporosis.

DIET THERAPY

Increasing the intake of calcium-rich foods is recommended in adult life as a possible preventive measure. Calcium supplementation can also be used. Maintaining physical activity in adult life should be recommended.

NURSING IMPLICATIONS

- Decreased intake of phosphorus may combat calcium losses because of the reciprocal relationship between these two minerals. This therapy is effective only for short periods and is used in the initial stages of prolonged immobilization.
- Liberal intake of fluid should accompany increased intake of calcium to prevent hypercalcemia and the formation of renal calculi.
- Milk is the best dietary source of calcium. It can be used as a beverage or in cooking. Dry skim milk powder can be added to many foods. Cheese is an alternative source of calcium.

Progressive Muscular Dystrophy

PATHOPHYSIOLOGY

Muscular dystrophy is a hereditary condition characterized by progressive degenerative changes in the muscle fibers. These changes lead to muscle weakness and atrophy. The muscles primarily affected are those of the girdle, proximal portions of the limbs, and eyes. In the Duchenne type of muscular dystrophy, the muscles of the face may be involved, resulting in an inability to suck, close the lips, bite, chew, or swallow. This type of muscular dystrophy begins in childhood. Poor hand-to-mouth coordination may also be present and affects food intake.

TREATMENT

There is no specific treatment. The patient is encouraged to lead a life as active as possible as long as possible. Exercise programs are recommended to prevent contractures.

DIET THERAPY

A low-Calorie diet is frequently prescribed to prevent obesity, which may develop as a result of reduced activity. Obesity complicates care and may impose increased restrictions on activity.

Foods that are easy to chew and swallow may be helpful for patients with the Duchenne type of muscular dystrophy. Pureeing or softening foods in a blender may permit greater ease in feeding and provides variety.

NURSING IMPLICATIONS

- Encourage patients to avoid constipating foods because gastric dilatation and fecal impaction frequently occur in muscular dystrophy.
- Encourage the use of muscles in eating activities to forestall atrophy.
- Encourage activities, other than eating, as sources of enjoyment. Using food as a substitute for other pleasurable pursuits can lead to obesity.

Extended Immobilization

PATHOPHYSIOLOGY

Patients with orthopedic injuries may lose from 15 to 20 pounds. This weight loss occurs as a result of bed rest, immobilization, stress, and trauma. Nitrogen losses lead to a negative nitrogen balance. Immobilization can result in deossification and osteoporosis of bones and hypercalcemia. Hypercalcemia predisposes the patient to kidney and bladder stones. Symptoms of hypercalcemia are more common in patients with low serum levels of albumin because albumin normally binds calcium and keeps it in the bloodstream.

Hypercalcemia is a special problem in children because of their accelerated rate of bone metabolism. Immobilized adolescents also experience problems related to hypercalcemia.

TREATMENT

Early ambulation is the best treatment when it is possible. Generous intake of fluids is recommended to aid in excretion of the excess calcium. Diuretics are sometimes used to prevent urinary stasis.

DIET THERAPY

The diet for a patient who is immobilized for extended periods should provide adequate quantities of high-biologic-value proteins to promote a positive nitrogen balance. An intake of 1.2 grams of protein per kilogram of ideal body weight is recommended. A positive nitrogen balance aids in the prevention of decubiti, infections, and skin breakdown.

A low-calcium diet does not result in hypocalcemia. Increased intake of phosphorus does reduce serum levels of calcium for the first few weeks after immobilization. Excessive intake of calcium should be discouraged but an adequate intake is necessary. A high-protein diet raises the calcium requirements of the body. Increased intake of fluids and urinary acidifiers provides protection against calcium stones.

NURSING IMPLICATIONS

- Monitor the calcium intake of patients on who are on liquid diets or tube feedings for long periods.
- Provide adequate sources of vitamin C to protect against skin breakdown.
- Treat urinary tract infections promptly; the nuclei of the calculi may be bacterial debris.
- See Chapter 11 for acid-ash foods.
- Provide increased roughage in the diet to prevent constipation.
- A negative nitrogen balance can result in decreased synthesis of plasma proteins and can contribute to anemia and clotting problems.

References

Barber, J., Stokes, L., & Billings, D. *Adult and child care* (2nd ed.). St. Louis: C. V. Mosby Company, 1977.

Brunner, L., & Suddarth, D. *Textbook of medical-surgical nursing* (4th ed.). Philadelphia: J. B. Lippincott Company, 1980.

Golovin, S. The endocrine system and skeletal disorders. In R. Howard & N. Herbold, *Nutrition in clinical care*. New York: McGraw-Hill Book Company, 1978.

Howe, P. *Basic nutrition in health and disease* (6th ed.). Philadelphia: W. B. Saunders Company, 1976.

Hunt, S., Groff, J., & Holbrooks, J. *Nutrition: Principles and clinical practice*. New York: John Wiley & Sons, 1980.

Jarrett, R. (Ed.). *Nutrition and disease*. Baltimore: University Park Press, 1979.

Krause, M., & Mahan, L. *Food, nutrition, and diet therapy* (6th ed.). Philadelphia: W. B. Saunders Company, 1979.

Luckmann, J., & Sorensen, K. *Medical-surgical nursing: A psychophysiologic approach* (2nd ed.). Philadelphia: W. B. Saunders Company, 1980.

Mitchell, H., Rynbergen, H., Anderson, L., et al. *Nutrition in health and disease* (16th ed.). Philadelphia: J. B. Lippincott Company, 1976.

Mourad, L. *Nursing care of adults with orthopedic conditions*. New York: John Wiley & Sons, 1980.

Thiele, V. *Clinical nutrition*. St. Louis: C. V. Mosby Company, 1976.

Watson, J. *Medical-surgical nursing and related physiology* (2nd ed.). Philadelphia: W. B. Saunders Company, 1979.

Whaley, L., & Wong, D. *Nursing care of infants and children*. St. Louis: C. V. Mosby Company, 1979.

Williams, S. *Nutrition and diet therapy* (3rd ed.). St. Louis: C. V. Mosby Company, 1977.

17
Diet Therapy in Deficiency Diseases

Classical cases of vitamin deficiencies are now rarely seen in North America. Increased interest and understanding of the vitamin requirements of the body, coupled with widespread fortification and enrichment of common foods, have led to the reduction of vitamin deficiency diseases. Vitamin deficiencies that resemble the textbook pictures are seen in areas where modern medicine is practiced only in cases of self-neglect due to psychiatric problems, age, alcoholism, or ignorance. Because of their low incidence, vitamin deficiencies are rarely suspected as possible diagnoses in modern medical practice. Borderline vitamin deficiencies, on the other hand, may be common when inadequate diets are followed for prolonged periods.

Vitamin A Deficiency

PATHOPHYSIOLOGY

Lack of vitamin A, either as preformed vitamin A (retinol) or as provitamin A (carotenoids), which is converted into retinol, disturbs the mucous membranes, the visual process, and development of teeth and bones. Retinol is a constituent of retinal visual purple, which is needed for vision in dim light. Deprivation of vitamin A can lead to drying and thickening of the surfaces of the conjunctivae and corneas (xerophthalmia), which is the leading cause of blindness in children in underdeveloped countries.

TREATMENT

The treatment of vitamin A deficiency involves supplying commercial vitamin A, orally or parenterally. The dosage varies with age and severity of the symptoms. Oral preparations are usually more effective as long as absorption is adequate. Vitamin E is sometimes given in conjunction with vitamin A to promote effective storage and to prevent hypervitaminosis A.

DIET THERAPY

A well-balanced diet with adequate amounts of vitamin A is used as an adjunct to vitamin supplementation and as protection against recurrence of the deficiency. Sufficient intake of proteins is essential because protein binds to vitamin A and transports it to the cells.

Good sources of vitamin A include whole milk, whole milk products, eggs, leafy green vegetables, and yellow fruits and vegetables. When skim milk, skim milk products, and margarine are used, they should be fortified with vitamin A.

Vitamin A is stable at the usual cooking temperatures; however, a covered pan is recommended for cooking vegetables. Cooking at a high temperature for a short period is preferable to cooking at a low temperature for a long period to prevent vitamin A loss in preparation of vegetables. Processing and advance preparation cause minimal loss because vitamin A is insoluble in water. Mashing, cutting, or pureeing may increase the availability of carotenes by rupturing cell walls within the foods.

NURSING IMPLICATIONS

- Very-low-fat diets lead to decreased absorption of vitamin A.
- Vitamin A supplementation should be provided for patients with chronic liver diseases, especially alcoholics.
- Skim milk and skim milk products lose all their vitamin A content when the fat is removed; fortification restores the vitamin A.
- Protein deficiency worsens vitamin A deficiency because vitamin A must be bound to proteins for transport throughout the body.
- Be alert for vitamin A deficiency in patients with conditions that reduce fat absorption, such as celiac disease, cystic fibrosis, obstructive jaundice, and infectious hepatitis.
- Vitamin A absorption depends on the presence of bile acids in the intestinal tract.
- Vitamin A is highly toxic in excessive doses (1,000 to 3,000 International Units per kilogram of body weight per day for children and adults), which may occur in overtreatment of deficiencies, food fads, and megavitamin therapy over long periods.
- Excessive intake of carotenes is not harmful but may cause a yellowish discoloration of the skin.

Beriberi

PATHOPHYSIOLOGY

A deficiency of vitamin B_1, thiamine, causes beriberi. Beriberi affects the nervous system and the heart. Thiamine is needed for key reactions in carbohydrate metabolism; intake requirements are based on caloric intake. Older people appear to use thiamine less efficiently, so that requirements remain high despite decreased energy intake.

Dietary inadequacy of thiamine causes polyneuritis, mental confusion, muscular weakness, ataxia, tachycardia, and eventually cardiac enlargement. Severe thiamine deficiency in infants may appear suddenly as cardiac failure. Beriberi is now rare in developed countries because of the enrichment of white flour and rice.

TREATMENT

Thiamine deficiency is treated by thiamine supplementation. Treatment usually consists of administration of vitamin B complex preparations because deficiencies of the vitamin B group tend to occur together.

DIET THERAPY

A high-protein, high-Calorie diet that is rich in sources of thiamine is recommended as an adjunct to vitamin supplementation. Good sources of thiamine include pork, beef, organ meats, whole grains, and vegetables. Thiamine is widely distributed in foods but not in high concentrations, so intake from many sources is necessary.

Thiamine is soluble in water; soaking vegetables or cooking them in large amounts of water results in losses. Thiamine is best preserved when food sources of the vitamin are cooked in an acid medium; both neutral and alkaline media destroy thiamine. Rice should not be washed before cooking or drained after cooking. Rice should be cooked in a small amount of water so that all the water is absorbed in the cooking process.

NURSING IMPLICATIONS

- Anorexia and nausea may prevent oral intake in the beginning of treatment. Thiamine and vitamin B complex are available for intravenous administration.
- Thiamine should be given to all alcoholics and other hospitalized patients who are unable to eat or who have conditions that increase their metabolic rates.

- Patients who are maintained on long-term intravenous therapy should have vitamin B complex added to one intravenous solution daily.
- Patients with chronic febrile conditions may suffer from thiamine deficiency as a result of increased metabolism.
- Converted rice contains more thiamine than do other types of rice.

Riboflavin Deficiency

PATHOPHYSIOLOGY

Riboflavin, vitamin B_2, is essential for growth and is thought to have numerous functions in the production of corticosteroids, red blood cells, and glucose from noncarbohydrate substrates and in the regulation of thyroid enzymes. Deficiency of riboflavin, ariboflavinosis, causes cheilosis (cracks at the corners of the mouth), scaly desquamation around the mouth, glossitis, eye irritation, photophobia, and corneal irritation.

TREATMENT

The treatment of ariboflavinosis is riboflavin supplementation, orally or intramuscularly. Intravenous administration of riboflavin causes a decreased pulse rate and is rarely used. Vitamin B complex is frequently prescribed because vitamin B deficiencies usually occur concomitantly.

DIET THERAPY

A well-balanced diet that includes good sources of riboflavin is recommended. Foods rich in riboflavin include milk, milk products, liver, eggs, meats, and leafy green vegetables.

NURSING IMPLICATIONS

- Urinary excretion of riboflavin is related to the body's nitrogen balance. Increased excretion of riboflavin occurs after burns and surgical procedures that involve extensive protein loss. Decreased excretion of riboflavin occurs during growth periods, lactation, and convalescence.
- Riboflavin is only partially water soluble. Losses in the preparation of vegetables can be minimized if they are steamed. Baking soda should not be used in cooking to preserve color because it increases loss of riboflavin.

- Suspect riboflavin deficiency in patients who exist on marginal diets, devoid of animal protein and leafy vegetables.
- Strict vegetarian diets that prohibit meats, eggs, and milk are likely to be low in riboflavin.
- The use of opaque milk containers has reduced riboflavin loss from milk due to exposure to sunlight. Reconstituted dry milk should also be stored in opaque containers.
- Any condition that causes an increased metabolic rate, stress, or malabsorption increases the need for riboflavin.
- Achlorhydria, lack of gastric secretion of hydrochloric acid, may precipitate riboflavin deficiency. Riboflavin is destroyed by alkaline substances. Achlorhydria occurs in pernicious anemia and stomach cancer. Older people tend to have decreased concentrations of hydrochloric acid in their gastric secretions.

Pellagra

PATHOPHYSIOLOGY

Pellagra results from a deficiency of niacin or its percursor tryptophan. Niacin is needed by all body cells because it participates in many metabolic functions, including glycolysis, fat synthesis, and tissue repair. Pellagra is characterized by weakness, lassitude, anorexia, and indigestion; these symptoms progress to dermatitis, diarrhea, and dementia in severe cases.

TREATMENT

Pellagra is treated by nicotinamide, an amide of niacin that does not produce flushing. Vitamin B complex is also used because deficiencies of B vitamins rarely occur in isolation.

DIET THERAPY

A well-balanced diet that includes good sources of niacin and tryptophan is prescribed. Tryptophan is an essential amino acid that is found in abundance in high-biologic-value proteins. Good sources of niacin or tryptophan (or both) include liver, whole grains, yeast, lean meats, and poultry. Milk is a poor source of niacin but a moderately good source of tryptophan.

Patients with pellagra are usually started on a liquid diet because of glossitis, anorexia, and gastrointestinal disturbances. As these symptoms respond to therapy, patients are advanced to a soft and, eventually, to a high-protein, regular diet.

NURSING IMPLICATIONS

- Niacin is stable in foods; it can withstand reasonable periods of cooking, heat, and storage.
- Because niacin is water soluble, liquids in which niacin-rich foods are cooked should be used to make soups, sauces, or stews when possible.
- Pellagra is rare in developed countries because of enrichment of bread.
- In countries where modern medicine is practiced, pellagra is a disease seen only in alcoholics, elderly recluses, and others with bizarre eating habits.

Vitamin C Deficiency

PATHOPHYSIOLOGY

Lack of vitamin C, ascorbic acid, results in scurvy; this vitamin deficiency is characterized by red, swollen, bleeding gums; poor wound healing; capillary fragility; and subcutaneous hemorrhages. Vitamin C has numerous enzyme functions and appears to be necessary for the functioning of all body cells.

TREATMENT

The treatment of vitamin C deficiency consists of oral or parenteral doses of ascorbic acid. Massive oral doses can cause gastrointestinal distress.

DIET THERAPY

A well-balanced diet with generous amounts of foods rich in vitamin C is used to prevent or treat scurvy. Good sources of ascorbic acid include fresh, canned, or frozen citrus fruits; tomatoes; white and sweet potatoes; leafy vegetables; strawberries; cantaloupes; broccoli; and green peppers.

NURSING IMPLICATIONS

- Vitamin C deficiency is rare in developed countries but occurs in cases of self-neglect due to psychiatric problems, advanced age, alcohol, or ignorance.

- Vitamin C deficiency may occur in artificially fed infants who do not receive vitamin supplements.
- Vitamin C is destroyed by heat, exposure to air, and storage.
- To preserve the vitamin C content of foods, avoid prolonged cooking at high temperatures. When preparing frozen vegetables, boil the water first, then add the vegetables and cook quickly. Cut fresh vegetables just before use, and cook by steaming.
- Vitmin C is destroyed by alkaline media, dehydration, and lengthy exposure to copper and iron utensils.
- Prepare only the amount of vegetables needed for one meal; leftover vegetables lose their vitamin C.
- Vitamin C may be added when foods are processed.
- Breakfast drinks, even if high in vitamin C, often contain a large amount of sugar. They are usually more expensive than are canned or frozen orange juice.

Vitamin D Deficiency

PATHOPHYSIOLOGY

A deficiency of vitamin D decreases the absorption of calcium and phosphorus. A decreased serum level of calcium stimulates the parathyroid glands to release parathyroid hormone. This hormone increases resorption of bone and excretion of phosphates, leading to increased serum levels of calcium. A decrease in serum levels of calcium inhibits calcification, resulting in soft bones. Affected children suffer from rickets and delayed dentition; adults show osteomalacia.

TREATMENT

The treatment of vitamin D deficiency is oral administration of one of the active metabolites of vitamin D_3 or a synthetic analogue. Adequate amounts of calcium are also provided.

DIET THERAPY

Vitamin D deficiency rarely develops from nutritional inadequacies; fortification of milk and margarine has been helpful in this respect. Lack of exposure to sunlight or interference with the absorption of dietary vitamin D is more apt to be responsible for the deficiency.

NURSING IMPLICATIONS

- Rickets may occur in breast-fed infants who do not receive vitamin supplemention.
- Milk given to children should be checked to ensure that it is fortified.
- Deficiencies can occur in patients who have inborn errors of vitamin D metabolism or intestinal malabsorption of fats. Exposure to substances that are toxic to the gastrointestinal tract or kidneys may also lead to vitamin D deficiency.
- Patients with chronic renal failure or renal tubular defects may have vitamin D deficiency.
- Corticosteroids and phenytoin (Dilantin) interfere with absorption of vitamin D. Patients on long-term therapy with these drugs should be assessed for the possibility of deficiency.
- Patients who adhere to the ethnic practice of shielding children and women from sunlight should alert the nurse to the possibility of deficiency.
- The melanin in dark-skinned people may prevent as much as 95% of the vitamin D from reaching the deeper skin layers to be metabolized into its active form. Dietary sources of vitamin D are of special importance to such people, particularly in the northern parts of the country.

Marasmus

PATHOPHYSIOLOGY

Marasmus is a condition in which losses of body fat and weight occur over a long period. Marasmus is due to inadequate caloric intake. Severe fat and muscle wasting occurs, but body function is maintained. Patients with chronic conditions that interfere with food intake or absorption may suffer from marasmus.

TREATMENT

The aim of treatment is to provide the required caloric intake by whatever means best suits the clinical situation. The use of parenteral nutrition and hyperalimentation should lead to a decrease in the incidence of marasmus among hospitalized patients.

DIET THERAPY

Oral intake of nutrients is the best method of supplying the body's caloric needs. When food cannot be taken by mouth, tube feedings can be used.

When the enteral route is not feasible, parenteral nutrition can be given.

Dietary management of marasmus is influenced by the presence of dehydration, electrolyte imbalances, vitamin deficiencies, and concurrent conditions or infections. Fluid and electrolyte imbalances should be corrected immediately. Oral or parenteral glucose provides a quick energy source. Initial enteral feedings must be limited in both amount and caloric content because the digestive capacity is reduced. Diluted skim or breast milk is frequently used in the early phase of therapy. Solid foods are added gradually as tolerance develops. High-biologic-value proteins in adequate amounts, often up to 5 grams per kilogram of body weight, are indicated. Caloric intake sufficient to prevent ingested protein from being used as an energy source is essential. Vitamin and mineral supplements are required.

NURSING IMPLICATIONS

- Inadequate intake should not be permitted to persist more than 48 hours.
- Nurses should take the initiative in suggesting alternative feeding modes for anorectic patients.

Kwashiorkor

PATHOPHYSIOLOGY

Kwashiorkor is protein malnutrition that may occur with adequate caloric intake. This condition was originally described in Africa. The term kwashiorkor was applied to the situation in which a child is removed from breast-feeding to permit a newly born sibling to nurse. The deposed child then receives a high-carbohydrate, low-protein diet. Kwashiorkor is now recognized as occurring when children are given a starchy, low-protein diet during growth periods. It also can occur in hospitalized children and adults who are unable to eat and who are under increased stress because of injury or surgical intervention.

Kwashiorkor is characterized by sharp decreases in the serum level of albumin, lymphocyte count, and transferrin level. Easily pluckable hair, edema, and delayed wound healing are symptoms of kwashiorkor.

TREATMENT

The treatment is to provide high-quality protein in the diet. Tube feedings, intravenous amino acids, and hyperalimentation may be needed to ensure adequate intake of proteins. Fluid and electrolyte imbalances must be corrected. Both potassium and magnesium levels may be depressed.

Vitamin A also should be provided because lack of protein will restrict transport of vitamin A (vitamin A must be bound to proteins for transport).

DIET THERAPY

Oral feedings consist of milk or a protein-rich milk substitute; the diet then advances to one that is rich in high-biologic-value proteins. Skim milk may have to be used in the early phases of treatment because fat is poorly tolerated. Adequate amounts of vitamins and minerals should be supplied by the diet or by supplementation.

NURSING IMPLICATIONS

- Nurses should be alert to situations in which acute stress is coupled with inadequate intake of proteins. Patients suffering from major trauma, sepsis, or burns and those who have undergone major surgical procedures are potential candidates.
- Nurses should monitor both the quality and the quantity of food intake.
- Patients should not be maintained solely on clear fluids or 5% dextrose and water intravenous feedings for prolonged periods.

Hyponatremia

PATHOPHYSIOLOGY

Hyponatremia is a condition in which there is a decreased concentration of sodium in the blood. Patients on low-salt diets do not show an immediate reduction of the serum levels of sodium and chloride because the kidneys are able to conserve sodium until the output is almost zero. Within 4 to 5 days, however, the serum levels of sodium and chloride fall, causing hypovolemia. In response to the low serum level of sodium and hypovolemia, secretion of aldosterone is stimulated. Aldosterone, an adrenocortical hormone, induces retention of sodium and water and excretion of potassium. Hyponatremia and hypovolemia inhibit the release of antidiuretic hormone. The body attempts to compensate for the potassium loss by shifting potassium out of the cells. Urinary output decreases, leading to oliguria and anuria.

Reduced tonicity of the extracellular fluid allows fluid to move into the cells by osmosis. Swelling of the brain cells causes muscle twitching and convulsions.

TREATMENT

The treatment of hyponatremia is replacement of sodium as quickly as possible without producing an extracellular fluid volume excess. When blood volume is normal or increased, 3 to 5% sodium chloride is usually given intravenously. When the blood volume is low, 0.9% saline is given intravenously.

DIET THERAPY

Hyponatremia may occur as a result of decreased intake of sodium, decreased absorption of sodium, increased excretion of sodium (diaphoresis, diarrhea), or increased urinary loss of sodium. Decreased intake may be the result of overzealous adherence to a low-sodium diet. In such cases, the diet prescription and the patient's interpretation of it should be carefully reviewed. Additional sodium is easily provided for patients who are able to take oral food or fluids by the addition of salt and salty foods to the diet.

NURSING IMPLICATIONS

- Patients receiving vigorous diuretic therapy, especially with thiazide diuretics or furosemide (Lasix), may lose sodium out of proportion to water loss and experience hyponatremia.
- Hyponatremia should be suspected in any situation in which the normal sodium and water balance is altered, such as increased output and decreased intake of sodium or decreased output and increased intake of water.
- Many instances of hyponatremia are related to replacement of water and sodium losses by water alone.
- When nasogastric suction tubes are irrigated, air or isotonic saline should be used.
- Patients undergoing nasogastric suction who are permitted sips of water or ice chips should be carefully monitored for the amount of intake.
- Excessive use of 5% destrose in water or other electrolyte-free intravenous solutions leads to hyponatremia.
- Repeated tap water enemas may lead to hyponatremia.
- Forcing fluids into patients with increased secretion of antidiuretic hormone can lead to hyponatremia. Secretion of this hormone is increased during the early postoperative period, posttrauma periods, and after frequent injections of morphine sulfate.

- Reduced secretion of aldosterone leads to increased excretion of sodium.
- Chronic wasting diseases may be associated with reduced serum levels of sodium.
- Schizophrenic patients may drink excessive amounts of water during periods of hallucination.

Hypokalemia

PATHOPHYSIOLOGY

Hypokalemia is a decrease in the serum level of potassium. Reduced intake or increased loss of potassium quickly leads to a drop in the serum level of potassium because the kidneys continue to excrete potassium at the usual rate for some time. Compensatory measures fail to return the serum level to normal. The body attempts to compensate by shifting potassium out of the cells in exchange for sodium or hydrogen. As a result of the intracellular hydrogen shift and urinary loss of hydrogen, metabolic alkalosis develops. In chronic potassium depletion, the kidneys lose their ability to respond to antidiuretic hormone because they have lost the ability to concentrate urine.

TREATMENT

The treatment of hypokalemia is replacement of potassium losses. Oral potassium liquids or tablets may be used. In emergency situations or when oral administration is prohibited, intravenous replacement is used. Intravenous potassium can be given only when urinary output is adequate. Complete replacement of serious potassium losses may take up to 1 week. Oral replacement is safer than intravenous replacement because hyperkalemia is less likely to develop.

DIET THERAPY

Nonlethal potassium deficits can be corrected by ingestion of potassium-rich foods. Potassium is widely distributed in all foods, except pure fats and oils. Good sources of potassium include meats, bananas, orange juice, potatoes, tomatoes, coffee, tea, cola beverages, and chocolate. Salt substitutes that contain potassium (Co-Salt, Neocurtasal) may be prescribed as part of the diet plan.

NURSING IMPLICATIONS

- Be alert for hypokalemia in patients who are taking diuretics, particularly the thiazide type, because they retard reabsorption of potassium.

- Potassium is lost in vomitus, diarrhea, and fistula drainage fluid from the small intestine and colon.
- Gastric and intestinal suction lead to potassium losses.
- Hypokalemia accompanies diabetic acidosis.
- Watch for potassium loss in patients receiving digitalis. Be particularly alert for hypokalemia in patients who are taking digitalis along with thiazide diuretics. Potassium antagonizes the action of digitalis.
- Potassium loss occurs in severe trauma. Crushing injuries release intracellular potassium.
- Patients undergoing corticosteroid drug therapy have increased potassium losses.
- Alcoholics and others with poor food intake may suffer from hypokalemia.
- Because potassium is an intracellular electrolyte, it is not easily destroyed by food preparation or processing.

Hypocalcemia

PATHOPHYSIOLOGY

Hypocalcemia results from insufficient intake, malabsorption, or excessive losses of calcium or vitamin D. Calcium influences neuromuscular irritability and participates in the formation of teeth and bones and the clotting of blood. Acute hypocalcemia causes tetany and can lead to death from laryngospasm.

Calcium is absorbed in the duodenum. Conditions that increase intestinal motility can reduce absorption of calcium.

TREATMENT

The treatment of calcium deficiency involves administration of calcium orally or intravenously. In emergency situations, 10% calcium gluconate is administered intravenously for tetany and convulsions. Vitamin D supplementation may be used as adjunctive therapy to promote absorption of calcium.

DIET THERAPY

The best dietary source of calcium is milk. Providing adequate amounts of calcium in the diet without ingesting milk or milk products is extremely difficult. A high-protein diet is recommended to increase absorption of calcium from good dietary sources.

An increased need for calcium occurs in vitamin D deficiency, pancreatic insufficiency, intestinal malabsorption, and chronic renal failure. Pregnancy and lactation increase the dietary need for calcium as well.

NURSING IMPLICATIONS

- Leafy green vegetables are good sources of calcium.
- The ethnic practice of cooking soup bones in vinegar releases calcium from the bones into the stock.
- Advise older patients to include milk in their diets. If milk is not acceptable as a beverage, advise patients to use milk in cooking or to include milk products, such as yogurt and cheese, in the diet.
- Nonfat dry milk can be used as an economical, low-Caloric source of calcium.
- Hypocalcemia is more likely to occur in patients with low serum levels of albumin. Calcium is bound to protein in the blood for transport to cells.
- Antacid and laxative abuse reduce absorption of calcium by altering the pH of the gastrointestinal tract. Calcium is most soluble in an acid medium. Laxatives also increase intestinal motility and reduce absorption.
- Watch for hypocalcemia in patients receiving citrated blood transfusions. Citrate and calcium bind together to form a complex, thus reducing the serum level of available calcium.

Hypomagnesemia

PATHOPHYSIOLOGY

Magnesium is needed for cellular metabolism, enzyme activation, and protein metabolism. Deficiencies of magnesium adversely affect the neuromuscular system and the heart. Hypomagnesemia is usually the result of poor absorption or increased excretion of magnesium.

TREATMENT

Hypomagnesemia is usually treated with intramuscular or intravenous magnesium sulfate.

DIET THERAPY

Hypomagnesemia is rarely due to poor dietary intake. Foods rich in magnesium may be added to the diet to assist in raising the serum level or in preventing recurrences of the deficiency. Magnesium-rich foods include meats, green vegetables, whole grains, nuts, seafood, soybeans, and legumes. Magnesium is a component of chlorophyll, which gives green vegetables their color.

NURSING IMPLICATIONS

- Avoid maintaining patients on magnesium-free intravenous solutions for prolonged periods.
- Be alert for hypomagnesemia in alcoholics, severely malnourished patients, and patients with severe, chronic diarrhea.
- Hypomagnesemia may occur in patients with intestinal malabsorption, hypoparathyroidism, or during the diuretic phase of renal failure.

References

Brunner, L., & Suddarth, D. *Textbook of medical-surgical nursing* (4th ed.). Philadelphia: J. B. Lippincott Company, 1980.

Goodhart, R., & Shils, M. (Eds.). *Modern nutrition in health and disease* (6th ed.). Philadelphia: Lea & Febiger, 1980.

Howard, R., & Herbold, N. *Nutrition in clinical care.* New York: McGraw-Hill Book Company, 1978.

Krause, M., & Mahan, L. *Food, nutrition and diet therapy* (6th ed.). Philadelphia: W. B. Saunders Company, 1979.

Luckmann, J., & Sorensen, K. *Medical-surgical nursing: A psychophysiologic approach* (2nd ed.). Philadelphia: W. B. Saunders Company, 1980.

Metheny, N., & Snively, W. *Nurses' handbook of fluid balance* (3rd ed.). Philadelphia: J. B. Lippincott Company, 1979.

Robinson, C., & Lawler, M. *Normal and therapeutic nutrition* (15th ed.). New York: Macmillan Publishing Company, 1977.

Whaley, L., & Wong, D. *Nursing care of infants and children.* St. Louis: C. V. Mosby Company, 1979.

Williams, S. *Nutrition and diet therapy* (3rd ed.). St. Louis: C. V. Mosby Company, 1977.

18
Diet Therapy in Inborn Errors of Metabolism

Phenylketonuria

PATHOPHYSIOLOGY

Phenylketonuria is a congenital defect in phenylalanine metabolism. Phenylalanine is an essential amino acid found in all natural foods. Patients with phenylketonuria lack the hepatic enzyme phenylalanine hydroxylase, which is needed for the conversion of tyrosine from phenylalanine. In the absence of this enzyme, phenylalanine must be metabolized by pathways other than those leading to tyrosine. This alternative metabolism results in rising serum levels of phenylalanine and phenylpyruvic acid and accumulation phenylketone bodies in the urine. Abnormal amounts of unmetabolized phenylalanine interfere with normal brain development and may cause severe mental retardation. Lack of tyrosine results in reduced production of the pigment melanin and the hormones epinephrine and thyroxine.

TREATMENT

Phenylketonuria is treated by dietary restriction of phenylalanine to maintain serum levels between 2 and 10 milligrams per 100 milliliters. Early recognition and treatment are essential to prevent mental retardation.

DIET THERAPY

The dietary treatment plan is designed to control intake of phenylalanine, to provide limited amounts of tyrosine and protein, and to ensure

250

adequate intake of Calories, minerals, and vitamins for normal growth and development. The mainstay of the diet for patients with phenylketonuria is Lofenalac, a synthetic powder with low phenylalanine content. Lofenalac provides 85 to 90% of the protein in the diet. The rest of the protein comes from 1% protein fruits and vegetables, tapioca, cornstarch, and butter.

Lofenalac is prepared as a formula for infants; a small amount of milk is added to the powder to provide the needed amount of the essential amino acid phenylalanine. Exchange lists have been developed to assist in providing variety. Foods in the exchange lists contain the equivalent of 15 milligrams of phenylalanine. As the child grows, Lofenalac can be used to make puddings and cookies. Another synthetic product, Phenyl-Free, a powder that can be reconstituted as a beverage, contains no phenylalanine but provides amino acids, carbohydrates, fats, vitamins, and minerals. Phenyl-Free allows more latitude in the diet of older children, but this powder should never be used as the sole diet.

The diet is extremely restrictive. Breads, meats, fish, poultry, cheeses, milk, legumes, nuts, and eggs must be eliminated. Special low-protein flour can be used to make bread and other bakery products. The question of how long the diet should be followed has not been answered. Some authorities suggest that the diet can be relaxed after 6 years of age, when brain development is nearly complete. This timing coincides with school attendance, when parental control of the diet is necessarily reduced. Other authorities cite studies relating reduced intelligence quotients to relaxed dietary control. If dietary controls are lifted, they must be reimposed for affected women before and during pregnancy. Phenylalanine crosses the placental barrier, and increased fetal serum levels of phenylalanine can result in congenital mental retardation.

NURSING IMPLICATIONS

- Routine height and weight assessments are useful in monitoring the adequacy of the diet.
- Lofenalac provides 454 Calories, 15 grams of protein, 60 grams of carbohydrate, and 18 grams of fat per 100 grams of powder. Lofenalac is best prepared by mixing with diluent in a blender.
- Hemoglobin levels should be carefully monitored because of the severe restriction of protein intake.
- Intake of manganese, zinc, and niacin may be low when the primary protein source is synthetic.
- Tyrosine is an essential amino acid for patients with phenylketonuria because their bodies cannot produce it.
- Growth increases the need for phenylalanine.

- Febrile illnesses increase the need for phenylalanine and require increased intake.
- Inadequate intake of phenylalanine leads to the catabolism of body protein and a temporary increase in the serum level of phenylalanine.
- Signs of inadequate intake of phenylalanine include anorexia, vomiting, and listlessness.
- Natural protein contains 2 to 5% phenylalanine. High-biologic-value proteins are high in phenylalanine.
- Many sweets, jams, jellies, and some candies contain no phenylalanine and can be used to increase caloric intake and to flavor the synthetic foods.
- During illness, increased intake of fluids, carbohydrates, and fruit juices is indicated.
- The diet should include different textures and types of food to encourage self-feeding. Foods that require chewing are important for jaw development and speech.
- Lofenalac and Phenyl-Free are expensive in the amounts needed for children with phenylketonuria. Families may need direction to sources of financial assistance.

Maple Syrup Urine Disease (Branched-Chain Ketoaciduria)

PATHOPHYSIOLOGY

Maple syrup urine disease results from an inborn error of metabolism in which the enzyme oxidative decarboxylase, normally found in white blood cells, is defective or absent. Without this enzyme, the body is unable to remove the carboxyl group in the second step of the breakdown of the amino acids valine, leucine, and isoleucine. (Valine, leucine, and isoleucine are also referred to as branched-chain amino acids.) Consequently, these amino acids and their ketoacid derivatives accumulate in the blood and urine, leading to neurologic damage, respiratory difficulty, and mental retardation. The incomplete metabolism of these amino acids causes the sweat, earwax, and urine of patients to give off an odor resembling maple syrup.

TREATMENT

The treatment of maple syrup urine disease is dietary restriction of valine, leucine, and isoleucine to control the serum levels of these amino acids. Some types of maple syrup urine disease respond to high doses of thiamine pyrophosphate, which increases the activity of oxidative decarboxylase.

DIET THERAPY

The diet used in maple syrup urine disease provides specifically controlled amounts of valine, leucine, and isoleucine. The basic diet is supplemented with fruits, vegetables, and cereals and is low in protein. Two synthetic products are available to meet the body's protein needs without providing any restricted amino acids: MSUD-Aid, which provides Calories, protein (exclusive of branched-chain amino acids), vitamin B complex, and minerals; and MSUD Diet Powder, which provides all the nutrients of MSUD-Aid plus fats. The leucine allowed by the diet can be provided by adding controlled amounts of milk or milk solids. The amounts of valine and isoleucine provided by the milk allowance are inadequate for growth. Pure solutions of isoleucine and valine are available.

NURSING IMPLICATIONS

- Maintaining the serum levels of the branched-chain amino acids within safe levels is not easy. Small fluctuations in intake produce wide fluctuations in serum concentrations. Rigid dietary control is essential.
- A 50-milliliter syringe is used to measure milk allowance, formula, and pure solutions of the branched-chain amino acids to ensure accuracy.
- Gelatin contains small amounts of the branched-chain amino acids and can be used as a base. Amino acids are added to this base to maintain nitrogen balance.
- Infection leads to tissue catabolism, which increases the serum levels of the branched-chain amino acids. When infections occur, intake of sweetened, low-protein fruit juices should be encouraged to reduce tissue catabolism.
- Low-protein fruits and vegetables, sucrose, glucose, and products made from gluten-free flour add variety to the diet. Low-protein fruits include apples, apricots, bananas, oranges, peaches, pears, pineapples, and strawberries. Low-protein vegetables include asparagus, green and yellow beans, beets, cabbage, carrots, lettuce, tomatoes, potatoes, spinach, and squash.
- Formulas that contain pure solutions of amino acids and saccharides should be sterilized by the aseptic method. Terminal sterilization alters the formula.

Galactosemia

PATHOPHYSIOLOGY

Galactosemia is a condition that results from the deficiency of the hepatic enzyme galactose-1-phosphate uridyl transferase. This enzyme is one of the three enzymes required for the conversion of galactose to glucose. Absence of the enzyme results in increased serum and urinary levels of galactose. Galactosemia causes physical and mental retardation, cataracts, portal hypertension, and cirrhosis.

TREATMENT

The treatment of galactosemia is dietary modification. Cataracts can be treated surgically.

DIET THERAPY

Galactose does not occur in free form in foods; it is the result of intestinal hydrolysis of lactose. The diet for galactosemia is a lactose-free diet. Milk, milk products, and lactose-containing products are eliminated from the diet. Casein hydrolysate, soy milk, or meat-based formulas can be used. It is important to check labels for lactose. Any product that contains dry milk solids, casein, whey, whey solids, or curds also contains lactose and should not be used. Products that contain lactate, lactic acid, and lacto-albumin are safe to use. A lactose-free diet requires calcium and ribo-flavin supplementation.

The diagnosis of galactosemia can be established prenatally, and affected pregnant women should be placed on lactose-free diets for the duration of their pregnancies. Breast-feeding is contraindicated for infants with galactosemia.

NURSING IMPLICATIONS

- Patients must remain on milk-free diets for life; breads may be permitted after affected children reach school age.
- All unprocessed fish and animal products (except brains and muscles) contain no lactose. Liver, brain, and pancreas store galactose and are avoided.
- Fresh fruits and vegetables (except peas) are allowed.
- Creamed cheeses contain lactose; cheddar cheeses are permitted.
- Cracked wheat and Vienna breads usually do not contain milk; however, all labels should be examined carefully.
- Some artificial sweeteners and foods made with them contain lactose.

- Many medication tablets have a lactose base.
- See Chapter 6 for additional information related to lactose-free diets.

Glycogen Storage Disease Type I (Gierke's Disease)

PATHOPHYSIOLOGY

In Gierke's disease, the enzyme glucose-6-phosphatase, which is required for reconversion of glycogen to glucose, is absent. Dietary glucose is normally removed from the circulation by the liver and stored as glycogen. Patients with Gierke's disease are unable to reconvert the stored glycogen to glucose and thus show hypoglycemia and increased gluconeogenesis from proteins and fats. Hypoglycemia suppresses secretion of insulin and leads to growth failure. Lipid metabolism is increased, leading to fat deposits and xanthomas (lipid deposits in the skin). Such patients also produce large amounts of lactic acid, which causes lactic acidosis.

TREATMENT

The treatment of Gierke's disease is primarily dietary intervention. Oral sodium bicarbonate is used to treat the lactic acidosis. Portacaval shunts to divert glucose-rich blood from the liver to the periphery have been employed successfully.

DIET THERAPY

The aims of diet therapy are to maintain glucose homeostasis, to prevent hypoglycemic reactions, and to provide sufficient protein and Calories for a positive nitrogen balance and growth. Milk is eliminated from the diet because of its lactose content. Sucrose and sugar-containing foods are avoided. Formulas that contain glucose are permitted. Pregestimil is a formula that contains glucose. CHO-Free formula with added glucose may also be used.

The diet consists of small glucose feedings as the carbohydrate source, normal amounts of proteins, and reduced intake of fats. Medium-chain triglycerides may be substituted for fats to reduce xanthoma formation. Frequent feedings and protein meals are used to prevent hypoglycemia.

NURSING IMPLICATIONS

- Glycogen storage disease abates with age. The patient may not have symptoms after adolescence.

- Twenty-five percent glucose may be given by nasogastric tube to prevent nocturnal hypoglycemia.
- Excessive caloric intake is avoided to reduce the accumulation of fat and glycogen in the liver.

Wilson's Disease (Hepatolenticular Degeneration)

PATHOPHYSIOLOGY

Wilson's disease is a derangement of copper metabolism. There is a deficiency of the plasma protein ceruloplasmin, which normally binds most of the copper in the blood. In the absence of ceruloplasmin, copper is loosely bound to albumin in the serum. Copper deposits accumulate as the patient ages, producing degenerative changes in the liver and brain. Kidney stones may also develop.

TREATMENT

The treatment of Wilson's disease is a combination of a low-copper diet and D-penicillamine drug therapy. D-Penicillamine is a chelating agent that binds copper to itself for urinary excretion.

DIET THERAPY

The diet for Wilson's disease eliminates foods high in copper content. The following foods would be restricted:

Liver
Kidney
Oysters
Mushrooms
Chocolate
Poultry
Whole-grain cereals
Brain
Nuts
Dried fruits
Dried legumes
Shellfish

NURSING IMPLICATIONS

- The diet is unappetizing and stringent. Durg therapy is more effective.
- Breast milk contains more copper than does cow's milk.
- The patient's water supply should be checked for copper content. Distilled water can be used in areas where the water supply is high in copper.
- Copper utensils should not be used in food preparation.
- Watch caloric intake to prevent obesity.
- D-Penicillamine should be taken orally before meals.

References

Cowie, V. Diet in pregnancy reduces danger. *Nursing Mirror,* September 6, 1979, *149,* 10.

Goodhart, R., & Shils, M. (Eds.). *Modern nutrition in health and disease* (6th ed.). Philadelphia: Lea & Febiger, 1980.

Gracey, B. Quick diagnosis preserves a life. *Nursing Mirror,* November 23, 1978, *147,* 21.

Howard, R., & Herbold, N. *Nutrition in clinical care.* New York: McGraw-Hill Book Company, 1978.

Hunt, S., Groff, J., & Holbrook, J. *Nutrition: Principles and clinical practice.* New York: John Wiley & Sons, 1980.

Kelly, J. Wilson's disease. *Nursing Mirror,* February 22, 1979, *148,* 8.

Krause, M., & Mahan, L. *Food, nutrition and diet therapy* (6th ed.). Philadelphia: W. B. Saunders Company, 1979.

Marlow, D. *Textbook of pediatric nursing* (5th ed.). Philadelphia: W. B. Saunders Company, 1977.

Reyzer, N. Diagnosis: PKU. *American Journal of Nursing,* November 1978, *78,* 11.

Robinson, C., & Lawler, M. *Normal and therapeutic nutrition* (15th ed.). New York: Macmillan Publishing Company, 1977.

Scipien, G., Barnard, M., Chard, M., et al. *Comprehensive pediatric nursing* (2nd ed.). New York: McGraw-Hill Book Company, 1979.

Suitor, C., & Hunter, M. *Nutrition: Principles and application in health promotion.* Philadelphia: J. B. Lippincott Company, 1980.

Thiele, V. *Clinical nutrition.* St. Louis: C. V. Mosby Company, 1976.

Whaley, L., & Wong, D. *Nursing care of infants and children.* St. Louis: C. V. Mosby Company, 1979.

Williams, S. *Nutrition and diet therapy* (3rd ed.). St. Louis: C. V. Mosby Company, 1977.

19
Diet Therapy in Cancer

Cancer and Food Intake

Cancer is a complex variety of disorders with diverse etiologies. Therapies that destroy cancer cells also destroy normal body cells, especially cells undergoing rapid growth. Improved nutrition has been related to an increased neoplastic growth rate in laboratory animals; however, the more rapid growth increases the susceptibility of the cancer cells to treatment modalities. Improved nutritional status may make patients suitable candidates for therapy previously denied them. Improved nutritional status enhances the patient's response to therapy and tends to reduce side effects of the treatment. Patients who receive optimal nutritional care have increased survival rates and adapt better to rehabilitation programs. For any patient with cancer, good nutrition can improve the quality of life.

Despite the diversity of diseases represented by the term cancer, several commonalities exist. Most cancers are treated by surgical procedures, radiation therapy, chemotherapy, immunotherapy, or by a combination of these therapies. Cachexia (extreme weight loss, weakness, and severe wasting of tissues) is associated with advanced cancer and is related to anorexia, taste changes, accelerated metabolism, treatment reactions, and depression. Malnutrition in the cancer patient does not have to be accepted; most patients can be adequately nourished if all available feeding methods are used appropriately.

In planning nutritional care for the cancer patient, all the factors involved must be assessed. The dietary assessment suggested in Chapter 3 serves as a basis; factors associated with the location of the cancer and treatment are added. Nutritional care should be planned and implemented early in the course of the disease. It should be altered as indicated by changes in treatment or response to treatment. Continuity of nutritional care is essential when patients change units, facilities, or are cared for at home.

Nurses should not complacently accept anorexia or cachexia in their patients with cancer. They should use the variety of information available to them to increase oral intake. When oral feedings are inadequate to maintain the nutritional status, the nurse should make sure that the physician is aware so that other options (tube feedings, intravenous nutrition, hyperalimentation) may be considered. Nurses must also remember the psychologic aspects related to food intake and their effect on the patient's emotional status. Food is associated with nurture and comfort. Eating is related to health, and offers of food express caring and concern.

DIET THERAPY

Taste abnormalities occur with extensive neoplastic disease and metastases. There is decreased ability to taste salt and even greater loss of taste acuity for sugar. The lower taste threshold for urea may cause a profound aversion to meats in some patients; such patients also say that meat smells rotten. The substitution of milk, eggs, and cheeses provides protein sources when meat is rejected.

Many cancer patients experience early satiety. They do not lose their appetites but become satisfied after a small amount of food is consumed. For such patients, frequent, small meals and snacks may be helpful. Many patients are able to eat better early in the day and find their appetites decreasing as the day progresses. Such patients may find that a large breakfast, followed by smaller and smaller meals as the day progresses is a better way of handling food intake.

Some patients deny loss of appetite but decrease their food intake. A diet diary is helpful in assessing actual food intake and in planning nutritional modifications. Diet therapy for the cancer patient consists of encouraging adequate intake of proteins, carbohydrates, fats, vitamins, and minerals in whatever manner is most effective for each patient.

NURSING IMPLICATIONS

- Fever, surgical intervention, and stress increase the production of corticosteroids and catecholamines, which, in turn, increases catabolism of body protein and gluconeogenesis. Depression may also trigger the release of catecholamines.
- Alcohol may be used as an appetite stimulant if the physician permits.
- Sugar may be added to foods when the taste threshold for sugar is increased to make them more palatable and increase caloric intake. Sugar should not replace essential nutrients.
- Cold foods are better accepted by cancer patients than are hot foods.

Common favorites include cold, clear fluids, carbonated beverages, ices, jello, watermelons, grapes, and peeled cucumbers. Cold protein plates of egg or meat salad may be preferable to warm meals. Ice cream and salted nuts combine cold with added salt and protein and make an appealing snack.

- Many foods can be made more appealing through the addition of salt, sugar, lemon juice, or spices.
- Deep breathing, ice chips, or sips of carbonated beverages may allay nausea.
- Patients who tire easily should not be served foods that require intensive chewing.
- In hospitals, treatment may interrupt meals. Evening may be the best time to catch up on food intake. A well-stocked unit kitchen may help increase intake.
- Pain medication may be given before meals, or intake of food may be encouraged when pain is at its lowest level.
- The importance of making trays and the environment attractive should not be forgotten.
- Social eating may improve intake. Visitors could be encouraged to bring and share gifts of food.
- When taste is affected, the appearance and aroma of food become even more important.
- Patients who are responsible for preparing their meals should take advantage of periods when they feel well to prepare extra food. Having food ready to eat may make eating less of a chore when patients do not really feel hungry.
- Elemental diets require an intact duodenum and jejunum for proper absorption.
- Total parenteral nutrition (TPN) provides sources of nitrogen and amino acids, Calories, electrolytes, minerals, and vitamins when oral intake is not possible. TPN is usually a long-term treatment; unless it is continued for 10 days, it is usually not worth the possible danger of the procedure and the risk for infection.
- It is important for cancer patients to eat adequately, and measures to tempt their appetites are more effective than are constant verbal reminders of the importance of eating. Many factors that affect food intake are beyond the patient's control and are best overcome by ingenuity and the available strategies to increase food intake.

Radiation Therapy and Food Intake

Radiation (the emission of waves or particles of radiant energy) is used externally, internally, and systemically as therapy for cancer. The aim of radiation therapy is to destroy the rapidly dividing neoplastic cells. Radiation also destroys the normal cells that divide rapidly (hair follicles, bone marrow, gastrointestinal mucous membrane). The nutritional status of the patient influences the dose of radiation therapy that can be tolerated. Radiation therapy may affect nutrition in the following ways:

- General loss of appetite
- Nausea and vomiting
- Malabsorption due to mucosal damage

Radiation sickness, which is no longer a common complication of therapy, is directly related to the dose of radiation and to the extent of the cancer. Radiation sickness may cause nausea, vomiting, and diarrhea. Inflammation of the mouth and throat may occur in upper-body irradiation. Radiation sickness is treated by providing adequate fluid intake and frequent, small feedings of high-protein, high-Calorie foods. Acid fluids and spices are avoided when the mouth and throat are inflamed. Highly seasoned foods and extremes of temperature can also irritate inflamed mouths and throats.

Radiation therapy may be given for periods ranging from 1 month to 1 year. The anorexia that accompanies the treatments usually subsides within several weeks after the last radiation dose. Direct and indirect exposure of the gastrointestinal tract destroy mucosal cells in the tract lining and affect digestion.

Irradiation of the oropharyngeal region can have a profound effect on food intake. Loss of taste may follow irradiation of a region of the body that includes the taste buds. Salivation is decreased, leading to dryness of the mouth and difficulty in swallowing. Some patients complain of a burning sensation in their mouths. Dental problems and loss of teeth may further complicate food intake. When food becomes tasteless, aroma and appearance become more important. Moist foods are helpful when chewing and swallowing are difficult. The use of sauces and gravies should be encouraged. Sipping fluids throughout the meal may provide additional moistness.

Irradiation of the lower portion of the neck may lead to esophagitis and dysphagia. Abdominal and pelvic irradiation may result in malabsorption, diarrhea, obstruction, or fistulas. Diarrhea may respond to a low-residue diet. Adequate fluids are important to prevent dehydration.

NURSING IMPLICATIONS

- Frequent mouth care is essential when oral inflammation occurs. Commercial mouthwash solutions are generally too astringent and are usually replaced by bland mixtures, such as normal saline and bicarbonate of soda.

- Loss of taste acuity usually results in the rejection of meats, fish, poultry, and eggs. Milk and cheeses become more important as protein sources.
- Cold foods, such as ice cream and ices, are often acceptable to a patient whose mouth is inflamed because of their numbing effect.
- Fruit nectars may replace citrus fruit juices when the mouth is inflamed. Check the adequacy of vitamin C intake when citrus fruits are eliminated from the diet.
- Lidocaine (Xylocaine) may be used as a mouth rinse to numb painful mouths and increase food intake.
- Placing liquid under the tongue may ease swallowing and may prevent aspiration when swallowing is difficult.
- It may be easier to swallow liquids sipped through a straw. Dipping the straw in the fluid and reversing it may help initiate sucking.
- Sugarless gums and mints may stimulate salivation. Some patients find that gum disintegrates in their mouths.
- Tilting the head back may ease swallowing.

Surgical Intervention and Food Intake

Four types of surgical procedures are used in the treatment of cancer patients: diagnostic, radical, prophylactic, and palliative. Much of the information in Chapter 9 is equally applicable to cancer patients preoperatively and postoperatively. However, some radical surgical procedures used in the treatment of cancer have profound effects on food intake.

Radical resections of the oropharyngeal area lead to chewing and swallowing difficulties; tube feedings may be required. Patients with laryngectomies can progress to oral feedings.

Esophagectomy and vagotomy result in gastric stasis, hypochlorhydria, steatorrhea, and diarrhea. Medium-chain triglycerides may be used as a source of fats to combat steatorrhea. A low-residue diet is used to relieve diarrhea.

Gastrectomy leads to the dumping syndrome, malabsorption, achlorhydria, lack of intrinsic factor, and hypoglycemia (see Chapter 6). Intestinal resection of the jejunum results in decreased absorption. Resection of the ileum leads to vitamin B_{12} deficiency, bile salt losses, and diarrhea. Vitamin B_{12} can be given intramuscularly or subcutaneously. Medium-chain triglycerides may relieve diarrhea even without replacement of bile salts. Massive bowel resection can lead to life-threatening malabsorption, metabolic acidosis, and malnutrition. Total parenteral nutrition may be lifesaving for such patients.

The judicious use of feeding techniques can aid the patient in maintaining nutrition despite radical surgical procedures. The oral route, when possible, is preferred. When chewing and swallowing are impaired but digestion and absorption remain intact, tube feedings can be used. If digestion is impaired but absorption is intact, elemental diets can be used. Intravenous nutrition through a peripheral vein can be used when the gastrointestinal tract is temporarily unable to handle nutrient intake. Total parenteral nutrition offers an alternative route for long-term gastrointestinal dysfunction.

NURSING IMPLICATIONS

- The psychologic aspects of feeding remain important despite the feeding method. Sometimes the pleasant aroma of foods, such as the aroma of coffee, can make a tube feeding more pleasant.
- Liquid diets may presents problems for the elderly, who do not usually tolerate large amounts of fluid well.
- Tube feedings should be individualized and modified to suit concurrent cardiovascular, renal, or endocrine problems.
- Nasogastric tube feedings should be given slowly, at room temperature, to prevent gastric distress.
- Family foods prepared in a blender are sometimes recommended for tube feedings. Daley (1979) has pointed out that the amount of fluid needed to reduce the solids to the proper consistency may result in excessive volume.

Effects of Chemotherapy and Food Intake

The goal of chemotherapy in cancer treatment is to destroy all malignant cells without destroying an excessive number of normal cells. Chemotherapy involves the use of drugs that destroy rapidly dividing neoplastic cells. Chemotherapy also destroys the rapidly dividing normal cells of the hair follicles, bone marrow, and gastrointestinal mucous membrane. Chemotherapy has systemic effects, in contrast to the local effects of radiation therapy and surgical procedures. Most of the widely used chemotherapeutic agents cause anorexia, nausea, vomiting, stomatitis, diarrhea, and sloughing of the colonic mucosa. Anorexia usually starts on the day of treatment and lasts for several days. When chemotherapeutic agents are administered once per month, the patient has 3 weeks without anorexia in which to build up nutrient intake. More frequent administration reduces this symptom-free period accordingly. When the medication is given every day, timing the administration so that the peak action occurs during sleep has proven helpful in increasing food intake.

Frequent, small meals during nausea-free periods are helpful in the management of nausea and vomiting. High-protein, high-Calorie foods and fluids should be selected. Cold foods may be more acceptable, particularly for patients who find that food odors trigger their nausea. Ice cream and ices may be accepted because of the numbing effect of the cold temperature. Carbonated beverages and ice chips are often effective in relieving nausea. Oral hygiene is important, particularly after a vomiting episode. A soft toothbrush and nonirritating solution is recommended. If the mouth is too sensitive to allow toothbrushing, mouth irrigations may be substituted.

Antiemetics are most effective when they are started the night before chemotherapy and continued at 6-hour intervals while the symptoms persist. The rationale for this regimen is that it weakens the vomiting center's response to the stimuli (Beaupre, 1980).

Stomatitis is managed by frequent oral hygiene routines using nonirritating solutions. Lidocaine (Xylocaine) mouth rinses before meals may relieve discomfort temporarily and improve food intake. A soft, bland diet is usually the most acceptable. Hard foods, hot spicy foods, and alcohol should be avoided.

Diarrhea is managed by the use of a low-residue diet and constipating foods, such as boiled skim milk and applesauce. Tea and broth are used to replace potassium losses. Adequate fluids are needed to replace fluid lost in the diarrheal stools.

The folic acid antagonist methotrexate interferes with the utilization of folic acid. Alternate courses of folic acid and methotrexate may be given to prevent severe folic acid deficiency. Folic acid antagonists also cause a spruelike condition in which absorption of carbohydrates, proteins, and fats is decreased.

The plant alkaloid vincristine may cause acute jaw pain and interfere with food intake. Vincristine therapy may also result in paralytic ileus. Fruit juices and fluids may be accepted by straw when jaw pain is present. Paralytic ileus necessitates introduction of drug therapy. Plant alkaloids tend to be constipating; increased intake of fluids and fiber may prevent this problem.

The antibiotic mithramycin, which is used in cancer therapy, may precipitate hypocalcemia; increased intake of milk might help prevent this imbalance. The corticosteroid hormones cause gastric irritation and fluid retention. Antacids or milk may be prescribed with the medication or the patient may be directed to take the drug with meals to reduce gastric irritation. Retention of fluid should not be confused with an increase in body tissue; edema often masks malnutrition.

NURSING IMPLICATIONS

- Taste alterations may occur with chemotherapy. Patients frequently complain of a metallic taste. Hard candy may relieve this symptom.

- Suggestions have an important role in the patient's response. All measures that are used to relieve symptoms should be presented positively. Patients should be asked what measures have been effective in the past in coping with similar symptoms. If these measures are not contraindicated, they should be tried.
- Tetrahydrocannabinol (the active principle of marihuana) relieves nausea, vomiting, and anorexia in patients undergoing chemotherapy. This substance is becoming more available for cancer patients in some states and is reported to be effective.

Immunotherapy and Food Intake

Immunotherapy is under investigation as a modality for managing cancer. The goal of immunotherapy is to strengthen the immune response of the patient to help the body destroy neoplastic cells. Immunotherapy may be active, passive, or adaptive. In active immunotherapy, antigens prepared from tumor cells or BCG (bacillus Calmette-Guérin) are injected into the patient. In passive immunotherapy, donor antibodies, lymphocytes, or lymphoid cells are used. Adaptive immunotherapy involves the transfer of donor cells and the subsequent development of active antibodies.

It is an established fact that malnutrition reduces the immune response. Good nutritional care should be adjunctive therapy for patients undergoing immunotherapy. Side effects of immunotherapy include nausea, vomiting, abdominal pain, and fatigue. All these symptoms reduce food intake and necessitate nursing intervention to promote nutrition.

References

Beaupre, C. Nursing care implications of cancer chemotherapy. In *Professional nurse continuing education*. New York: Le Jacq Publishing, 1980.

Butterworth, C. New concepts in nutrition and cancer: Implications for folic acid. *Contemporary Nutrition*, December 1980, 5, 12.

Copeland, E., Van Eys, J., & Shils, M. *Nutrition and cancer*. New York: American Cancer Society, 1978.

Cullen, P. Patients with colorectal cancer: How to assess and meet their needs. *Nursing 76*. September 1976, 6, 9.

Daley, K. Oral cancer everyday concerns. *American Journal of Nursing*, August 1979, 79, 8.

Donovan, M., & Pierce, S. *Cancer care nursing*. New York: Appleton-Century-Crofts, 1976.

Glucksberg, H., & Singer, J. *Cancer care.* Baltimore: Johns Hopkins University Press, 1980.

Gullo, S. Chemotherapy: What to do about special side effects. *RN,* April 1977, *40,* 4.

Hartley, H. National conference on nutrition in cancer. *Nutrition Today,* September/October 1978, *13,* 5.

Howard, R., & Herbold, N. *Nutrition in clinical care.* New York: McGraw-Hill Book Company, 1978.

Hunt, S., Groff, J, & Holbrook, J. *Nutrition: Principles and clinical practice.* New York: John Wiley & Sons, 1980.

Krause, M., & Mahan, L. *Food, nutrition and diet therapy* (6th ed.). Philadelphia: W. B. Saunders Company, 1979.

Luckmann, J., & Sorensen, K. *Medical-surgical nursing: A psychophysiologic approach* (2nd ed.). Philadelphia: W. B. Saunders Company, 1980.

Morra, M., Suski, N., & Johnson, B. *Eating Hints: A handbook for cancer patients.* New Haven, Conn.: Yale University Press, 1979.

Rose, J. Nutritional problems in radiotherapy patients. *American Journal of Nursing,* July 1978, *78,* 6.

Ross Laboratories. *Nutrition: A helpful ally in cancer therapy.* Columbus, Ohio, January 1978.

Schreier, A., & Lavenia, J. The nurses' role in nutritional management of radiotherapy patients. *Nursing Clinics of North America,* March 1977, *12,* 1.

Shils, M. Nutrition and neoplasia. In R. Goodhart & M. Shils (Eds.), *Modern nutrition in health and disease* (6th ed.). Philadelphia: Lea & Febiger, 1980.

Suitor, C., & Hunter, M. *Nutrition: Principles and application in health promotion.* Philadelphia: J. B. Lippincott Company, 1980.

Valencuis, J. Nutritional support of the cancer patient. In C. Kellog, & B. Sullivan (Eds.), *Current perspectives in oncologic nursing.* St. Louis: C. V. Mosby Company, 1978.

Whitworth, F. Feeding the cancer patient. In consultation. *Nursing 78,* October 1978, *8,* 10.

20
Diet Therapy in Relation to Religious and Cultural Customs

The influences of religion and culture on a patient's attitude toward food and dietary modification are often overlooked in the delivery of health care. Refusal to eat or to comply with a diet regimen is attributed to anorexia or lack of understanding. Nurses readily accept lack of appetite; it is a common symptom to them. Health educators intensify their teaching when they think that a patient does not understand the need for a dietary change. Interpreters are sought when language appears to be a barrier to understanding. The health care worker rarely inquires if the problem is related to religious or cultural food habits.

It is not possible to be familiar with the dietary practices of all religions and cultures. There is a paucity of published information on the subject. However, health care personnel can be alert to the possibility that the refusal of a particular food or diet is related to cultural or religious beliefs. Once aware of the possibility, health care workers can make suitable inquiries and revise their dietary offerings. When planning therapeutic diets for patients of other cultures, the cultural pattern should be considered. Ethnic foods should be included if the patient prefers them and if they are appropriate in the therapeutic diet. When ethnic dishes are included in the diet, the nurse should know their ingredients. If a particular ingredient is contraindicated, there should be a willingness to experiment with acceptable substitutes.

Nurses are accustomed to treating patients as though they shared the same background and value system as themselves. Recently, more interest and concern have been expressed in understanding the backgrounds and beliefs of individual patients as a basis for health teaching. Many patients of various ethnic backgrounds have adopted American food habits, others cling to their cultural patterns, and still others have a mixed pattern that combines a little of both. Older patients often prefer the traditional cultural practices. Some patients may revert to the cultural patterns of their childhoods when ill. Whatever the situation, it is worthwhile to consider culture as a possible reason for food refusal or dietary noncompliance. The food patterns of some religions and cultures are discussed to provide some insight into the kinds of food practices that might influence a patient's behavior toward diet.

Black Americans

Black Americans have a higher infant mortality and a shorter life expectancy than do Americans in general. Children less than 5 years of age have one-half the chance of survival of their white counterparts, due primarily to deaths in the first year of life (Martin, 1976). Hypertension is a particular problem in black Americans. Tuberculosis is three times as prevalent and childhood disease six times as prevalent in the black community.

DIETARY PRACTICES

The food intake of black Americans may not differ from typical American fare. There are, however, variations in food habits that are reflections of ancestry and the part of the country in which the person grew up. What is known as "soul food" stems from the dietary habits of Southern blacks, who economized in their cooking by making a variety of dishes from such foods as chicken wings, bacon ends, ribs, and chitterlings (chitlins—hog intestines that are boiled and then fried) and such field animals as rabbit and squirrel. The fat from pork products was saved and used to fry foods. Collard and other greens were usually combined with pork and thus cooked for long periods. The food was prepared with feeling—or from the soul—and the term now applies more to the emotional manner in which food is prepared than to the food itself.

Some West Indian blacks still practice voodoo beliefs that may influence their reactions to particular foods. One belief is that certain food mixtures cause serious illness. Watermelon and whiskey are considered a harmful combination. Penicillin is considered dangerous if injected after a drink of whiskey. Fish and milk or ice cream are thought to cause problems if eaten at the same meal. The combination of milk and cherries is also avoided. Milk is not given to patients with fevers, particularly young patients.

Black patients may find hospital food flavorless because they may be accustomed to well-seasoned foods. Instructions related to low-sodium diets should consider the importance of condiments, barbeque sauces, smoked meats, salt pork, and pickled foods in the traditional black American diet. When possible, suggestions for substitute seasonings are preferable to the elimination of well-liked dishes if the manner of preparation is the only factor that makes the food unacceptable in the diet. Some blacks believe that hypertension is caused by pork. This belief may be related to the elimination of bacon, sausage, and salt pork from low-sodium diets.

The diets of some black Americans may contain excessive starch and sodium. Protein is apt to be lacking in adequate amounts because protein sources tend to be expensive. Many black children are deficient in iron, folacin, vitamin A, and Calories. Obesity is a common finding in black women because of an intake that is high in highly refined carbohydrates, fats, and Calories. Many adult blacks are lactase deficient and avoid milk. Calcium is obtained from liberal use of greens and from buttermilk, used as a beverage or in cooking.

NURSING IMPLICATIONS

- Buttermilk, yogurt, and fermented cheeses are frequently tolerated by lactase deficient patients.
- When dietary teaching is done, be sure to include all people responsible for food selection and preparation. Children are often involved in this activity.
- Nurses need to be aware that black children tend to have lower hemoglobin readings even though they may not be nutritionally deficient, and assessing black children according to established normal values may lead to erroneous conclusions.

American Indians

There are more than 300 Indian tribes in the United States, each having its own culture; however, some generalizations are possible. Reservation life has interfered with the Indian's ability to ingest traditional foods, which in many instances were preferable to the highly refined foods now available to them. Health problems of American Indians include the development of hypertension, gastric ulcer, and cirrhosis at a younger age than for the American population in general. Infant mortality is high. There is an increased incidence of malnutrition and tuberculosis. Children often exhibit serious protein deficiencies. Diabetes mellitus is a particular problem, especially in pregnant women. Indians tend to remain asymptomatic with blood levels of glucose higher than 500 milligrams per 100 milliliters. Diabetic Indians may not follow their diets during feasts because it is a social, and sometimes religious, requirement that everyone join in the feasting.

DIETARY PRACTICES

The protein deficiency in children may be related to the lack of milk and cheeses in the typical diet. A large proportion of American Indians have lactase deficiency.

American Indians regard Anglo foods as bland and unattractive. The addition of traditional spices makes some Anglo foods more acceptable. Green chili is a favorite spice that is a rich source of vitamin C.

NURSING IMPLICATIONS

- If a Navaho Indian needs to increase potassium intake, instant tea and coffee are more available and acceptable than the frequently recommended orange juice and bananas.
- The traditional Navaho diet does not include fish, chicken, pork, or vegetables (Wauneka, 1962), and some Navahos reject these foods.
- The diets of American Indians tend to be deficient in Calories, calcium, riboflavin, vitamin C, and vitamin A.

Chinese

Traditional Chinese beliefs about food reflect the Yin-Yang concept. The Chinese feel that health is the result of balance between yin and yang forces. Foods and diseases are categorized as yin (cold) or yang (hot); the hot and cold designations have no relationship to temperature. Yang conditions affect the external body, the skin, and the hollow organs. Yin conditions are those that tend to draw a person inward, cause cold feelings, or lack of appetite. Yang conditions are characterized by excess energy, fever, dry throat, gritty eyes, or a crusted nose. Yin conditions are treated by yang foods, and vice versa, to restore balance. A sore throat with fever is an example of a yang condition; treatment consists of the yin foods, watercress soup and watermelon, while salads (yang) would be avoided. Cancer is a yin condition; ear infections are yang.

DIETARY PRACTICES

Pregnancy and birth are yin conditions. The prescribed diet includes special dishes that require long cooking periods and that are rich in proteins, calcium, and minerals. Ginseng is given in the seventh to eighth months of life. Soy sauce is avoided during pregnancy because it is thought to make babies dark. Pregnant women may refuse to take prescribed iron supplements because they believe that the iron will harden the fetal bones and make delivery difficult.

A yang diet is prescribed for the first month postpartum. Raw and cold foods are avoided; meats, liver, rice, eggs, and chicken soup are included. The soup is made with pig's knuckles and vinegar; the process of cooking bones in an acid solution increases the calcium content of the soup. Rice wine may be given after 2 weeks postpartum; before that time it is avoided because it is thought to stimulate uterine bleeding. The traditional diet may be constipating and necessitate increased intake of fluids and fiber. Hospital diets may be refused if they are not balanced in terms of yin and yang foods.

The Chinese favor moderation; extreme diets (all raw fruits and vegetables, or all cold or all hot foods) are rejected. Ginger is believed to counteract the toxins in foods. Ginger root can be added to foods to increase the yang content. Garlic is believed to rid the body of yang conditions. Herbs are used with prescribed drugs as broths. Chinese are not accustomed to milk or milk products; lactose intolerance is common. The stir-fry method of food preparation is used, which retains nutrients. Some Chinese are vegetarians. When meat is used, it is usually in limited amounts. The typical Chinese diet may be low in proteins, calcium, and vitamin D.

NURSING IMPLICATIONS

- Milk is rarely used as a beverage but may be accepted in Ovaltine or in custards.
- Tofu (soybean curd) is a good source of protein and iron. If calcium salts are used to precipitate the curd, tofu is also a good source of calcium.
- Cooked fruits and vegetables are preferred to raw ones. Raw vegetables are often refused completely.
- Ice water is thought to shock the system; hot drinking water may be preferred.
- Concentrated sweets are rarely used.
- Soy sauce is a favorite condiment, and Chinese patients would be more likely to comply with a low-sodium diet if soy sauce is limited rather than completely eliminated.
- Rice and tea are staples in the Chinese diet and should be included in prescribed diets when possible.

Cubans

DIETARY PRACTICES

The traditional Cuban diet consists of meats, fish, poultry, eggs, legumes, milk, and cheeses as protein sources. Black beans are the favorite legumes and are frequently served mixed with rice. Fruits and vegetables are used liberally. Plantains (starchy roots) are used; they resemble potatoes in nutrient content. Fruits are the basis for sweets. Flan (a custardlike dessert) is popular.

Meats are usually fried; lard is the preferred shortening. Breakfast tends to be inadequate, consisting of sweetened coffee and bread or Cuban crackers. Coffee and carbonated beverages are popular in the adult diet; milk and carbonated beverages are popular in the children's diet.

NURSING IMPLICATIONS

- The Cuban food intake is easily adapted to therapeutic diets. Spanish versions of exchange lists are available for use in diet planning.
- The practice of mixing black beans and rice provides a complete protein source and should be encouraged.
- The calcium intake of the diet could be increased by the use of calcium-rich vegetables, such as spinach and broccoli. The addition of cheese to breakfast would improve the Calorie content of the meal as well as the calcium intake.
- The decreased use of carbonated beverages and the substitution of vegetable oils for lard would improve the diet without undue change of custom.

Filipinos

The Filipino concept of disease is a combination of American medicine and folk practices. Filipino folk medicine is based on three basic beliefs:

- The body may contain impurities;
- A balance between hot and cold is desirable for health;
- Treatment involves natural and supernatural forces.

Flushing is used to rid the body of impurities. Flushing is accomplished by stimulation of perspiration, vomiting, flatus, or menstrual flow. In the case of a chest cold or fever, vinegar is used to flush, A combination of vinegar, water, salt, and hot pepper is used to produce diaphoresis. A mixture of ginger and lemon fried in olive oil is used to aid in expelling mucus. Corn silk boiled in water produces a liquid used as a diuretic.

The balance of hot and cold resembles the Chinese Yin-Yang concept. Heat may be required to maintain internal temperatures. A tea made of ginger and sugar is used for cold diseases (sore throat, hoarseness). Ginger is also considered a general stimulant that restores strength. Ginger also has a carminative effect.

Belief in the supernatural causes of illness leads to the need for protection from outside forces. Physicians are unable to cure illnesses of supernatural origin according to Filipino belief.

DIETARY PRACTICES

Rice is the staple of the traditional Filipino diet; it is usually served at every meal. Rice is frequently mixed with meat and vegetables. Pork, beef, and chicken are commonly used. They are prepared in a vinegar and garlic sauce. Pork and pork organ meats are spiced with whole peppers. The diet tends to be high in sodium, and salt is used generously. Soy sauce and patis (a salty liquid made from fish) are also used.

NURSING IMPLICATIONS

- Major adaptations would be necessary to prepare a low-sodium diet that would be acceptable to a patient accustomed to the traditional Filipino diet.

Greeks

DIETARY PRACTICES

The traditional Greek diet uses lamb as the preferred meat; organ meats, poultry, fish, eggs, and legumes are also used. Milk and cheeses are popular; adults favor yogurt; children are given hot, boiled milk with added sugar. Maize, rice, and wheat are the predominant grains in the Greek diet. Bread is served at every meal. Vegetables are well cooked, often with broth, tomatoes, onions, parsley, and olive oil. Vegetables and legumes are frequently the main dish. Peeled, raw fruits are served as desserts. Eggs are included in the diet but usually not at breakfast.

NURSING IMPLICATIONS

- Adaptation of the Greek diet to a low sodium intake would pose problems; feta cheese and olives, two favorite foods, are high is sodium.

- Vegetables should be cooked for shorter periods to preserve the vitamin content.
- Unpeeled fruits would increase the fiber in the diet.
- The practice of adding sugar to the children's milk should be discouraged to reduce empty Calorie intake and prevent dental caries.

Italians

DIETARY PRACTICES

Italians usually eat a light breakfast, a large noontime meal, and a smaller evening meal. Bread and pasta are basic to the traditional diet. Sources of protein include chicken, veal, beef, fish, sausage, and pork products. Milk is rarely used as a beverage, but cheeses are used widely and provide the needed calcium source. Vegetables are frequently served in thick soups. Fruits are well liked. Garlic, wine, olive oil, and tomato puree are used to flavor foods.

NURSING IMPLICATIONS

- Adaptation to special diets is easier if some pasta is permitted.
- Sausage and cold cuts need to be eliminated from low-sodium diets.
- The use of wine, garlic, and unsalted tomato puree should be encouraged to replace high-sodium seasonings in sodium-restricted diets.

Japanese

DIETARY PRACTICES

Rice and fish are staples in the traditional Japanese diet. Raw fish is considered a delicacy. Meat is used in small amounts, usually mixed with vegetables and grains. Milk is included in the children's diet. Cheese is rarely eaten; eggs are popular. Soybean products are an important source of protein. Tofu (soybean curd) is used extensively. When soybean curd is precipitated by calcium salts, it also is a good source of calcium. Commonly used vegetables include seaweed, bamboo shoots, and bean sprouts. Fruits are eaten as desserts. Butter and cream are rarely used; soy and rice oils are the shortenings in the typical Japanese diet.

NURSING IMPLICATIONS

- Foods are prepared by the stir-fry method, which preserves vitamins.

- The heavy use of salt, pickled vegetables, and high-sodium sauces (soy and teriyaki) in the Japanese diet may pose some difficulties if there is need to adapt to a low-sodium diet. This dietary transition would be easier if alternative seasonings were suggested as part of the dietary teaching. Spices, herbs, and lemon juice are frequently used as flavor enhancers.
- The limited use of milk in the adult diet may be related to the high incidence of lactose intolerance among the Japanese.

Jews

The impact of Jewish dietary practices is influenced by whether the patient is an Orthodox, Conservative, or Reform Jew. The kashruth are strictly observed by the Orthodox Jew, nominally observed by the Conservative Jew, and minimally observed by the Reform Jew. The kashruth are Jewish dietary laws. The term kosher is used to describe foods that are fit, proper, and in accordance with the kashruth.

DIETARY PRACTICES

Jewish dietary laws restrict the use of meats to animals with cloven hooves that chew cuds. Only the forequarter of such animals can be used for food unless the hip sinew and thigh vein are removed from the hindquarter. This restriction permits the intake of lamb, beef, venison, and goat meat but forbids pork and rabbit. All animals must be free of disease and killed according to ritual in a manner that causes the least pain to the animal. As much blood as possible must be removed from the carcass; the meat is then soaked or salted to remove the remaining blood. Fish that have both fins and scales are permitted; shellfish and eels are not allowed.

According to dietary law, foods are classified as:

- Inherently kosher (pareve) in their natural state, namely, grains, fruits, vegetables, tea, and coffee;
- Requiring some processing to make kosher, namely, meats, poultry, and cheese; or
- Inherently not kosher, namely, pork, shellfish, and eel.

Waste products are not used. Cream of tartar is considered a waste product and is forbidden.

Dietary laws prohibit serving meat and dairy products at the same meal. Milk or milk products may be consumed before a meal. After meat is eaten, 3 to 6 hours must elapse before any dairy product is ingested. Fish or eggs may be eaten with dairy products or meat meals. Two separate sets of utensils are needed to cook and serve meat and dairy products if the dietary laws are strictly observed. Eggs that contain blood spots may not be eaten.

The traditional Jewish diet tends to be high in saturated fats and cholesterol. Jewish people have a high incidence of diabetes mellitus, obesity, lactose intolerance, and ulcerative colitis. Special diets can be tailored to observe the dietary restrictions. Hospitalized Jewish patients should be consulted about their dietary practices; nurses should ensure that these practices are not violated.

NURSING IMPLICATIONS

- The meat and poultry used in hospitals is not considered kosher. A complete line of kosher frozen foods is available to medical facilities.
- The fish and eggs on hospital menus may be used freely.
- Foods may be cooked in foil and served on disposable plates to eliminate the need for separate cooking and serving utensils for meat and dairy meals.
- The designation pareve used in labeling processed foods means that the product does not contain dairy products, meat, or poultry.

Mexicans

Some Mexican people practice folk medicine and believe in a supernatural basis for certain diseases. Health practices may be a combination of modern medicine and folklore. Tea brewed from fresh orange leaves is thought to prevent insomnia and nervousness. Rice, bananas, and greasy, fried foods may be avoided to ensure good health. Apples, tamales, and coffee are not considered healthy when served at the evening meal. To some extent, Mexicans ascribe to a hot and cold food theory.

DIETARY PRACTICES

The traditional Mexican diet includes meat a few times per week; examples include chicken, pork chops, frankfurters, hamburgers, and cold cuts. Eggs and dried beans are other important protein sources. Milk and cheese are used in limited amounts because of their cost. When milk is available, it is frequently made into custard. Corn is the basic grain and is used to make the popular tortillas. When tortillas are made from corn that has been soaked in lime (calcium oxide), they become a good source of calcium. Fresh fruits and vegetables may be difficult to obtain. Potatoes, red and green peppers, tomatoes, and onions are used extensively. Foods are usually fried in lard, salt pork, or bacon fat. Chili peppers, onions, and garlic are used as seasonings. Coffee is a popular beverage for adults and children. The food intake of Mexicans tends to be high in fats and sodium and low in calcium and folacin.

NURSING IMPLICATIONS

- The vitamin content of the diet should be evaluated when spicy foods are restricted for medicinal reasons because peppers are used for seasoning. Chili peppers are a good source of vitamin A; red and green peppers are rich in vitamin C.

Mormons

DIETARY PRACTICES

The Mormon religion prohibits the intake of alcohol and stimulant beverages. Water and milk are the predominant beverages.

NURSING IMPLICATIONS

- The major implication of Mormon dietary practices would be for patients on liquid diets. Black coffee and clear tea would not be acceptable to Mormons on clear liquid diets.
- Broth, ginger ale, jello, and strained and diluted fruit and vegetable juices are acceptable.

Muslims

DIETARY PRACTICES

The Muslim religion prohibits the ingestion of pork and all pork products. All animals to be consumed must be slaughtered in the name of Allah. Kosher meats are acceptable, as are fish, shellfish, and fowl. Alcohol is prohibited, and stimulant beverages are discouraged. Animal shortenings are avoided. Only kosher gelatins should be used; this restriction eliminates marshmallows, gelatin desserts, and many candies.

Foods considered healthy by Muslims include pure honey, dates, meats (except pork), seafood, and sweets. Vegetable oil should be used in food preparation.

NURSING IMPLICATIONS

- Compliance with the Muslim restrictions should not present problems if kosher frozen foods are available.
- Adaptations to special diets require only the recognition of the prohibited foods and appropriate substitutions.

• Nurses should be aware that Muslim patients desire to wash their hands and clean their mouths in some manner before meals.

Poles

DIETARY PRACTICES

The traditional Polish diet is based on the foods that grow well in Poland. These foods include as protein sources milk, cheese, sour cream, eggs, pork, and fish. Rye, millet, barley, buckwheat, maize, and potatoes are the major sources of carbohydrate. Popular vegetables include cabbage, onions, beets, turnips, beans, mushrooms, and cucumbers. Fruits and berries are widely used. Bread is served at every meal; it is considered the holiest of foods and is never wasted. Bread crumbs are used to line pans, thicken gravies, and as a vegetable topping. In Poland, salt, sugar, coffee, and tea had to be imported and were not widely available.

Poles still favor pork and luncheon meats but have increased their intake of beef. Meat soups are popular. Polish meals tend to be highly seasoned and salted. Sweets are popular. The diet tends to be high in saturated fats and high in total fats, salt, and sugar.

NURSING IMPLICATIONS

• Suggest steaming vegetables to retain vitamin content.
• Encourage use of whole-grain breads and cereals.
• Stress the importance of reducing the intake of saturated fats, salt, and sugar.

Puerto Ricans

Puerto Ricans have a high incidence of infant mortality, tuberculosis, malnutrition, and parasitic infestations. They follow the hot-cold food-disease concept to some extent. Belief in the supernatural etiology of disease and folk medicine exist along with acceptance of modern medical practices.

DIETARY PRACTICES

The poor, island Puerto Ricans exist on a diet in which red kidney beans mixed with rice is the main source of protein. Milk, eggs, and leafy green vegetables are rarely used. When Puerto Ricans come to the United States, their diet continues to be basically high in starch with liberal use of inexpensive fats. Rice and beans in combination provide a complete protein source. Dried, salted codfish is used extensively. Viandas (starchy roots, such as plantains and green bananas) are used in place of bread, they are similar in nutritional value to bread or potatoes. Beans and viandas are rich sources of vitamin B complex and iron. Meats are expensive and are used mainly to flavor stews. Milk is also considered too expensive for general use; heavily sugared coffee is a favorite beverage. Children and pregnant women drink malta, a beverage made from caramel, malt extract, and sugar. Malta is not very nutritious; it provides some vitamin B complex from the small amount of malt used in its preparation.

The typical Puerto Rican diet consists of a breakfast of coffee and bread, lunch of rice and beans and a salad, and a dinner of leftovers from lunch. Desserts usually consist of fruits and fruit preserves. The diet lacks a variety of fruits, vegetables, and adequate amounts of proteins and vitamins A and C.

NURSING IMPLICATIONS

- Calcium may be lacking in the diet. Cheese is well accepted, and its use should be encouraged because milk is not often used.
- Pregnant women may need to increase their intake of folic acid to prevent megaloblastic anemia. Sources of folic acid include fish, legumes, and whole grains.
- Obesity may be a problem because of the large amount of fat used in food preparation and the high intake of sugar.

Seventh Day Adventists

DIETARY PRACTICES

Seventh Day Adventists generally avoid all flesh foods, although this practice is not a tenet of their faith. They may be ovolactovegetarians. Ovolactovegetarians avoid, meat, poultry, and fish but consume milk and eggs. Alcohol and stimulant beverages are avoided, and the use of highly seasoned foods and condiments is discouraged. An interval of 5 to 6 hours between meals is practiced, with between-meal feedings discouraged. The main meal of the day is usually served in the middle of the day. The vegetarian diet of Seventh Day Adventists is highly developed and makes use of combinations of proteins to ensure adequate intake of essential amino acids. Vegetarian diets tend to be low in saturated fats and cholesterol and high in fiber, which is probably compatible with good health.

NURSING IMPLICATIONS

- A hospitalized vegetarian would have difficulty selecting a well-balanced diet from the usual hospital menu.
- Special diets may be adapted to vegetarian intake.
- The vegan diet, which eliminates milk and eggs as well as meat, may present problems in ensuring adequate intake of essential amino acids, particularly to meet the needs of growing children and pregnant women.

Vietnamese

DIETARY PRACTICES

The Vietnamese diet uses poultry and pork back but little beef. Fish is a regular part of the diet. Fish is also used to make a sauce that is served with many other foods. Rice is a diet staple; soybeans and peanuts are also eaten. Vegetables, such as cabbage, sweet potatoes, squash, watercress, and spinach, are used. Coconut and raw sugar are consumed as sweets. Little fresh milk is used; tea is the principal beverage. The Vietnamese diet reflects both Chinese and French influences.

NURSING IMPLICATIONS

- The high salt content, particularly of Vietnamese fish sauce, is an important consideration when intake of sodium is restricted.
- The use of milk in cooking should be encouraged because milk provides calcium.
- Cheese, yogurt, and greens are alternative sources of calcium that may be accepted.

References

American Dietetic Association. *Cultural food patterns in the U.S.A.* Chicago, 1976.

Baca, J. Some health beliefs of the Spanish speaking. *American Journal of Nursing,* October 1969, *69,* 10.

Bauwens, E. *The anthropology of health.* St. Louis: C. V. Mosby Company, 1978.

Berkowitz, P., & Berkowitz, N. The Jewish patient in the hospital. *American Journal of Nursing,* November 1967, *67,* 11.

Branch, M., & Paxton, P. *Providing safe care for ethnic people of color.* New York: Appleton-Century-Crofts, 1976.

Brink, P. (Ed.). *Transcultural nursing.* Englewood Cliffs, N.J.: Prentice-Hall, 1976.

Campbell, T., & Chang, B. Health care of the Chinese in America. *Nursing Outlook,* April 1973, *21,* 4.

Chang, B. Some dietary beliefs in Chinese folk culture. *Journal of the American Dietetic Association,* May 1974, *64,* 5.

Chung, H. Understanding the Oriental maternity patient. *Nursing Clinics of North America,* March 1977, *12,* 1.

Community outlook. Asian diet fact sheet. *Nursing Times,* November 10, 1977, *73,* 45.

DeGracia, R. Cultural influences on Filipino patients. *American Journal of Nursing,* August 1979, *79,* 8.

Gonzales, H. Health needs of the Mexican-American. In *Ethnicity and health care.* New York: National League for Nursing, 1976.

Herbold, N. Community nutrition. In R. Howard & N. Herbold, *Nutrition in clinical care.* New York: McGraw-Hill Book Company, 1978.

Hongladarom, H., & Russell, M. An ethnic difference—Lactose intolerance. *Nursing Outlook,* December 1976, *24,* 12.

James, S. When your patient is black West Indian. *American Journal of Nursing,* November 1978, *78,* 11.

Kolasa, K. I won't cook turnip greens if you won't cook kielbasa; food behavior of Polonia and its health implications. In E. Bauwens, *The anthropology of health.* St. Louis: C. V. Mosby Company, 1978.

Krause, M., & Mahan, L. *Food, nutrition and diet therapy* (6th ed.). Philadelphia: W. B. Saunders Company, 1979.

Leininger, M. *Transcultural nursing.* New York: John Wiley & Sons, 1978.

Martin, B. Ethnicity and health care: Afro-Americans. In *Ethnicity and health care.* New York: National League for Nursing, 1976.

Natow, A., Heslin, J., & Raven, B. Integrating Jewish dietary laws into a dietetic program. *Journal of the American Dietetic Association.* July 1975, *67,* 7.

Primeaux, M. Caring for the American Indian patient. *American Journal of Nursing,* January 1977, *77,* 1.

Rotkovitch, R. Ethnicity and health care: The Jewish heritage. In *Ethnicity and health care.* New York: National League for Nursing, 1976.

Sakr, A. Dietary regulations and food habits of Muslims. *Journal of the American Dietetic Association.* February 1971, *58,* 123.

Smith, G. Multicultural components of nursing. In *Ethnicity and health care.* New York: National League for Nursing, 1976.

Suitor, C., & Hunter, M. *Nutrition: Principles and applications in health promotion.* Philadelphia: J. B. Lippincott Company, 1980.

Wauneka, A., Helping a People to Understand. *American Journal of Nursing,* July 1962, *62,* 7.

Williams, R. (Ed.). *Textbook of black-related diseases.* New York: McGraw-Hill Book Company, 1975.

Williams, S. *Nutrition and diet therapy* (3rd ed.). St. Louis: C. V. Mosby Company, 1977.

Wong, R. Chinese-Americans and health care. In *Ethnicity and health care*. New York: National League for Nursing, 1976.

Wood, R. The American Indian and health care. In *Ethnicity and health care*. New York: National League for Nursing, 1976.

Yohai, F. Dietary patterns of Spanish-speaking people living in the Boston area. *Journal of the American Dietetic Association*, September 1977, *71*, 9.

21

Dietary Considerations Throughout the Life Span

The beginning influence of diet in life is difficult to identify. The dietary influence on the outcome of pregnancy is well recognized. The nutritional status of the mother before and at the time of conception is also of prime importance; however, the establishment of sound nutritional practices that will be followed throughout life starts with the newborn infant.

Infancy

The newborn infant's average birth weight is 7 to 7½ pounds. Growth in the first year of life is rapid, tapering off slightly in the last 6 months. An infant usually doubles his or her birth weight at 4 to 5 months and triples it at 1 year. Energy requirements are high: 117 kcal per kilogram of body weight during the first 6 months, 108 kcal per kilogram during the second 6 months. A term newborn infant is able to digest and absorb proteins, simple carbohydrates, and a moderate amount of fat. The starch-splitting enzyme amylase is not produced until later. A newborn infant has a higher fluid requirement in relation to body size than does an older child or adult.

DIET

The ideal food for infants is breast milk. The current recommendation is breast milk as the only source of nutrients for the first 6 months of life. There are several advantages to breast milk. Breast-feeding avoids the early introduction to the gastrointestinal tract of antigens often present in infant formulas and solids and reduces the incidence of infantile allergy.

283

Breast milk supplies protective maternal antibodies while the infant's immune system is maturing. Breast-feeding promotes bonding. The lipids present in breast milk are absorbed better than are the lipids in other infant feedings. Breast milk has a higher linoleic (essential fatty acid) content. There is some indication that breast-feeding prevents infantile obesity. The breast milk at the end of the feeding period, hind milk, has a higher fat content, which provides satiety and signals the infant to stop nursing. Breast milk has a higher cholesterol content than do commercial formulas; some authorities believe that this increased concentration may promote the development of efficient pathways for the metabolism of cholesterol throughout life as well as provide cholesterol for the production of nerve tissue and bile.

Breast-fed infants need other sources of vitamin C, vitamin D, fluoride, and iron. Vitamin C can be provided by introducing dilute orange juice at 1 to 2 months and gradually increasing the proportion of orange juice to water until the infant is receiving full-strength juice. Vitamin D is given as a vitamin supplement. Fluoride may also be given as a supplement if the water supply is not fluoridated or if the infant does not drink sufficient water to meet his or her fluoride needs. Newborn infants usually have an abundant supply of red blood cells at birth; the destruction of excess cells provides an adequate source of iron for 4 to 6 months. The small amount of iron present in breast milk is well absorbed. After 4 months, infants need dietary sources of iron. Premature infants who have not had the opportunity to store iron need an iron source earlier; such infants appear to absorb iron better than do term infants.

Cereal is usually the first solid food given to breast-fed infants. Cereal provides iron, calcium, phosphorus, thiamine, riboflavin, and niacin. Meat is sometimes selected as the first solid food for the breast-fed infants because of its iron and protein contents.

Infants who are not breast-fed are usually given 5 to 10% glucose 4 hours after birth. Advocates of reduced intake of refined sugar question this early introduction of sugar in the diet. Formulas that simulate human milk and that are fortified with minerals and vitamins may be selected for artificially fed infants. A formula that consists of evaporated whole milk, water, and corn syrup is an inexpensive and adequate source of nutrients when supplemented with a multivitamin preparation. Undiluted cow's milk and skim milk should not be used as a basis for an infant's formula. Cow's milk contains too much protein and requires dilution. Skim milk lacks the essential fatty acid linoleic acid. Fluoride supplementation is needed if the local water supply is not fluoridated.

Newborn infants cannot swallow voluntarily until 10 to 12 weeks of age. Before that time, swallowing must be stimulated by sucking. Sucking follows a rhythmic pattern, with bursts and pauses. If an infant is stimulated to suck during the pauses (e.g., by stroking the cheek), there is decreased likelihood that sucking will be resumed and increased likelihood that the length of the pause will be increased. Infants should not be expected to suck constantly throughout feeding time; pauses should be allowed. Bottle-fed infants are expected to finish the formulas in their bottles; the amount of milk that a breast-fed infant receives is usually not known. Bottle-fed infants may be given a bottle whenever they fuss. Bottle-fed infants are usually given solid foods at an early age.

Developmentally, infants cannot swallow without previous sucking until 2½ to 3 months. The flow of saliva needed to manage solid foods increases at about 3 months. The extrusion reflex, in which infants push food out of their mouths with their tongues, lasts until about 4 months. The sense of taste is not developed until 3 to 4 months. Spoon-feeding is not developmentally sound until 4 to 6 months. Infants begin to sleep through the night, regardless of diet, at about 9 weeks.

At one time, newborn infants doubled their weights at 6 months and tripled their weights at 1 year; birth weight now doubles at 4 to 5 months but still triples at 1 year. The end result of the earlier weight gain is a heavier infant to be lifted and carried and, possibly, the beginning of obesity. *Nutrition Reviews* (1979) reports that one-third of all infants who were above the 90th percentile in weight for the first 4 to 6 months became obese during adult life. Bottle-fed infants should be given the opportunity for nonnutritive sucking. Boiled water can be given between feedings, the natural pattern of sucking should be recognized and pauses permitted, and nonsweetened pacifiers should be used. Satisfying the infant, not emptying the bottle, should become the goal at feeding time.

Bottle-fed infants should be given dilute orange juice at 1 to 2 months. Vitamin C supplements replace orange juice for infants with family histories of allergy. Enriched rice cereal, the first solid, should be introduced at 4 to 6 months. Other grain cereals can be introduced later. Vegetables follow at 7 months, fruits at 8 months. Meats and cottage cheese can be given to bottle-fed infants at 9 months; early use of meats for bottle-fed infants can result in excessive intake of protein.

Infants should be exposed to a variety of food textures and do not need teeth to handle the early forms. The usual progression is from strained to mashed to minced to chopped to cut table foods. Teeth begin to emerge at 4 months, although teething is highly variable. Once infants begin to teethe, they will enjoy munching toast, crackers, and zwieback.

When bottle-fed infants are 4 to 6 months old, they may be given whole milk. Sterilization of feedings is no longer necessary. Infants may become constipated initially due to the change in curd tension.

Weaning from the bottle or breast may begin in the second half of the first year. At 5 to 6 months, infants are able to approximate their lips to a cup. At 1 year, they are able to hold a cup and drink from it with assistance. The weaning process should be gradual and accomplished by 2 years. Breast-fed babies may be weaned directly to a cup. Bottle-fed babies may accept juice or water from a cup but cling to the bottle for milk feedings.

"Nursing bottle caries," tooth decay related to the practice of putting babies to bed with a bottle of milk or juice, can be prevented by reducing the sugar content of the formula when teeth erupt and by discontinuing nocturnal milk or juice bottles. When fluids that contain sugar are given at bedtime, the fluids pool around the teeth. The sugar in such fluids is converted to lactic acid by the bacteria in the mouth. The lactic acid mobilizes calcium from the teeth, resulting in decay of the enamel. Water may be used in the nocturnal bottle, or the infant's mouth may be rinsed with water after a prebedtime feeding.

Home preparation of baby food is acceptable if there is scrupulous cleanliness in all aspects of preparation. Sugar and salt should be withheld from the family foods until after the infant's portion is prepared. Foods prepared in advance should be frozen. Carrots, spinach, and beets have a high nitrate content that may be converted to nitrites before consumption. These vegetables should not be prepared in advance and stored but may be used fresh at infrequent intervals.

Commercially prepared baby foods are safe and no longer contain salt and other additives. Sugar has been removed from most baby foods, except the desserts.

NURSING IMPLICATIONS

- Commercially prepared mixed dinners and baby soups have a high water content and contain little meat. Selecting meats and vegetables separately provides better nutritional value. Baby desserts that contain too much refined sugar are not needed in the infant diet; fruits can be used as desserts. Egg yolk can be given after 8 months; baby desserts should not be used as a source of egg yolk in the diet.

- When new foods are introduced into the diet, they should be served in small amounts (1 teaspoon) and given one at a time to allow better recognition of allergic responses.

- Foods rejected at one time can be reintroduced at another time.

- A variety of foods should be encouraged, but stringy foods, nuts, raisins, and popcorn, all of which might cause choking, should be avoided.

- Milk intake should not exceed 1 quart daily to prevent refusal of other foods and the possible development of milk anemia.

Childhood

TODDLERS

Toddlers, 1 to 3 years of age, are struggling for autonomy; they are more interested in their environment and their growing motor skills than in eating. The growth rate of toddlers slows, and they need fewer Calories but more protein per kilogram of body weight. At 1 year, the average toddler needs 1,000 kcal, at 3 years, 1,300 to 1,500 kcal (90 kcal per kilogram). Protein intake should be 2 grams per kilogram of body weight, with half the amount supplied by high-biologic-value proteins.

At least 16 ounces of milk should be included in the toddler's diet. Milk provides protein, calcium, riboflavin, and vitamins A and B_{12}. Fortified milk provides vitamin D. Whole milk should be used until 2 years to provide linoleic acid, which is contained in the milk fat. Fortified soybean milk can be used in vegan diets. Yogurt, cheese, and buttermilk contribute to milk intake. Toddlers who drink more than 24 ounces of milk per day do not have sufficient intake of other foods and may suffer from milk anemia. Milk anemia has a peak incidence at 18 months. Lean red meat as part of the recommended 1 to 3 ounces of foods from the meat group can be a source of iron. Bite-sized pieces of meat are often acceptable as snacks. Whole-grain or enriched breads and cereals should be used.

Four servings of fruit and vegetables daily are recommended. One serving daily should consist of citrus fruit or tomato to provide vitamin C. Leafy green and yellow vegetables should be served frequently. Toddlers tend to prefer raw vegetables served as finger foods. Raw carrots should be avoided because they can cause choking. Although salads usually are not popular because they are mixtures, individual salad ingredients served separately are often accepted.

Toddlers should have three or four servings from the bread group. These selections can include cereals and pastas. Whole-grain or enriched foods should be used. Infant cereals are often continued because of their iron content; sugar-coated cereals should be avoided. Factors to consider in selecting cereals include the total amount of sugar, fiber content, additives, and coloring. Dry cereals are often taken as finger-fed snacks.

In addition to the basic four food groups, toddlers should have 1 to 2 teaspoons of margarine or butter for its vitamin A content. Desserts, such as puddings, ice cream, and custards, are better for toddlers than are cakes, cookies, and pies. Homemade cookies that contain oatmeal, carrots, raisins, molasses, or chopped nuts provide essential nutrients and are also treats.

NURSING IMPLICATIONS

- The toddler's struggle for autonomy may be manifested in refusal of food, mealtime negativism, and ritualism. Toddlers should be allowed their rituals.
- Parents should avoid mealtime arguments over their toddler's refusal to eat. Toddlers will not starve but may develop poor dietary habits as the result of constant pressure from their parents to eat. A relaxed attitude on the part of the adult is difficult but important.
- Toddlers should not be bribed to eat nor rewarded for eating. Food

has its own values and should not be manipulated by the parents or children.

- A readily available supply of finger foods and frequent serving of the toddler's favorite foods may increase intake, if necessary.
- In general, toddlers like hamburgers, French-fried potatoes, chicken, spaghetti, and macaroni. They tend to refuse casseroles, salads, and other mixed dishes.

PRESCHOOLERS

Preschoolers, 3 to 6 years of age, gain an average of 2 kilograms of body weight and 6 to 8 centimeters in height per year. By 6 years, the child has doubled his or her weight at 1 year (42 pounds) and increased his or her height at 1 year by one-half (42 inches). Growth in the preschool period proceeds at a slower rate, but energy requirements for the endless walking, running, and climbing are high. Preschoolers are asserting their independence and using their developing vocabulary to express food likes and dislikes.

DIET

Protein needs continue to be high, with high-biologic-value protein still providing half of the approximately 40 grams needed daily. Intake of calcium and iron is important. Intake of vitamins A and C may be low; fruits and vegetables should be encouraged as snacks and finger foods. Appetites continue to be poor. Five small meals per day may be more acceptable than the traditional three. The evening meal should be kept light because a tired child is apt to be negative toward food.

Preschoolers should receive 16 ounces of milk daily, 1 to 3 ounces of selections from the meat group, four servings from the fruit and vegetable group (including a source of vitamin C daily and liberal use of leafy green and dark yellow vegetables for vitamin A), and four servings from the cereal group, with whole grains preferred.

NURSING IMPLICATIONS

- Preschoolers generally prefer raw vegetables and reject those with strong flavors. Tough and stringy foods are also disliked.
- Preschoolers tend to prefer single foods, served lukewarm.
- Different foods served on the same plate should not be allowed to touch one another.
- Finger foods continue to be popular.
- Food jags occur and should be handled in a relaxed manner.

SCHOOL-AGE CHILDREN

School-age children, 6 to 12 years old, are in a latent period of growth; the rate is slow and steady. Compared to previous periods, changes occur slowly. There is a gradual decline in food requirements per unit of body weight. The average yearly gains are 3 to 5 kilograms in weight and 6 centimeters in height, ending with the growth spurt of puberty.

DIET

School-age children retain their likes and dislikes of earlier years and imitate family food preferences. Exposure to other family patterns as the result of eating at friends' houses may reverse former food dislikes and increase the variety of foods enjoyed.

Breakfast for the school-age child may be inadequate. The school-age child may suffer from school phobia and be unable to eat. Many school-age children must make their own breakfasts and may not have the time or desire to make proper selections. Lunch is eaten at school, and intake is at the child's discretion despite what may be packed or available at the lunch counter. Parents have little direct knowledge of their child's food intake, except for the evening and weekend meals.

The appetites of school-age children have improved, and food intake is more varied. Two servings from the milk group are recommended daily, although such children usually take more. Recommended intake includes 2 to 3 ounces from the meat group, which includes eggs, poultry, fish, legumes, and peanut butter, good sources of proteins, vitamins, and minerals. Fruit and vegetable (three to four servings) choices should include a source of vitamin C daily, and leafy green or dark yellow vegetables three or four times weekly. Whole-grain breads and cereals (three to four servings daily) and 1 to 2 tablespoons of margarine or butter are recommended. The diet should be assessed for adequate contents of proteins, vitamin A, and vitamin C.

NURSING IMPLICATIONS

- After-school snacks are an important part of the food intake. Working parents should have nutritious snacks prepared in advance so that they are ready to eat. Fruits, raw vegetable sticks, and peanut butter sandwiches are popular.
- Sweetened carbonated beverages should not be available because unsupervised children usually select them instead of milk or juices.
- Sources of empty Calories and foods high in refined sugar should be eliminated; dental caries and childhood obesity are common problems.

Adolescence

DIET

Childhood ends with the growth spurt of adolescence, when physiologic age is a better guide to nutritional needs than is chronologic age. Caloric needs increase greatly to meet the increased metabolic demands of adolescence. Girls need approximately 2,000 to 2,500 kcal per day; boys need 2,500 to 3,000 kcal per day. Protein needs increase to 50 to 60 grams per day. Calcium intake is essential for bone growth. Iron intake is important, especially to replace menstrual losses in girls. The adequacy of calcium and iron intake is a major dietary concern. An adequate source of iodine is needed to support increased thyroid activity; iodized salt should be used. B vitamins are needed for the increased metabolic activity. There may be few sources of vitamins A and C in the typical adolescent diet.

Many aspects of adolescence, other than the growth rate, influence diet. Adolescents are concerned about the changes in their bodies and must adjust to changing body images. The striving for independence may lead to rejection of family ideas about nutrition as well as other values. There may be increased interest in sports participation and concern about food intake for maximal performance. Many teenagers develop an interest in diet that is based on scientific as well as unscientific information.

Adolescents should receive the following items from the basic four food groups:

- 3 or more cups of milk or the equivalent from the milk group
- 2 or more servings of meat, poultry, legumes, fish, or eggs
- 4 or more servings of fruits and vegetables, including a source of vitamin C daily, and leafy green or dark yellow vegetables three or four times per week; potato or a substitute daily
- 2 to 6 or more servings of bread or cereal, with emphasis on whole grains
- 1 to 2 tablespoons or more of butter or margarine

Adolescent girls, who are particularly concerned about their rapid weight gain and physiologic fat deposits, frequently go on crash diets. Nutritionally unsound diets not only deprive adolescent girls of nutrients needed for growth but also interefere with the building of reserves needed for future childbearing. Foods that are frequently eliminated by dieting teenage girls include milk, eggs, bread, cereal, and butter or margarine. The use of oral contraceptives by teenage girls increases their need for folic acid, vitamin B_6 and, to lesser degrees, vitamin C, thiamine, and riboflavin. The use of an intrauterine device increases menstrual flow and intensifies the need for iron.

Adolescent boys are also at risk nutritionally because of their increasing energy needs and rapidly expanding muscle mass. They especially need adequate sources of Calories, protein, iron, folic acid, B vitamins, and iodine. Adolescent athletes should have prudent, well-balanced diets. They have increased needs for energy, water, and salt but not for protein. Emphasis on protein intake above the normal requirements for athletes is unnecessary and expensive. Serum levels of cholesterol start to rise during adolescence, and curtailing excessive intake of saturated fats may be desirable.

Acne affects approximately 80% of the adolescent population. Acne results from increased activity of androgenic hormones, which causes hyperkeratosis of the hair follicles and sebaceous glands, leading to blockage by sebum; secondary infection usually follows. Acne usually occurs on the face, neck, shoulders, back, and upper part of the chest. The treatment is frequent, careful cleansing of the involved areas, followed by application of antibacterial ointment. Astringents, cryoslush, ultraviolet light, and hormones are also used in treatment.

NURSING IMPLICATIONS

- Diet has no effect on the progress of acne, despite long-standing admonitions to avoid chocolate, fried foods, nuts, and sweets. Teenagers with acne should select well-balanced diets.
- Chocolate and fried foods may be eliminated, but their absence will have more effect on body weight and serum levels of cholesterol than on acne.

Pregnancy

DIET

Poor nutrition in pregnancy can result in inadequate maternal weight gain and intrauterine malnutrition, leading to the birth of an infant with low birth weight and a decreased chance of survival. Generally, the fetus grows at the expense of the mother, even if she is mildly undernourished. When the mother is severely malnourished, the fetus is at risk because it cannot use what is not available. The nutritional status of the mother before conception is important in terms of nutrient reserves and basic eating habits.

Caloric intake during pregnancy is related to body weight and activity. A weight gain of 22 to 28 pounds (10 to 15 kilograms) is recommended. A gain of 2 to 4 pounds (1 to 2 kilograms) should occur in the first trimester with a 1-pound (0.4 kilogram) gain per week throughout the rest of the pregnancy. During the first trimester, the mother should have balanced portions of essential nutrients, with emphasis on quality, not on quantity, of food intake. Caloric intake during pregnancy should be sufficient to meet energy needs so that protein is spared for anabolic requirements. An increase of 300 kcal per day or a 14 to 15% increase over prepregnancy intake is usually adequate. Inadequate weight gain is not desirable, even in the presence of obesity. Every mother needs to gain the recommended 22 to 28 pounds. Excessive weight gain (more than 28 pounds) is not desirable; if such a gain occurs, the diet should be evaluated to eliminate Calories without sacrificing essential nutrients. Pregnant women should be cautioned against periods of fasting. Fasting leads to ketoacidosis, which can be dangerous to the fetus.

Protein intake during pregnancy is increased by 30 grams, or 65 to 68% over the woman's prepregnancy requirements. This two-thirds increase is for normal pregnancies; high-risk mothers are advised to double their protein intake. Protein requirements can also be calculated on the basis of 1.3 grams per kilogram of ideal body weight for a mature woman. Protein is needed for the development of the fetus, uterus, mammary glands, placenta, blood, amnionic fluid, and for storage reserves. Two-thirds of the protein intake should be provided by high-biologic-value proteins.

Calcium intake should be increased by 0.4 gram (50%), a recommended intake of 1.2 grams per day for a mature woman. Calcium is needed for development of fetal teeth and bones and for blood clotting. Calcium intake is critical in the third trimester, when fetal bones are mineralized. Good sources of calcium include milk and milk products, and leafy green vegetables.

The iron needs of pregnant women are increased by 30 to 60 milligrams per day. The amount of iron needed cannot be provided by the typical diet, and supplementation is required. Iron is needed to correct possible deficiencies, to provide for increased maternal blood volume, for fetal blood storage (a 3- to 4-month supply is stored in the liver), and for blood loss during delivery.

Iodine needs are increased by 25 micrograms (15 to 17%) to meet the increased needs generated by increased activity of the thyroid gland. Iodized salt should be used in food preparation and seasoning. Fish and the iodates used to condition bread dough are other sources of iodine.

The vitamin A requirements are increased by 1,000 International Units, or 200 retinol equivalents, an increase of 20 to 25% over prepregnancy needs. Vitamin A is needed for cell development, maintenance of epithelial tissue, and development of teeth and bones. Sources of vitamin A include liver, egg yolks, butter, fortified margarine, dark green and yellow vegetables, and fortified milk.

The vitamin B requirements are increased as follows:

- Thiamin by 0.4 milligram, or 40%
- Riboflavin by 0.3 milligram, or 20 to 25%

- Niacin equivalents by 0.2 milligram, or 15 to 17%
- Vitamin B_6 by 0.6 milligram, or 30%
- Folic acid by 400 micrograms, or 100%
- Vitamin B_{12} by 1.0 microgram, or 30%

The B vitamins are needed for the production of enzymes to handle the increased metabolic activity. Folic acid is particularly important because it is needed for DNA synthesis and maturation of red blood cells. Inadequate intake of folacin may lead to megaloblastic anemia. This type of anemia is commonly seen in women who have had multiple pregnancies.

Vitamin C requirements are increased by 20 milligrams, or 30%. Vitamin C is needed to produce the intercellular cement in connective and vascular tissues and to enhance absorption of iron. Sources of vitamin C include citrus fruits, berries, melons, and cabbage.

Vitamin D is needed to promote absorption of calcium and phosphorus. The prepregnancy requirement is increased by 5 micrograms of cholecalciferol, or 100%. Sources of vitamin D include fortified milk and margarine, butter, liver, and egg yolks.

A pregnant woman's diet should include at least 1 quart of milk daily to provide calcium, phosphorus, riboflavin, and vitamin D. One pint of milk provides 18 grams of protein, or 60% of the additional protein required. Milk substitutes, such as yogurt and cheeses, may replace some of the milk.

Pregnant women should eat 4 ounces or more of food selected from the meat group, which includes organ meats, fish, poultry, meats, eggs, nuts, and legumes. From the fruit and vegetable group, they should select five to seven or more servings. A citrus fruit and a potato should be included daily, with leafy green or dark yellow vegetables (for vitamin A and folacin) three or four times weekly. Two to four or more daily servings from the bread and cereal group are recommended, with emphasis on whole grains and enriched cereals and pastas. At least 1 to 2 tablespoons of butter or margarine are recommended. Pregnant women should have at least 6 to 8 glasses of water daily. They should avoid saccharin, alcohol, excessive intake of caffeine, and all drugs not specifically prescribed by their obstetricians.

Vegans can satisfy their protein requirements by using complementary plant proteins. The elimination of animal proteins from the diet may necessitate calcium and vitamin B_{12} supplementation. Iron absorption may be compromised in the absence of heme iron. Heme iron is supplied by meats. Pregnant vegetarians should be encouraged to include milk in their diets.

Women who are lactose intolerant may be able to substitute yogurt and buttermilk for milk. When milk is restricted, they need to find alternative sources of vitamins A and D.

Diet can be helpful in the management of some complications of pregnancy. Morning sickness, a mild and transitory nausea and vomiting that occurs in the first trimester, may be relieved by frequent, dry meals consisting of easily digested carbohydrates. Fluids should be taken between meals rather than at mealtimes. Crackers or dry popcorn eaten before arising in the morning may allay nausea. Food odors may trigger nausea; if a pregnant woman does not have to prepare her food, she may be able to eat. Nutritional reserves, from sound preconceptual nutrition, help pregnant women nourish their fetuses despite such periods of nausea and vomiting.

Heartburn, the regurgitation of gastric contents into the esophagus through a relaxed cardiac sphincter, may also be relieved by dry meals. Pregnant women should also be counseled to avoid fried, strongly flavored, and highly spiced foods.

Constipation develops as the enlarging uterus presses on the lower intestinal tract. A relaxation of the gastrointestinal tract also occurs in pregnancy. Constipation may be prevented or relieved by increased intake of fluids and the inclusion of laxative foods in the diet. Laxative foods include whole grains, bran, prunes, figs, fruits, and fruit juices.

Eclampsia is characterized by hypertension, proteinuria, and edema occurring after the twentieth week of gestation. The treatment of eclampsia no longer involves sodium restriction and diuretics. Pregnant women need sodium and iodine from iodized salt. The kidneys are efficient during pregnancy and capable of maintaining sodium balance. Eclamptic women are usually hospitalized for bed rest and management of hypertension. Self-imposed salt restriction or the use of nonprescription "water pills" shoud be vigorously discouraged as unnecessary and dangerous.

NURSING IMPLICATIONS

- Patients should be cautioned against fasting before prenatal appointments to reduce weight. Fasting leads to acidosis, which can cause fetal damage.
- Pregnant women sometimes ingest clay or starch. Clay is believed to relieve morning sickness and hunger pains. Clay has no food value but can interfere with absorption of iron. Cornstarch contains 465 kcal per cup and no other nutritive value. Laundry starch is also eaten.

Pregnancy in Adolescence

Pregnancy occurring before physical maturity presents numerous problems. Pregnant teenagers must meet their own nutritional needs for growth and development as well as the additional nutritional demands of pregnancy. The growth spurt in American girls occurs between 10½ and 13 years and is usually complete by 17 years. Pregnancy occurring within 4 years of the menarche places the mother-to-be at biologic risk because of anatomic and physiologic immaturity. The greatest risk of adolescent pregnancy is to the fetus, who has an increased incidence of low birth weight, malformation, and mortality. There is an increased incidence of eclampsia in pregnant adolescents.

The rapid increase in the incidence of adolescent pregnancies will lead to more scientific knowledge of the nutritional needs of the mother and fetus. At present, nutritional recommendations are based on the RDAs for the woman, which depend on her age plus the established increases for pregnancies. Diets for pregnant adolescents should include adequate Calories for a 24- to 30-pound weight gain, usually an increase of 300 kcal per day. The protein requirements are 1.7 grams per kilogram of ideal body weight for girls less than 15 years of age and 1.5 grams per kilogram for those more than 15 years of age. The recommended milk intake is 6 cups per day, or the equivalent from the milk group for protein and calcium needs.

Diet counseling may be difficult. Most teenage girls do not want to gain weight. Every attempt should be made to modify their usual diets to meet the demands of pregnancy. Suggestions like the substitution of a cheeseburger for a hamburger are more likely to be effective than are rigid directions about protein intake. Tofu is a good source of protein and calcium and a food that might appeal to pregnant adolescents. Pregnant adolescents should be encouraged to substitute needed nutrients for empty Calories; milk beverages could replace carbonated beverages. The eating habits of pregnant adolescents should be respected; frequent snacking is fine. Suggestions for snacks might include peanuts, raw vegetable sticks, cheese, and dry popcorn. A pregnant adolescent's interest in food should be used to teach good nutrition. The diet of a pregnant adolescent is most apt to be deficient in calcium, iron, vitamin A, and vitamin C.

Lactation

DIET

Lactation imposes a greater physiologic stress on women than does pregnancy and necessitates further increases in nutritional support. The energy requirements are increased by 300 kcal per day over the pregnancy needs or 500 kcal per day over the nonpregnancy needs. It takes 400 kcal per day to produce breast milk; the milk produced contains 20 kcal per ounce. Protein requirements are increased by 20 grams over nonpregnancy requirements, a reduction of 10 grams from the requirements of pregnancy.

Calcium needs are the same as for pregnancy. Calcium is no longer needed for formation of bones; it is now needed as a component of breast milk. The RDAs for energy, vitamin A, niacin, riboflavin, iodine, and zinc are higher than for pregnancy. The RDAs for protein, folacin, and iron are less than for pregnancy. The RDAs for vitamins C, D, E, B_6, B_{12}, thiamine, calcium, phosphorus, and magnesium remain the same as the pregnancy recommendations.

Colostrum, the initial postpartum secretion from the maternal breasts, contains 67 kcal per 100 milliliters (21 kcal per ounce); colostrum contains more protein, sodium, potassium, chloride, vitamin A, niacin, tocopherol, and antibodies than does breast milk. Breast milk cannot be perfectly synthesized in the laboratory. It is composed of more than 100 constituents, including nutrients, enzymes, hormones, and antibodies. Breast milk protects against respiratory infections, enteric infections, and allergies (Beal, 1980). Nutritionally it contains one-third of the protein of cow's milk. The carbohydrate of breast milk is mainly lactose, and the content is higher than cow's milk. The fat content of breast milk is variable and accounts for about 50% of the Calories. Breast milk contains the essential fatty acid linoleic acid. The calcium to phosphorus ratio is 2:1, which is optimal for calcium absorption. Breast milk produces a small curd that is easy to digest and absorb.

Infants may be breast-fed within 6 hours of delivery, when general anesthesia has not been used. Early initiation of breast-feeding promotes bonding and stimulates production of milk. Breast-feeding should be on a demand basis to promote production and flow of milk. If supplemental feedings are necessary, they should be given after the nursing period, not before or in place of. Breast milk can be expressed manually and frozen for future use.

The diet for a lactating woman should be a continuation of the recommended diet for pregnancy, with the following additions. The increased intake of Calories should come from sources of vitamins A and C, niacin, riboflavin, and zinc (leafy green vegetables, citrus fruits, whole grains, milk, meats, and poultry). The daily quart of milk or equivalent requirement continues; the total fluid intake is increased to 3 quarts per day from milk, water, and juices. The diet should contain an increased amount of citrus fruit, leafy green and dark yellow vegetables, and iodized salt.

NURSING IMPLICATIONS

- After the first month of nursing, there may be a disparity between supply and demand. This disparity usually adjusts itself within 24 hours with more frequent feedings. It should not be taken as an indication of the need for supplemental feedings or weaning.

- There is no need to restrict intake of chocolate or spicy foods; they have been shown to be nonirritating to the infant's gastrointestinal tract.
- Coffee, alcohol, and drugs are excreted in breast milk and should be used only under a physician's direction.

Young Adulthood (18 to 40 Years)

With the end of the growth period, the demand for most nutrients is reduced. Food intake in mature adults is needed to provide nutrients for the maintenance and repair of body cells. The life-style of young adults usually changes. They may leave the parental home, establish an independent home, and assume responsibility for food slection and preparation. The type of employment may influence eating habits, particularly when cocktails and business lunches are the established procedure. Young adults without the time or interest to prepare meals rely heavily on eating out or convenience foods, both of which often contribute excessive amounts of salt and refined sugar to the diet. A young mother at home with young children may develop the habit of finishing her child's meal to avoid waste. Obesity may gradually become a problem as a more sedentary life-style is adopted.

Young adult women who use oral contraceptives need extra folacin, vitamin C, riboflavin, vitamin B_6, and vitamin B_{12}. Young adult women who use intrauterine devices need extra iron and vitamin C to compensate for increased menstrual losses.

The recommended daily selections from the basic four food groups for young adults include:

- Milk group: 2 or more servings
- Meat group: 2 or more servings
- Vegetable and fruit group: 4 or more servings. The need for citrus fruit each day continues as does the recommendation for leafy green and dark yellow vegetables three or four times weekly.
- Bread and cereal group: 4 or more servings
- 1 to 2 tablespoons of butter or margarine

Middle Adulthood (40 to 65 Years)

Adults in their middle years usually are more sedentary and need to reduce caloric intake accordingly. Improved financial status may increase the intake of rich foods and the frequency of dining out. Business or social lunches may be an important aspect of a middle-aged adult's lifestyle. Food may be used as consolation for business failure or family desolation. Body image may become a less important influence on weight control.

The middle-aged adult's selections from the basic four food groups are the same as the young adult's selections; the need for Calories is reduced.

Older Adulthood (65 + Years)

DIET

Older adults have decreased needs for energy and for niacin, thiamine, and riboflavin, which are related to energy requirements. The need for iodine is reduced because the activity of the thyroid gland decreases. There are no increased needs.

Income is probably the most important influence on diet. Many older adults must limit the amount of their fixed income that is spent on food to meet other financial obligations. Food shopping may be difficult because of physical disability or lack of transportation. Living alone and dining alone decrease the pleasure of preparing and eating meals. Therapeutic diets necessitated by medical conditions may not be appealing. Loss of teeth makes chewing difficult. One-half of the 65-year-olds are edentulous. Two-thirds of 75-year-olds have no teeth. Dentures increase bitter and sour taste sensations. There is a normal altering of taste because of a reduction of the number of taste buds. Older adults have decreased secretion of gastric acid, which results in less efficient digestion.

The diets of older adults are typically high in breads, cakes, and cereals. Intake of proteins may be decreased because meats are difficult to chew and expensive. Intake of iron and calcium may be inadequate. Older adults should be encouraged to eat whole-grain cereals and breads and to substitute cheeses, eggs, and peanut butter for meats, if necessary as sources of proteins, and to continue intake of milk, if possible, as a source of calcium and proteins. In general, the diet of older adults should be low in fat, high in fiber and iron, with good sources of vitamin B_{12} and calcium. The selections from the basic four food groups are the same as those for young adults. Older adults may wish to avoid hard, sticky foods that are difficult to chew.

NURSING IMPLICATIONS

- Older adults should be discouraged from abusing laxatives and should increase their intake of fiber and fluids instead.

- Anemic older adults who drink tea should be advised to use tannin-free tea because the tannin in tea inhibits absorption of iron.

References

Abrams, B. Helping pregnant teenagers eat right. *Nursing 81,* March 1981, *11,* 3.

Aftergood, L., & Alfin-Slater, R. Women and nutrition. *Contemporary Nutrition,* March 1980, *5,* 3.

Beal, V. *Nutrition in the life span.* New York: John Wiley & Sons, 1980.

Busse, E. Eating in later life: Physiologic and psychologic factors. *Contemporary Nutrition,* November 1979, *4,* 11.

Carruth, B. Adolescent pregnancy and nutrition. *Contemporary Nutrition,* October 1980, *5,* 10.

Combs, K. Preventive care in the elderly. *American Journal of Nursing,* August 1978, *78,* 8.

Flynn, K. Iron deficiency anemia among the elderly. *Nurse Practitioner,* November 1978, *3,* 11.

Heslin, J. Milk—Which one is best for baby? *American Baby,* February 1980, *42,* 3.

Howard, R., & Herbold, N. *Nutrition in clinical care.* New York: McGraw-Hill Book Company, 1978.

Lockhart, J. Breast milk. *Contemporary Nutrition,* January 1979, *4,* 1.

Nutrition Reviews. *The development of adipose tissue in infancy. Nutrition Reviews.* June 1979, *37,* 6.

Price, J. Nutrition for the elderly. *Journal of Nursing Care,* April 1979, *12,* 3.

Ripa, L. Nursing habits and dental decay in infants: "Nursing bottle caries." *Contemporary Nutrition,* May 1978, *3,* 5.

Runyan, T. *Nutrition for today.* New York: Harper & Row Publishers, 1976.

Scarpa, L., & Kiefer, H. (Eds.). *Sourcebook on food and nutrition* (2nd ed.). Chicago: Marquis Academic Media, 1980.

Suitor, C., & Hunter, M. *Nutrition: Principles and application in health promotion.* Philadelphia: J. B. Lippincott Company, 1980.

Swanson, J. A toddler's eating habits. *Pediatric Nursing,* January/February 1979, *5,* 1.

Williams, S. *Nutrition and diet therapy* (3rd ed.). St. Louis: C. V. Mosby Company, 1977.

Wills, B. Food becomes fun for children. *American Journal of Nursing,* December 1978, *78,* 12.

Winick, M. Nutrition and aging. *Contemporary Nutrition,* June 1977, *2,* 6.

Woodruff, C. Supplementary foods for infants. *Contemporary Nutrition,* January 1981, *6,* 1.

Worthington, B., Vermeersch, J., & Williams, S. *Nutrition in pregnancy and lactation.* St. Louis: C. V. Mosby Company, 1977.

Wurtman, J. What do children eat? *Journal of Nursing Care,* June 1978, *11,* 6.

22
Enteral Nutrition

Some patients have difficulty ingesting sufficient nutrients to meet their bodies' needs. Patients are fed orally, enterally, or parenterally. The oral route is the route of choice when possible. However, some patients are unable or unwilling to eat enough to meet their needs. If the intestinal tract is functional, it should be used. Enteral nutrition can provide adequate intake in many situations in which oral feedings are insufficient or medically contraindicated. Enteral feedings may be the only feeding technique used or may serve as a supplementary method.

Feedings are given via nasogastric tube (a feeding tube inserted through the nose into the stomach). This method is employed when patients have extreme anorexia, lesions of the mouth, after oral surgery, or difficulty swallowing. Patients who are unconscious, extremely weak, or psychotic may also be fed in this manner. The food administered is usually a liquid or semiliquid similar in consistency to foods that have been chewed and swallowed. Digestion and absorption take place in the normal manner. Tubes may also be placed directly into the esophagus (esophagostomy), stomach (gastrostomy), or jejunum (jejunostomy) by surgical incision. These tubes are sutured in place. In a cervical pharyngostomy, a feeding tube is placed in the hypopharynx through a stab incision in the neck; the tube is guided into the stomach and anchored with a suture at the incision.

Tube feedings may be given intermittently (bolus feedings) or by slow, continuous drip. Bolus feedings more closely resemble the normal pattern of food ingestion and permit the patient more freedom of activity. The maximal amount given in a bolus feeding is usually 300 milliliters. Fine polyethylene nasogastric feeding tubes reduce nasal discomfort and permit the delivery of the feeding by slow, continuous drip. Continuous drip feedings flow by gravity or are controlled by a pump. The continuous feeding improves absorption and reduces diarrhea, which is frequently associated with tube feedings. Continuous-drip feedings are regulated in the same manner as intravenous infusions. If the rate slows, catching up by increasing the rate is not permitted because it leads to cramping and diarrhea. Patients who receive constant-drip feedings sometimes experience gastric stasis. They should be watched closely for gastric distention, which can lead to gastric rupture. Other symptoms of gastric distention include epigastric and left upper quadrant pain and increasing abdominal girth. Gastric distention can be relieved by periodically disconnecting the tube from the infusion set.

Patients who receive bolus tube feedings may have their stomachs aspirated before each feeding to check for gastric residual. The usual rule is to withhold the feeding if more than 150 milliliters are aspirated. The gastric residual is reinstilled (up to 150 milliliters) because it contains useful gastric secretions and electrolytes. Infants and young children are especially vulnerable to electrolyte imbalance. Consistent residuals in excess of 150 milliliters should prompt reassessment of the feeding regimen.

Tube feedings must be nutritionally adequate, well tolerated by the patient, and easy to digest. Traditionally, tube feedings were prepared with a milk or egg base. Concern about lactose intolerance and cholesterol content have made these feedings less popular. There is a wide variety of commercially prepared products available to meet the individual requirements of many types of patients. Meals mixed in a blender have also been used as tube feedings in an attempt to conform to a typical food intake. Patients are shown a tray of food, which is then liquefied and fed via the tube. Pureed baby foods are also used to prepare balanced meals mixed in a blender.

Commercial products offer ease of preparation and consistency of nutrient content. Compleat-B (Doyle) is an example of a milk-based tube feeding. It contains sucrose, corn oil, beef, fruits, vegetables, minerals, and vitamins in addition to the milk and supplies 1 Calorie per milliliter. Ensure (Ross) is a lactose-free tube feeding. Ensure contains caseinate and soy proteins, corn syrup, sucrose, corn oil, vitamins, and minerals.

Chemically defined diets, such as Vivonex Standard Diet (Norwich-Eaton) and Flexical Elemental Diet (Mead Johnson Nutritional), require little or no digestion, are totally absorbed, and leave minimal residue in the upper portion of the small intestine. Chemically defined diets are also called elemental or space diets.

There are three basic types of enteral feedings that differ in osmolarity, digestibility, caloric density, lactose content, viscosity, and fat content. Isocal Complete Liquid Diet (Mead Johnson Nutritional) and Ensure are polymeric preparations of proteins, fats, and carbohydrates. They have a high molecular weight and a low osmolarity. They require normal digestion for the protein and fat. They deliver 1 kcal per milliliter.

Vivonex Standard Diet and Flexical are hyperosmolar mixtures of amino acids and monosaccharides. They do not contain triglycerides or starch, are ready to be absorbed without digestion, and deliver 1 kcal per milliliter.

TABLE 22-1
COMMON TUBE FEEDINGS

Feedings (1,000 cu cm)	How Supplied	Preparation	Uses	Calories	Carbohydrate (grams)	Protein (grams)	Fat (grams)	Sodium (milligrams)	Potassium (milligrams)	mOsm/kg	Points of Interest
Ensure	Canned	None	May also be given by mouth flavored	1,060	144.5	37.1	37.10	740	1,270	450	Lactose free
Ensure Plus	Canned	None	May also be given by mouth flavored	1,500	199.0	55.0	53.30	1,060	1,900	600	Lactose free
Nutri 1000	Canned	None	Also by mouth	1,060	101.0	40.0	55.00	520	1,458	400	Lactose free
Osmolite	Canned	None	Also by mouth	1,060	143.0	37.0	38.00	541	875	300	Lactose free
Sustacal	Canned and powdered	1 packet to 1 cup of milk	Also by mouth	1,000	148.0	65.0	24.00	1,000	2,220	625	
Citrotein	Powdered	¼ cup to ¼ cup of water	Also by mouth	533	97.9	32.2	1.4	546	546	496	Lactose free, low residue
Flexical	Powdered	1½ cup to 3 cups of water	Also by mouth	1,000	152.5	22.5	0.34	350	1,250	805	Lactose free, low residue

Product	Form	Preparation	Route								Comments
Meritene	Powdered	4 tablespoons to 1 cup of milk	Also by mouth	922	103.2	59.9	30.00	832	2,564	560	
Portagen	Powdered	1½ cups to 28 ounces of water	Also by mouth	1,000	112.0	34.0	46.00	400	100	354	Lactose free, medium-chain, triglycerides
Precision LR	Powdered	1 packet to 1 cup of water	Also by mouth	1,080	215.0	21.0	0.70	600	1,500	600	Lactose free, low residue
Vipep	Powdered	1 packet to 8½ ounces of water	Also by mouth	1,000	175.5	25.0	25.00	750	850	520	Lactose free, low residue
Vital	Powdered	1 packet to 8½ ounces of water	Also by mouth	1,000	185.0	41.6	10.20	382	1,164	450	Lactose free, low residue
Vivonex	Powdered	1 packet to 8½ ounces of water	Also by mouth flavored	1,000	225.0	20.4	13.00	860	1,170	550	Lactose free, low residue
Vivonex HN	Powdered	1 packet to 8½ ounces of water	Also by mouth flavored	1,000	202.0	41.7	8.60	770	702	844	Lactose free, low residue

Source: Green, M., & Harry, J. Nutrition in contemporary nursing practice. New York: John Wiley & Sons, 1980, by permission of the publisher.

The third type of feeding is a high-density feeding for patients who have fluid restrictions. A small-volume, high-Calorie mixture is prepared from commercial protein and carbohydrate products to yield 2 kcal per milliliter. Oils or medium-chain triglycerides can be added to further increase the caloric content. See Table 22-1 for a comparison of common tube feedings.

Generally, 1,000 to 1,500 milliliters (1,000 to 1,500 kcal) of the feeding are given daily to maintain nutritional balance. In enteral hyperalimentation, 2,500 milliliters or more are given daily. Patients may be maintained on enteral nutrition for days or years. A wide variety of formulas and additives are available to allow individualization of feedings to satisfy a patient's specific requirements for Calories, fluid volume, replacement needs, and enzyme deficiencies.

Most tube feedings are hyperosmolar and can cause cramping and diarrhea, especially when given too rapidly. When enteral nutrition is started, the feeding is usually diluted to one-third to one-half strength and regulated to flow at 50 to 100 milliliters per hour. The feeding is increased to full strength gradually over a 3-day period. Gastric aspirations are performed every 4 hours to check for gastric stasis. Blood and urine are monitored for hyperglycemia and glycosuria, which can develop as a result of the carbohydrate load of the feeding. Blood urea nitrogen and serum albumin levels are watched to monitor protein intake. Fluid volume and electrolyte concentrations should be evaluated. Most patients who receive tube feedings need additional water. Intermittent feedings should be preceded and followed by ingestion of water. Patients who are permitted fluids by mouth should be encouraged to take them to aid in reestablishing oral intake as well as to increase fluid intake.

Patients who receive high-glucose, hyperosmolar feedings can experience hyperglycemic, hyperosmolar, nonketotic coma, which is a life-threatening complication. Hyperglycemic, hyperosmolar, nonketotic coma develops as a result of solute overload and inadequate hydration. The symptoms include polyuria, thirst, and changes in the level of consciousness. Blood and urinary levels of glucose should be monitored to permit early recognition of rising glucose levels. The treatment is insulin to lower blood glucose levels and hydration to reduce osmolarity.

NURSING IMPLICATIONS

- Nasogastric feeding tubes irritate the nares. The use of a small-caliber tube and frequent nasal care provide comfort.
- Oral hygiene is essential when patients are undergoing tube feeding, unless contraindicated by oral surgery.
- Cramping and diarrhea may be relieved by slowing the rate or reducing the concentration of the feeding.

- Diphenoxylate hydrochloride with atropine (Lomotil) or paregoric may be prescribed for persistent diarrhea.
- Pectin, applesauce, or banana may be added to the feeding to thicken the stools.
- Chemically defined diets produce little residue, and patients on such diets have bowel movements about once every 5 days.
- Ideally, patients should be tube fed when sitting up or with the head of the bed elevated 30 to 45 degrees to prevent aspiration.
- Ambulation should be encouraged when possible because active muscles make the best use of proteins. Physical therapy can be helpful for bedfast patients. Physical activity also improves the morale of such patients.
- Feedings should be prepared in 24-hour amounts and refrigerated until needed.
- Bolus feedings are usually administered at room temperature.
- Constant-drip feedings can be placed in ice packs to prevent spoiling. Some pumps and feeding tubes have attached containers for ice.

References

Butterworth, C., & Weinsier, R. Malnutrition in hospital patients: Assessment and treatment. In R. Goodhart & M. Shils (Eds.), *Modern nutrition in health and disease* (6th ed.). Philadelphia: Lea & Febiger, 1980.

Feldtman, R., & Andrassy, R. Meeting exceptional nutritional needs. 2. Elemental enteral alimentation. *Postgraduate Medicine,* September 1978, *63,* 3.

Green, M., & Harry, J. *Nutrition in contemporary nursing practice.* New York: John Wiley & Sons, 1981.

Griggs, B., & Hoppe, M. Update nasogastric tube feeding. *American Journal of Nursing,* March 1979, *79,* 3.

Heymsfield, S., Bethel, R., Ansley, J., et al. Enteral hyperalimentation: An alternative to central venous hyperalimentation. *Annals of Internal Medicine,* January 1979, *90,* 1.

Hunt, S., Groff, J., & Holbrook, J. *Nutrition: Principles and clinical practice.* New York: John Wiley & Sons, 1980.

Kaminski, M. Enteral hyperalimentation. *Surgery, Gynecology & Obstetrics,* July 1976, *143,* 7.

Krause, M., & Mahan L. *Food, nutrition and diet therapy* (6th ed.). Philadelphia: W. B. Saunders Company, 1979.

Metheny, N., & Snively, W. *Nurses' handbook of fluid balance* (3rd ed.). Philadelphia: J. B. Lippincott Company, 1979.

Mitty, W., Nealon, T., & Grossi, C. Use of elemental diets in surgical cases. *American Journal of Gastroenterology,* April 1976, *65,* 4.

Suitor, C., & Hunter, M. *Nutrition: Principles and application in health promotion.* Philadelphia: J. B. Lippincott Company, 1980.

Whaley, L., & Wong, D. *Nursing care of infants and children.* St. Louis: C. V. Mosby Company, 1979.

23
Peripheral Vein Intravenous Nutrition

Parenteral nutrition is nutrition that is delivered to the patient by routes other than the alimentary tract (enteral nutrition). *Subcutaneous* and *intravenous* administration are the two major parenteral routes. Subcutaneous fluid administration (hypodermoclysis), although easier to initiate and maintain, is used infrequently because of the limitations placed on the types of fluid that can be used. Fluids administered by hypodermoclysis must be similar in tonicity and electrolyte content to extracellular fluid.

When enteral feedings are contraindicated, intravenous feedings provide a rapid and controlled method of replacing body fluids and nutrients. A "keep vein open" (KVO) intravenous line is often used for drug administration or as a precaution against the possible need for intravenous access for fluids or electrolytes. Recently, amino acids, glucose, and emulsified fat have been used to provide nutrition through peripheral veins. Peripheral vein intravenous nutrition is safer than central vein intravenous nutrition, although it places limitations on the type and quantity of the solutions administered (central vein intravenous nutrition is discussed in Chapter 24).

Intravenous feedings are used as stopgap measures until oral feedings can be resumed. *Maintenance intravenous therapy* is used to sustain homeostasis in patients who are unable to take nourishment by mouth but who do not have any fluid, electrolyte, or nutritional deficit. Preoperative and postoperative patients are frequently placed on maintenance intravenous therapy. *Replacement intravenous therapy* provides fluids, electrolytes, and nutrients lost through disease processes. Intravenous feedings are prepared to satisfy a patient's individual needs.

307

Fluids

REQUIREMENTS

A wide variety of intravenous fluids are available to meet individual patient needs. Approximately 2,500 to 3,500 milliliters of fluid are needed daily to carry out normal body metabolism. These figures are predicated on normal kidney function and do not include provisions for increased fluid losses or hypermetabolic states. Inadequate kidney function reduces fluid requirements. Increased fluid losses (vomiting, diarrhea, diaphoresis, wound drainage) and hypermetabolic states (fever, hyperthyroidism) increase fluid requirements.

Normally, water constitutes 60 to 70% of adult body weight. A loss of 20 to 30% of body water is usually fatal. A 10% water loss is a serious disruption of homeostasis. Under normal conditions, adult fluid requirements are 30 milliliters per kilogram of body weight. Neonates and infants need 120 to 150 milliliters per kilogram, and children need 120 to 130 milliliters per kilogram.

Excessive administration of intravenous fluid can lead to overhydration, fluid overload, pulmonary edema, and water intoxication. Adults can usually tolerate 35 to 50 milliliters per kilogram, or 3 to 3.5 liters, per day without danger of overhydration. The range is considerably narrower for infants, children, and older people.

SOLUTIONS

Intravenous fluids are classified as isotonic, hypotonic, or hypertonic. An isotonic intravenous solution has the same tonicity (osmotic pressure) as blood. Isotonic fluids introduced intravenously remain within the vascular system; there is no fluid shift to or from the blood. When hypotonic solutions are administered intravenously, the fluid is drawn out of the blood vessels by osmosis into the interstitial spaces and body cells. Hypertonic intravenous solutions have greater osmotic pressure than does blood. Fluid is drawn from the interstitial spaces and cells into the bloodstream when hypertonic solutions are administered intravenously.

Hydrating solutions are composed of carbohydrates and water or saline. A mixture of 5% dextrose in water is considered nearly isotonic; however, the dextrose is metabolized as soon as it reaches the bloodstream, leaving a hypotonic solution to be drawn into the interstitial spaces and cells. When rapid fluid replacement is desirable, 5% dextrose solutions can be given as quickly as 8 to 10 milliliters per minute.

Balanced solutions (Ringer's, Butler's) contain water and electrolytes. The electrolyte concentration of a balanced solution is a balance between the minimal physiologic needs and the maximal tolerance. Specific electrolyte deficits can be corrected by adding concentrated electrolyte solutions to hydrating solutions.

NURSING IMPLICATIONS

- Fluid losses are more critical in very young and very old people. Fluid represents a higher percentage of body weight in infants and children. Older people have less fluid reserves.
- Sterile water should never be given intravenously; it causes hydrolysis of red blood cells.
- Hypertonic intravenous solutions cause sclerosis and phlebitis of infused veins.
- Hypertonic solutions are useful in providing Calories or electrolytes without excessive fluid to patients with reduced kidney function.
- Hypertonic solutions of dextrose and mannitol are used to reduce edema by creating osmotic diuresis (the hypertonic fluid pulls fluid from the interstitial spaces into the blood; the blood circulates to the kidney, where the increased blood volume and pressure increase urinary output).
- Hypertonic solutions must be given slowly and in carefully controlled amounts.

Carbohydrates

REQUIREMENTS

The addition of carbohydrates to intravenous fluids provides a source of Calories. Carbohydrates are metabolized for energy, sparing the body protein that is burned when there is inadequate oral intake of carbohydrates. Carbohydrate intravenous solutions increase the liver glycogen stores. Carbohydrates are metabolized into energy, carbon dioxide, and water. Carbohydrate solutions are electrolyte free, but pure electrolyte solutions may be added as required. Glycosuria results when carbohydrate solutions are administered too rapidly. The body is unable to use all the dextrose as quickly as it is being infused.

Only the monosaccharides glucose, fructose, and invert sugar can be administered intravenously and be absorbed from the bloodstream by the body cells. Disaccharides and polysaccharides cannot be used by the body when given intravenously. A 5% dextrose solution provides 50 grams of dextrose per liter. Dextrose supplies 3.4 kcal per gram; 1 liter of 5% dextrose provides 170 kcal. The basic caloric requirement of an adult on bed rest is estimated to be 1,600 kcal per day; this figure does not include the increased demands imposed by fever or hypermetabolism. To provide the 1,600 kcal using 5% dextrose, 9 liters per day would be required. This amount is almost three times the amount of fluid that can be safely given intravenously in a 24-hour period. Hypertonic dextrose solutions are sometimes used to increase the caloric content. Hypertonic solutions must be given slowly to avoid damaging the infused vein. Too rapid administration of hypertonic glucose also stimulates the production of insulin and can lead to hypoglycemic reactions when the intravenous infusion is discontinued. Insulin to cover the rise in blood glucose content is sometimes given with hypertonic glucose solutions to prevent this overstimulation of insulin production.

Hypertonic dextrose solutions (20 to 50%) are sometimes used in the treatment of patients who cannot tolerate large volumes of fluid because of kidney failure. These highly concentrated solutions must be given slowly into a large vein to avoid circulatory overload and damage to the infused vessel. Dextrans, polymers of glucose, are used as plasma volume expanders in the presence of hemorrhage. Dextrans are heavy enough to act as albumin and hold fluid when the blood loss does not exceed one-third of the circulating volume. Dextrans survive in the bloodstream for about 24 hours, after which time they are degraded and excreted. The caloric content of commonly used carbohydrate solutions is listed in Table 23-1.

NURSING IMPLICATIONS

- The maximal rate for a dextrose infusion is 0.5 gram per kilogram of body weight per hour (Metheny & Snively, 1979). Fructose and invert sugar can be administered at a slightly more rapid rate.
- Fructose solutions do not require insulin for utilization, but they can cause a rise in the serum level of lactic acid, leading to lactic acidosis.

TABLE 23-1
CALORIC CONTENT OF COMMONLY USED
CARBOHYDRATE SOLUTIONS

	Kilocalories per Liter
Isotonic solutions	
5% dextrose in water/saline	170
5% fructose	187.5
5% invert sugar	187.5
Hypotonic solutions	
2.5% dextrose in water/saline	85
Hypertonic solutions	
10% dextrose in water/saline	340
10% fructose	375
10% invert sugar	375
20% dextrose	680
50% dextrose	1,700

Proteins

REQUIREMENTS

The protein requirement of a healthy adult is 0.8 gram per kilogram of body weight per day. Children require 0.8 to 2.0 grams per kilogram per day. Intravenous carbohydrate solutions may slow the body catabolism for a short period; however, the ability to supply protein intravenously aids in the maintenance of a positive nitrogen balance or in the correction of a nitrogen deficit. Intravenous protein solutions provide 4 kcal per gram of protein and the eight essential amino acids.

SOLUTIONS

Amino acid solutions (crystalline amino acids) are supplied in a 3.5% solution, which provides 140 kcal per liter and the essential and nonessential amino acids. Crystalline amino acids do not have the polypeptide bonding present in protein hydrolysates. This bonding is the cause of some reactions to intravenous protein administration. The 3.5% solution is nearly isotonic. There appear to be few adverse physiologic effects with the use of crystalline amino acids. Intravenous protein is expensive, does not provide an adequate energy source, and cannot be used as the exclusive source of Calories for patients with limited fat stores.

Protein hydrolysates are derived from casein or fibrin. They contain a mixture of essential and nonessential amino acids bonded together as polypeptides. Peptides have been shown to cause nausea and vomiting. Protein hydrolysates are less expensive and more concentrated sources of nitrogen than are synthetic amino acids. Disadvantages of protein hydrolysates include hyperosmolarity and the presence of some nitrogen in the form of dipeptides or tripeptides. Dipeptides and tripeptides are used less efficiently by the body than are amino acids. Protein hydrolysates may cause allergic reactions and are not suitable as the exclusive source of Calories.

Nitrogen balance can be improved by the use of intravenous amino acids, either alone or in conjunction with intravenous dextrose and fat. The improvement in nitrogen balance is greater with the use of amino acids intravenously than with intravenous dextrose alone. The basis for the use of amino acids in preference to dextrose to improve nitrogen balance is the following theory: Intravenous glucose stimulates production of insulin; increased blood levels of insulin are thought to prevent lipolysis of fat stores; and lipolysis of fat stores provides a source of energy. When amino acids are administered intravenously, they do not stimulate production of insulin and permit the mobilization of fatty acids that can be metabolized for energy. Fat metabolism and ketogenesis are desirable methods of reducing protein waste only in patients who have adequate fat deposits.

Protein loss during stress is reduced by the use of amino acids. Amino acids administered during catabolism can be converted to glucose and used for energy and also spare body protein in the same manner as does dextrose. Visceral protein mass can be maintained by 1 to 1.5 grams of protein per kilogram of ideal body weight.

Intravenous protein must be administered slowly. Usually, 1 to 2 liters per day is the maximal amount in the initial days of therapy. If the blood urea nitrogen level remains below 30 to 40 milligrams per 100 milliliter, the blood level of glucose falls to 100 milligrams per 100 milliliters, and ketones appear in the urine; this amount can be gradually increased to 3 to 4 liters per day (Metheny & Snively, 1979). The initial rate for protein hydrolysates is less than 2 milliliters per minute to permit observation for untoward reactions (nausea, vomiting, fever, chills, urticaria, abdominal pain). A slow rate is also indicated for patients with hepatic insufficiency. Intravenous protein cannot be given to patients with renal impairment because the kidneys must be able to excrete the nitrogenous wastes. A significant increase in the blood urea nitrogen level that is maintained for 3 consecutive days would necessitate discontinuing intravenous protein administration. Amino acid solutions are supplied in 3.5% (nearly isotonic) solutions and in 5 and 7% hypertonic solutions for use in peripheral vein intravenous nutrition.

NURSING IMPLICATIONS

- All unused solutions, cloudy solutions, and solutions that contain a precipitate must be discarded promptly.
- Drugs and other mixtures must not be added to protein solutions.
- Protein solutions should be refrigerated until they are used.
- Aminogen and Aminosol are protein hydrolysate solutions. Examples of crystalline amino acid solutions include Aminosyn, Freamine II, Travasol, and Veinamine.

Fat Emulsions

Intravenous dextrose and amino acid solutions delivered into peripheral veins cannot provide the total caloric requirements. The volume of fluid required to deliver the Calories would be excessive. The formulation of a safe, effective, intravenous fat emulsion has made total parenteral nutrition through a peripheral vein possible. Fat emulsions supply concentrated Calories in an isotonic solution. A 10% fat emulsion provides 1.1

kcal per milliliter, or 1,100 kcal per liter, as compared to 170 kcal per liter from 5% dextrose or 140 kcal per liter from 3.5% crystalline amino acids.

SOLUTIONS

Intralipid 10% is a 10% fat emulsion prepared from soybean oil; it is 54% linoleic acid and contains no nitrogen. Liprosyn is a 10% fat emulsion prepared from safflower oil; it contains 77% linoleic acid. Both solutions also contain egg yolk phospholipid emulsifiers, glycerol to adjust tonicity, and water.

Fat emulsions cannot be mixed with amino acids or any other intravenous drug or solution. Amino acid solutions and fat emulsions can be given through a two-bottle setup with a Y-tube connection just before the venipuncture. The lipid solution should be hung higher than the amino acid solution to prevent the lipid emulsion from flowing back up into the other solution.

Intravenous fat emulsions have two major functions. They serve as sources of linoleic acid to prevent or correct essential fatty acid deficiencies, and they are capable of replacing up to 60% of the glucose needs of the body. No more than 60% of the total caloric intake should be supplied by fats. Fat emulsions encourage nitrogen retention, weight gain, and wound healing. They may also protect peripheral veins from the slight hypertonicity of dextrose and amino acids and may reduce osmotic diuresis.

Fat emulsions are not recommended for premature infants or neonates with low birth weights because of their poor ability to clear fats and because of the risk for hyperlipidemia. Patients who are receiving fat emulsions should be observed for:

Chills
Fever
Dyspnea
Cyanosis
Nausea
Vomiting
Headache
Flushing
Chest pain
Back pain
Diaphoresis

Liver function and blood lipids should be monitored. Heparin may be used to promote fat clearance; it is particularly helpful for patients with peristent hyperlipidemia.

Fat emulsions are started at a slow flow rate and increased as the patient's reaction dictates. In adults, the emulsions are usually regulated at 1 milliliter per minute for the first 15 to 30 minutes and increased gradually to 125 milliliters per hour. Infusions in children are started at 0.1 milliliter per minute for the first 10 to 15 minutes and gradually increased to 1 gram per kilogram of body weight per 4 hours (Metheny & Snively, 1979).

NURSING IMPLICATIONS

- Fat emulsions are expensive.
- Fat emulsions tend to increase serum levels of cholesterol and are contraindicated in patients with serious liver disease and hyperlipidemia.
- Patients with preexisting pulmonary or vascular disease may be at risk when fat emulsions are used.
- Fat emulsions should not be mixed with electrolytes or other nutrients. Nothing should be added to fat emulsions.
- Filters should not be used with fat emulsions because of the size of the fat particles.
- Partially used solutions should be discarded.
- Intralipid 10% must be refrigerated for storage. Liprosyn does not require refrigeration. Refrigerated emulsions should be removed from the refrigerator at least 30 minutes before use.
- Fat emulsions should not be shaken. If the oil solution has separated, it should not be used.

Alcohol

SOLUTIONS

Ethyl alcohol can be used in combination with carbohydrates as an intravenous solution. Alcohol and carbohydrates provide a good source of Calories, permit glycogen storage, spare body protein, and provide sedation. Absolute ethyl alcohol provides 7 kcal per gram. A hypertonic solution of 5% alcohol and 5% dextrose provides 450 kcal per liter. A hypertonic solution of 10% alcohol and 5% dextrose supplies 750 kcal per liter. Alcohol does not necessitate the use of insulin when administered peripherally. Giving 200 to 300 milliliters of 5% alcohol within a 1-hour period provides sedation without intoxication (Metheny & Snively, 1979). When the rate of administration is faster than the body's ability to metabolize the alcohol solution, restlessness, inebriation, and coma result.

Side effects of intravenous alcohol include:

- Dulling of memory
- Loss of ability to concentrate
- Increased sense of well-being
- Increased pulse and respiration rates
- Vasodilatation

NURSING IMPLICATIONS

- Intravenous alcohol is contraindicated in patients with shock or impending shock.
- Intravenous alcohol should not be used in patients with epilepsy, severe hepatic dysfunction, or coronary thrombosis.
- Hypertonic alcohol solutions can cause phlebitis.

Vitamins

REQUIREMENTS

Vitamins are essential for the utilization of nutrients whether the nutrients are taken orally or parenterally. Vitamin requirements are increased in patients with stress, infections, burns, trauma, and after surgical procedures and during convalescence. Parenteral vitamins should be provided when there is inadequate oral intake or when a patient is being supported on intravenous therapy for more than 2 to 3 days.

The dosage of intravenous vitamins is usually 10 times the minimal daily requirements because of large urinary losses of vitamins. Vitamin B complex and vitamin C are frequently added to intravenous solutions; however, all vitamins can be given intravenously. The water-soluble vitamins, B complex and C, and water-miscible forms of the fat-soluble vitamins, A, D, and E, are available as intravenous multivitamin preparations. Folic acid, vitamin B_{12}, and vitamin K must be added separately to intravenous solutions because they are not included in multivitamin preparations.

NURSING IMPLICATIONS

- Occasionally, patients sensitive to thiamine hydrochloride, vitamin B_1, experience anaphylactic reactions characterized by weakness and pulmonary edema. Large doses and rapid administration of intravenous vitamin B_1 should be avoided.
- Vitamin K may cause flushing, sweating, and chest tightness.

Minerals

REQUIREMENTS

Patients who are undergoing prolonged intravenous therapy may need parenteral minerals. Iron can be given intramuscularly or intravenously to correct anemia. Zinc, copper, iodine, manganese, and chromium may be present as contaminants in amino acid solutions, but contaminants cannot be considered dependable sources. Patients who are maintained on intravenous nutrition for prolonged periods need basal amounts of trace elements. The basal needs are moderately increased in depleted and anabolic states. Severe depletion and catabolic states greatly increase the needs for trace elements. A commercial cocktail, Addamel, provides basal amounts of eight minerals: calcium, magnesium, manganese, iron, zinc, copper, fluoride, and iodide.

Electrolytes

REQUIREMENTS

The practice of adding electrolytes to intravenous solutions is well established. Recently, the need for additional electrolytes has been identified. Saline is the most familiar electrolyte replacement solution; it provides sodium and chloride. A 0.9% solution is isotonic. Hypotonic half-strength normal saline, 0.45%, and quarter-strength normal saline, 0.225%, are available alone or in combination with dextrose or other electrolytes. Hypertonic saline solutions of 3 or 5% are used when sodium depletion is severe.

SOLUTIONS

Electrolyte solutions are considered isotonic when the total electrolyte content is approximately 310 milliequivalents per liter. Hypotonic electrolyte solutions have an electrolyte concentration below 250 milliequivalents per liter. Hypertonic electrolyte solutions have an electrolyte concentration above 375 milliequivalents per liter.

Ringer's solution is an isotonic solution that contains sodium, potassium, calcium, and chloride in amounts similar to those in extracellular fluid. Ringer's solution is available with carbohydrates added as sources of energy. Lactated Ringer's solution is an isotonic solution that contains sodium, potassium, calcium, chloride, and lactate; it is a routine electrolyte replacement solution. Lactated Ringer's solution is useful in correcting metabolic acidosis and in replacing fluid losses from bile drainage, diarrhea, and burns because it closely resembles extracellular fluid in electrolyte contents. Commercial electrolyte solutions are available in a wide variety of electrolyte combinations to correct specific imbalances or to serve as a base for individual electrolyte additives.

Intravenous solutions that contain potassium require careful administration. Potassium should always be diluted to 20 to 40 milliequivalents per liter for adult patients. The rate of administration should not exceed 20 milliequivalents per hour. Older patients should receive potassium at even slower rates. Patients who require potassium in more concentrated solutions or at more rapid rates should undergo cardiac monitoring during the infusion. Hyperkalemia (elevated serum levels of potassium) can lead to cardiac arrest.

Calcium is usually given in amounts that represent 10% of the physiologic level. Excessive amounts of calcium or too rapid administration of calcium can result in cardiac arrest. Some people are hypersensitive to calcium; a check for sensitivity should be carried out before calcium is administered intravenously. Solutions that contain calcium should be started at a slow flow rate to allow time to detect hypersensitivity reactions. Calcium should not be added to solutions that contain bicarbonate and phosphate because these ions bind to calcium to form calcium carbonate and calcium phosphate, respectively, rendering the solution unusable and dangerous.

Magnesium is excreted by the kidneys and probably should be withheld from oliguric patients. Magnesium-containing solutions should be carefully regulated; rapid administration produces a sensation of warmth and can lead to cardiac arrest. A respiratory rate slower than 12 respirations per minute or the absence of deep tendon reflexes is a sign of hypermagnesemia. Intravenous calcium gluconate is the emergency therapy for seriously elevated serum levels of magnesium.

NURSING IMPLICATIONS

- A slowing pulse rate is an early sign of cardiac arrest.
- Potassium should never be given directly into intravenous tubing or directly into a vein; it should always be well diluted.
- Potassium should never be given under pressure.
- Intravenous solutions that contain potassium should be labeled conspicuously and should never be to allowed to run with the flow rate control wide open.
- When potassium is added to a solution, it should be well mixed in sufficient fluid so that its concentration remains within the range of 20 to 40 milliequivalents per liter.
- Intravenous solutions that contain potassium should not be administered until adequacy of urinary output has been established.
- Calcium causes sloughing of tissues if calcium solutions infiltrate.

- Calcium solutions are usually contraindicated in patients who are receiving digitalis. Calcium potentiates the action of digitalis and could lead to digitalis intoxication.

Total Parenteral Nutrition

Total parenteral nutrition via a peripheral vein is suitable for patients who require nutritional maintenance for short periods. A typical total parenteral nutrition admixture via a peripheral vein for a stable adult weighing 70 kilograms would be composed of the following components:

- Intravenous amino acids: 700 milliliters of a 7% solution, which would provide 49 grams of protein equivalent and 196 kcal
- 1,500 milliliters of 10% dextrose, which would provide 152 grams of carbohydrate and 517 kcal
- 1,260 milliliters of 10% fat emulsion, which would provide essential fatty acids and 1,386 kcal
- Total fluid volume = 3.5 liters
- Total Calories = 2,000
- Potassium, sodium, chloride, magnesium, and calcium added in appropriate amounts based on blood chemistry levels
- A multivitamin additive once daily

The fat emulsion would be administered through a Y-tube injection site located as close as possible to the venipuncture site. Maintenance nutritional therapy could be provided in this manner temporarily until oral intake could be resumed or until total parenteral nutrition through a central vein was deemed necessary for prolonged support.

References

Coran, A. Total intravenous feeding of infants and children without the use of a central venous catheter. *Annals of Surgery*, April 1974, *179*, 4.

Guhlow, L., & Kolb, J. Pediatric IVs: Special measures you must take. *RN*, March 1979, *42*, 3.

Intravenous nutrition handbook. Berkeley, Calif.: Cutter Laboratories, 1978.

Jacobson, N. How to administer those tricky lipid emulsions. *RN*, June 1979, *42*, 6.

Jeejeebhoy, K. *The role of fat in parenteral nutrition.* Chicago: Abbott Laboratories, 1979.

Karran, S., & Alberti, K. (Eds.). *Practical nutritional support.* New York: John Wiley & Sons, 1980.

Krause, M., & Mahan, K. *Food, nutrition and diet therapy* (6th ed.). Philadelphia: W. B. Saunders Company, 1979.

Law, D. Medical cure—Nutritional disaster. *Consultant,* June 1979, *19,* 6.

Luckmann, J., & Sorensen, K. *Medical-surgical nursing: A psychophysiologic approach* (2nd ed.). Philadelphia: W. B. Saunders Company, 1980.

Metheny, N., & Snively, W. *Nurses' handbook of fluid balance* (3rd ed.). Philadelphia: J. B. Lippincott Company, 1979.

Profile of aminosyn. Chicago: Abbott Laboratories, 1981.

Shils, M. Parenteral nutrition. In R. Goodhart, & M. Shils (Eds.), *Modern nutrition in health and disease* (6th ed.). Philadelphia: Lea & Febiger, 1980.

Silberman, H., Freehauf, M., Fong, G., et al: Parenteral nutrition with lipids. *Journal of the American Medical Association,* September 1977, *238,* 9.

Stroot, V., Lee, C., & Schaper, C. *Fluids and electrolytes: A practical approach* (2nd ed.). Philadelphia: F. A. Davis Company, 1977.

Suitor, C., & Hunter, M. *Nutrition: Principles and application in health promotion.* Philadelphia: J. B. Lippincott Company, 1980.

Vanamee, P. Parenteral nutrition. In *Nutrition reviews' present knowledge in nutrition* (4th ed.). New York: Nutrition Foundation, 1976.

24

Central Vein
Intravenous Nutrition

Central vein intravenous nutrition is a procedure by which nutrients are delivered intravenously through a catheter introduced into the subclavian vein and guided into the superior vena cava. For the purposes of this chapter, the following definitions are used. *Parenteral nutrition* is the process of supplying nutrients intravenously when it is unwise, impossible, or hazardous to supply them enterally. *Total parenteral nutrition* is the administration of sufficient nutrients by venous catheter to maintain anabolism. With the formulation of intravenous fat emulsions, it is possible to provide total parenteral nutrition via a peripheral vein for short periods (see Chapter 23). *Intravenous or parenteral hyperalimentation* is the administration, via a central vein, of sufficient nutrients (above the basal requirements) to achieve tissue synthesis, a positive nitrogen balance, and anabolism. *Hyperalimentation* is usually taken to mean nutrients in excess of maintenance needs. Suitor and Hunter (1980) relate the *hyper* to the hypertonic solutions used to achieve caloric requirements in the intravenous solutions. There is a tendency to use the terms *total parenteral nutrition* and *hyperalimentation* interchangeably. This chapter discusses the use of a central vein to provide nutrition as opposed to the use of a peripheral vein. Peripheral vein intravenous nutrition is safer than central vein nutrition but places limitations on the quantity of nutrients that can be administered.

The aim of central vein intravenous nutrition is to provide nutrients to maintain or increase lean body mass over an extended period. To satisfy the caloric needs of the body, a mixture of hypertonic dextrose, amino acids, vitamins, minerals, and electrolytes is administered.

PROCEDURE

A large central vein is needed to provide rapid dilution of the hyperosmolar solution. The superior vena cava provides appropriate dilution. The approach to the vena cava is usually through the subclavian vein in

320

adults and older children and through the internal or external jugular vein in young children and infants. The catheter is inserted under strict aseptic conditions, with the patient in Trendelenburg's position. The patient is asked to hold his or her breath and bear down (Valsalva's maneuver) when the catheter is inserted to prevent the formation of air emboli. Nurses may be asked to apply pressure on the abdomens of patients who are unable to comply with oral requests. The position of the catheter is checked by means of a roentgenogram. Sterile occlusive dressings are applied and changed regularly according to strict procedures to reduce the possibility of contamination. Sterile technique is mandatory during dressing, tubing, and bottle changes. Infection is a constant concern, and it is the major reason for discontinuing this therapy. The high dextrose content of the solution makes it an excellent medium for bacterial growth. Solutions are prepared under a laminar flow hood. A 24-hour supply is prepared and refrigerated until needed. Intravenous tubing and filters are changed daily; dressings are changed every 48 to 72 hours and as necessary to prevent contamination. Large clinical facilities have a team of physicians, dietitians, pharmacists, and nurses to oversee all aspects of the therapy. Such institutions report a lower incidence of infection. The intravenous solution is usually prepared in the pharmacy; in some agencies, however, the nurse is responsible for preparation of the solution.

INDICATIONS

Central vein intravenous nutrition is used when extended intravenous nutritional support is anticipated. It is not usually initiated for periods of less than 2 weeks. Shils (1980) stressed the need for early recognition of patients who are obviously going to be unable to eat for protracted periods and patients whose hypermetabolic states make it impossible for them to meet their nutritional needs orally or enterally. Central vein intravenous nutrition is frequently prescribed for patients who:

- Have lost more than 10% of their body weights
- Are unable to tolerate oral intake within 1 week after surgical procedures
- Have hypermetabolic states: major infections, burns, cancer
- Have congenital gastrointestinal anomalies
- Have been on routine intravenous therapy for 3 weeks
- Have inflammatory bowel diseases that interfere with absorption

NURSING INTERVENTION

The goals of nursing action when central vein intravenous nutrition is being administered include prevention of infection, maintenance of the prescribed flow rate, continuous patient assessment, and emotional support. Each facility has its own protocol for dressing technique. Infection control is improved when special teams teach and oversee the dressing, tubing, and bottle changes. It is easier to detect subtle differences in the appearance of the incision when the same nurses are responsible for the dressings. The intravenous feeding line should never be used for any other purpose (blood samples, intravenous drugs, central venous pressure readings); its integrity must be maintained. The flow rate must be carefully monitored. Infusion pumps may be used, but they do not eliminate the need for constant vigilance. A rate slower than ordered can lead to hypoglycemia and undernutrition. A more rapid rate can result in hyperglycemia, fluid overload, and cellular dehydration. "Catch-up" is not permitted in central vein intravenous nutrition; if the infusion rate is behind schedule, a new flow rate must be prescribed. Indiscriminate increases in flow rate could lead to hyperglycemia and osmotic diuresis. The flow rate should be checked at least every hour. A check of the flow rate should be accompanied by a check of the level of solution in the bottle and by checks of the dressing, tubing, connections, and filter.

A patient who is receiving central vein intravenous nutrition needs emotional support. The central vein intravenous line is a source of stress, as is the condition that makes it necessary. The inability to take food by mouth is unusual and unpleasant. Patients may worry about losing their appetites, complain of being preoccupied with thoughts of food, and dream or hallucinate about food. They should be encouraged to verbalize their feelings and concerns and should be reassured that these reactions are not unusual.

REQUIREMENTS

The energy requirements of a patient receiving central vein intravenous nutrition are 30 kcal per kilogram of ideal body weight per day. Nitrogen requirements are 0.140 gram per kilogram per day for maintenance and 0.597 gram per kilogram per day for replacement. Solutions of 25 to 50% dextrose are used with 3.5 to 7% amino acid solutions and selected electrolytes, minerals, and vitamins in amounts individualized to meet the patient's specific needs for Calories, proteins, fluids, and electrolytes. Extra potassium is needed to aid the movement of glucose into the cells. Special vitamin and trace element preparations are usually added daily to one bottle of the feeding solution.

Intravenous fat emulsions can be given via central vein infusion but cannot be mixed with dextrose or amino acids. When fat is not needed as an energy source, fat emulsions are usually given twice weekly via a peripheral vein to provide essential fatty acids.

TERMINATION OF THERAPY

When central vein intravenous nutrition is discontinued (except in cases of sepsis), the procedure is accomplished gradually to prevent insulin shock. Prolonged use of hypertonic dextrose stimulates secretion of insulin. The hypertonicity of the dextrose is gradually reduced and eventually replaced by isotonic dextrose. Oral intake of dextrose in the tapering off period is helpful in maintaining homeostasis. The weaning period is usually 48 hours.

HOME CARE

Patients who cannot resume oral feedings may continue on central vein intravenous nutrition at home. Some patients have surgically made external arteriovenous fistulas similar to those used in renal dialysis; others continue their feedings with the subclavian catheters. Patients at home often infuse their solutions at night to permit them to work during the day. They may use a pump regulator or rely on the force of gravity to provide flow as they sleep. The nightly regimen may include Intralipid given 3 to 4 hours before bedtime, followed at bedtime with the dextrose, amino acid, vitamin, electrolyte, and mineral solution. Heparinized saline may be injected into the tube daily to maintain patency, or a heparin lock may be used. Such patients are living proof of the value of central vein intravenous nutrition.

NURSING IMPLICATIONS

- The nurse should assess baseline vital signs and determine body weight before the catheter is inserted. These measures are used to assess changes.
- Vital signs are evaluated every 4 to 6 hours after the procedure is established.
- Weights should be recorded daily under the usual rule for accurate weighing: same scale, same time, and same clothing. A weight gain in excess of ½ pound per day suggests fluid retention.
- Careful intake and output records and observations for edema and dehydration are helpful in evaluating the adequacy of the feeding solution.
- The nurse should monitor the laboratory test results for blood level of glucose, total protein, blood urea nitrogen, creatinine, and electrolytes.
- Testing urinary levels of glucose and acetone is a nursing responsibility.
- Oral hygiene is essential because patients receiving central vein intravenous nutrition are prone to oral inflammation and candidal infections.
- A variety of flavored mouthwashes should be used in oral hygiene to reassure patients that they have not lost their sense of taste.

References

Borgen, L. Total parenteral nutrition in adults. *American Journal of Nursing*, February 1978, *78*, 2.

Brunner, L., & Suddarth, D. *Textbook of medical-surgical nursing* (4th ed.). Philadelphia: J. B. Lippincott Company, 1980.

Colley, R., & Wilson, J. Meeting patients' nutritional needs with hyperalimentation, how to begin hyperalimentation therapy. *Nursing 79*, May 1979, *9*, 5.

Colley, R., & Wilson, J. Meeting patients' nutritional needs with hyperalimentation, managing the patient on hyperalimentation. *Nursing 79*, June 1979, *9*, 6.

Colley, R., Wilson, J., & Mabel, D. Meeting patients' nutritional needs with hyperalimentation, providing hyperalimentation for infants and children. *Nursing 79*, July 1979, *9*, 7.

Dudrick, D. A. patient on I.V. therapy need not starve! *Consultant*, February 1978, *18*, 2.

Howard R., & Herbold, N. *Nutrition in clinical care*. New York: McGraw-Hill Book Company, 1978.

Hunt, S., Groff, J., & Holbrook, J. *Nutrition: Principles and clinical practice*. New York: John Wiley & Sons, 1980.

Karran, S., & Alberti, K. (Eds.). *Practical nutritional support*. New York: John Wiley & Sons, 1980.

Krause, M., & Mahan, L. *Food, nutrition and diet therapy* (6th ed.). Philadelphia: W. B. Saunders Company, 1979.

Luckmann, J., & Sorensen, K. *Medical-surgical nursing: A psychophysiologic approach* (2nd ed.). Philadelphia: W. B. Saunders Company, 1980.

Metheny, N., & Snively, W. *Nurses' handbook of fluid balance* (3rd ed.). Philadelphia: J. B. Lippincott Company, 1979.

Parenteral nutrition guidelines. Chicago: Abbott Laboratories, 1981.

Shils, M. Parenteral nutrition. In R. Goodhart & M. Shils (Eds.). *Modern nutrition in health and disease* (6th ed.). Philadelphia: Lea & Febiger, 1980.

Suitor, C., & Hunter, M. *Nutrition: Principles and application in health promotion*. Philadelphia: J. B. Lippincott Company, 1980.

TPN—Total parenteral nutrition. *Nurses' Drug Alert*, September 1977, *1*, 16.

Vanamee, P. Parenteral nutrition. In *Nutrition reviews' present knowledge in nutrition* (4th ed.). New York: Nutrition Foundation, 1976.

Wilson, J., & Colley, R. Meeting patients' nutritional needs with hyperalimentation, teaching patients to administer hyperalimentation at home. *Nursing 79*, August 1979, *9*, 8.

Wilson, J., & Colley, R. Meeting patients' nutritional needs with hyperalimentation, administering peripheral and enteral feedings. *Nursing 79*, September 1979, *9*, 9.

25
Diet-Drug Interrelationships

Administering medications with meals is common practice to reduce gastrointestinal side effects, but this practice can also result in reduced, delayed, or altered drug action. Using food as a vehicle to administer crushed tablets or to disguise taste can also affect the drug's action if the food alters the pH or chelates (forms a chemical compound with) the drug. Oral medications are affected by food in the gastrointestinal tract, the pH of the stomach and small intestine, and the motility of the gastrointestinal tract.

Fatty foods and high-fat, low-fiber meals slow the emptying of the stomach by as much as 2 hours. The action of a drug administered with or after such a meal would be similarly slowed. High-protein meals increase gastric blood flow and increase the absorption of some drugs. Meals high in glucose cause a slight, transient decrease in blood flow to the gastrointestinal tract that tends to decrease drug absorption.

Alcohol, hot beverages, and antacids should not be given with sustained-release tablets or capsules because these substances can cause premature erosion of the pH-sensitive coating on the drug. Enteric-coated tablets should not be given with alkaline meals or antacids.

Many drugs, particularly central nervous system depressants, should not be taken in conjunction with alcohol because of a cumulative depressant effect. Other drugs combined with alcohol intake produce an effect similar to disulfiram (Antabuse), with an acute onset of facial flushing, dyspnea, nausea and vomiting, palpitation, headache, and hypotension. Alcohol consumed with some drugs increases the potential for gastric irritation and bleeding.

Most antibiotics are more effective if administered when the stomach is empty. Tetracycline should not be administered with milk or milk products because its effectiveness is reduced when it combines with the calcium in these foods. Some drugs deplete body stores of essential nutrients or interfere with their absorption.

Generalities cannot ensure proper drug administration. The remainder of this chapter contains specifics on diet-drug interrelationships for the nurse's aid in administering medications, preparing nursing care plans, and teaching patients. Drugs are listed alphabetically according to generic name. The generic name is followed by representative trade names. The drug classification is italicized. Information about the ideal administration time in regard to meals is provided. Drugs that can be taken with food or milk to minimize gastrointestinal side effects are identified. The effects of drugs on nutrient stores are also indicated.

ACETAMINOPHEN (Acephen, Aceta, Datril, Liquiprin, Tempra, Tylenol)

Analgesic

- Best administered in fasting state
- Food, especially carbohydrates, delays rate of absorption but does not prevent total absorption
- Foods that contain pectin delay absorption

ACETOHEXAMIDE (Dymelor)

Oral Antidiabetic

- Give immediately before breakfast for optimal control of blood levels of glucose and to reduce gastric distress
- Avoid alcohol; the combination produces disulfiram-type reactions (see page 325)

ACETOSULFONE SODIUM (Promacetin)

Antibacterial (leprostatic)

- Give in nonfasting state to reduce gastric distress

ACETYLSALICYLIC ACID AND ACETYLSALICYLIC ACID COMPOUNDS (A.S.A., Aspergum, Aspirin, Decapryn, Ecotrin)

Analgesic, Antipyretic, Antiinflammatory

- Food delays and decreases absorption but reduces nausea and gastric distress
- Administer with food, milk, crackers, or a full glass of water
- Functions as a folic acid antagonist
- Depletes body stores of vitamin C and vitamin K
- Avoid alcohol; the combination increases the risk for gastrointestinal bleeding

---

ADRENOCORTICOSTEROIDS (oral)

Hormone

- Administer in nonfasting state to reduce gastric distress
- Avoid alcohol; it increases the risk for gastric bleeding
- Decreases metabolism of vitamin D
- Causes increased urinary losses of zinc, vitamin C, calcium, potassium, and magnesium
- Decreases absorption of calcium, phosphorus, vitamin A, and vitamin B_6
- Increases blood levels of glucose, triglycerides, and cholesterol

---

ALLOPURINOL (Zyloprim)

Antigout

- Better tolerated when taken with or immediately after meals
- Maintain fluid intake to produce a urinary output of at least 2,000 milliliters per day
- May interfere with absorption of riboflavin, calcium, magnesium, and potassium
- Avoid alcohol; it reduces the effect of the drug

ALUMINUM HYDROXIDE GEL (Alu-Cap, Amphojel, Dialume, No-Co-Gel, Nutrajel)

Antacid

- Administer gel in half-glass of water
- Chew tablets before swallowing with milk or water
- Tends to cause constipation

- Decreases absorption of vitamin A
- Causes increased fecal excretion of phosphates, which may lead to phosphate depletion in patients on low-phosphate diets for management of urinary calculi
- May cause hypomagnesemia

AMBENONIUM CHLORIDE (Mytelase)

Cholinergic Acetylcholinesterase Inhibitor

- Most effective when given 30 to 40 minutes before meals

AMINOPHYLLINE (Aminophyllin, Somophyllin)

Sympathomimetic

- Administer with food or meals; food delays absorption but does not reduce total amount absorbed
- Food prevents gastric irritation

AMINOSALICYLIC ACID (Aminosalicylic Acid, PAS, Tubacin)

Antitubercular

- Administer in fasting state; food reduces absorption
- May be given with small amounts of food to reduce nausea and vomiting
- Tablet is enteric coated; do not give with milk
- Has a bitter aftertaste
- Functions as a folic acid antagonist
- Reduces absorption of fat and vitamin B_{12}

AMMONIUM CHLORIDE (Nodema)

Systemic Acidifier, Diuretic, Expectorant

- Give with or after meals to reduce gastrointestinal side effects
- Increases urinary excretion of magnesium

AMOXICILLIN (Amoxil, Polymox, Trimox, Utimox, Wymox)

Antibiotic

- Give in fasting state; food delays and reduces absorption

AMPHETAMINE SULFATE (Benzedrine)

Central Nervous System Stimulant, Anorexiant

- As anorexiant, give 30 minutes before meals
- Decreases sensitivity to sweet taste in some patients
- Increases sensitivity to bitter taste in some patients

AMPICILLIN (A-Cillin, Amcill, Omnipen, Penbritin, Polycillin, Principen)

Antibiotic

- Administer in fasting state, 1 hour before meals or 2 hours after meals; food reduces and delays absorption
- Do not administer with large amounts of fruit juice, beer, wine, or soft drinks because of acid content

ANISOTROPINE METHYLBROMIDE (Valpin)

Antispasmodic, Anticholinergic

- Administer before meals and at bedtime; food interferes with absorption

ASCORBIC ACID (Ascor, Cebid, Cecon, Cemill)

Vitamin

- Administer in nonfasting state to prevent gastric irritation

ATROPINE SULFATE

Anticholinergic

- Administer 30 minutes before meals to prevent interference with absorption

BELLADONNA AND BELLADONNA COMPOUNDS (Donabarb, Donnatal)

Cholinergic Blocker

- Administer in fasting state, ideally 30 minutes to 1 hour before meals; food interferes with absorption

BETHANECHOL CHLORIDE (Mitrol 10, Myotonachol, Urecholine)

Cholinergic

- Decreased incidence of nausea and vomiting when administered in fasting state

BISACODYL (Bicol, Biscolax, Bon-O-Lax, Dulcolax, Rolax, Vactrol)

Cathartic

- Swallow whole; do not bite or chew
- Do not administer within 1 hour of milk or milk products; alkaline foods disintegrate enteric coating

BUSULFAN (Myleran)

Antineoplastic

- Best administered in nonfasting state

CALCIUM CARBONATE, PRECIPITATED (Alka-2, Amitone, Dicarbosil, Tums)

Antacid, Calcium Supplement

- Administer 1 hour after meals for antacid action
- Administer with meals for calcium supplementation
- May cause rebound hyperacidity, constipation, flatulence, and hypercalcemia
- Long-term use, combined with a diet rich in vitamin D, may cause milk-alkali syndrome (nausea, vomiting, abdominal pain, headache, elevated serum levels of calcium and phosphorus, metabolic alkalosis, renal insufficiency)

CALCIUM CHLORIDE

Mineral

- Administer 1 hour to 90 minutes after meals for best absorption
- Administer with milk to reduce gastrointestinal irritation

CARBAMAZEPINE (Tegretol)

Anticonvulsant

- Administer with food; food increases absorption

CARBENICILLIN INDANYL SODIUM (Geocillin)

Antibiotic

- Administer in fasting state; food delays absorption
- Give with a full glass of water; drug has unpleasant taste
- High doses increase urinary excretion of potassium

CARISOPRODOL (Rela, Soma)

Skeletal Muscle Relaxant

- Administer in nonfasting state; food reduces nausea and vomiting
- Avoid alcohol; it potentiates the depressant effects on the central nervous system

CEPHALEXIN (Keflex)

Antibiotic

- Ideal administration time is 1 hour before or 2 hours after meals; food delays and reduces absorption

---

CEPHRADINE (Anspor, Velosef)

Antibiotic

- Administer in fasting state; food delays absorption

CHARCOAL, ACTIVATED (Charcodote, Darco 60)

Antidote, Adsorbent

- Mix powder with water, concentrated fruit juice, or chocolate powder; powder is tasteless
- Do not mix with ice cream or sherbet; antidotal efficiency is markedly reduced

---

CHLORAL HYDRATE (Aquachloral, Cohidrate, Noctec, SK-Chloral Hydrate, Somnos)

Sedative, Hypnotic

- Administer after meals to reduce nausea and vomiting
- Administer with full glass of water
- Avoid alcohol; it prolongs the hypnotic effect

CHLORAMBUCIL (Leukeran)

Antineoplastic

- Entire daily dose may be administered at one time
- Administer 1 hour before breakfast or 2 hours after evening meal to reduce nausea

---

CHLORAMPHENICOL (Amphicol, Chloromycetin, Mychel)

Antibiotic

- Avoid alcohol; the combination produces minor disulfiram-type reactions (see page 325)

- Decreases absorption of lactose
- Increases requirements for folic acid, riboflavin, vitamin B_6, vitamin B_{12}, vitamin A, and iron

CHLORDIAZEPOXIDE HYDROCHLORIDE
(Chlordiazachel, J-Liberty, Librium)

Antianxiety

- Best administered 30 minutes before meals
- Can be taken with or immediately after meals to reduce gastrointestinal distress
- Can be taken with milk to reduce gastric distress

CHLOROTHIAZIDE (Diuril, Ro-Chlorozide)

Diuretic

- Administer after meals to reduce gastric irritation
- Causes increased urinary excretion of magnesium

CHLOROTRIANISENE (TACE)

Synthetic Hormone

- Administer in nonfasting state to reduce nausea and vomiting

CHLORPROMAZINE HYDROCHLORIDE (Chlor-PZ, Klorazine, Promachlor, Promapar, Thorazine)

Antipsychotic, Antiemetic

- Administer with meals to reduce gastrointestinal side effects
- Long-term use may lead to hypercholesterolemia
- Avoid alcohol; the combination produces respiratory depression and reduces hepatic function

CHLORPROPAMIDE (Diabinese)

Antidiabetic

- Administer with breakfast for optimal control of hyperglycemia and to reduce gastrointestinal side effects
- Avoid alcohol; the combination produces minor disulfiram-type reactions (see page 325)

CHLORTHALIDONE (Hygroton)

Diuretic, Antihypertensive

- Administer with breakfast
- Avoid alcohol; it potentiates the hypotensive effect
- Avoid natural licorice; the combination produces severe hypokalemia
- Increases urinary excretion of zinc

CHOLESTYRAMINE (Questran)

Ion-Exchange Resin, Hypocholesterolemic

- Mix well with fluid; unpalatable taste may need to be disguised
- Reduces absorption of vitamin B_{12} and calcium
- Reduces absorption of fat and fat-soluble vitamins
- Impairs absorption of iron
- Reduces absorption of medium-chain triglycerides, glucose, xylose, and carotene

CIMETIDINE (Tagamet)

Histamine H_2-Receptor Blocker

- Administer with meals for peak serum levels and optimal inhibition of gastric secretion

CLINDAMYCIN (Cleocin)

Antibiotic

- Ideal administration time is 1 hour before or 2 hours after meals
- May be given without regard to food intake because absorption is not appreciably affected by food
- Food in the stomach at time of administration reduces gastric irritation

CLOFIBRATE (Atromid-S)

Antihyperlipidemic

- Causes reduced or altered sensations of taste
- Has an unpleasant aftertaste
- Reduces absorption of vitamin B_{12}, iron, glucose, carotene, and medium-chain triglycerides

CLOXACILLIN SODIUM MONOHYDRATE (Cloxapen, Tegopen)

Antibiotic

- Administer in fasting state, 1 to 2 hours before meals or 2 hours after meals; food decreases absorption
- Do not administer with fruit juices, beer, wine, or soft drinks

COLCHICINE (Colsalide)

Antigout

- Administer immediately before or after meals to reduce gastric irritation
- Reduces absorption of vitamin B_{12}, fat, lactose, nitrogen, carotene, and xylose
- Increases fecal excretion of potassium and sodium
- Decreases serum levels of cholesterol

CO-TRIMOXAZOLE (Bactrim, Septra)

Sulfonamide

- Best absorption occurs when administered 1 hour before meals or 2 hours after meals with a full glass of water
- Encourage fluid intake to prevent crystallization in urine
- Functions as folic acid antagonist

CYANOCOBALMIN (Kaybovite, Rhodavite, Vitamin B-12)

Vitamin

- Administer in nonfasting state; food increases absorption
- Excessive intake of alcohol may reduce absorption

CYCLACILLIN (Cyclapen)

Antibiotic

- Best administered with full glass of water 1 hour before or 2 hours after meals

CYCLANDELATE (Cyclanfor, Cyclospasmol, Cydel)

Vasodilator

- Best administered when the stomach is empty but can be given with milk or meals if gastrointestinal irritation occurs

CYCLOPHOSPHAMIDE (CTX, Cytoxan)

Antineoplastic

- Preferably administered when the stomach is empty
- May be given with meals to reduce gastrointestinal distress
- Encourage fluid intake to dilute drug concentration in urine

CYCLOSERINE (Seromycin)

Antitubercular

- Best administered just before meals
- May be administered after meals if gastric distress occurs
- Depletes body stores of vitamin B_6 and niacin
- Functions as a folic acid antagonist
- May decrease absorption of calcium, magnesium, and vitamin B_{12}

CYCRIMINE HYDROCHLORIDE (Pagitane)

Antiparkinson

- Administer in nonfasting state to prevent gastric irritation

CYPROHEPTADINE HYDROCHLORIDE (Cyprodine, Periactin)

Antihistamine, Antipruritic

- Administer in nonfasting state to prevent gastric irritation
- Encourage fluid intake to relieve dry mouth
- Avoid alcohol; the combination potentiates the depressant effects on the central nervous system

DEMECLOCYCLINE (Declomycin)

Antibiotic

- Administer in fasting state; food and milk reduce absorption
- Administer with full glass of water to prevent esophageal irritation

DIAZEPAM (Valium)

Antianxiety

- Administer in nonfasting state; food delays absorption but reduces nausea
- Avoid alcohol; the combination potentiates the depressant effects on the central nervous system

DICLOXACILLIN SODIUM (Dycill, Dynapen, Pathocil, Veracillin)

Antibiotic

- Best administered in fasting state, 1 hour before or 2 hours after meals
- Food reduces absorption
- Has an unpleasant taste

DIETHYLSTILBESTROL (Synestrin, DES)

Hormone

- Administer in nonfasting state to reduce nausea and vomiting

DIGOXIN (Lanoxin, Masoxin, SK-Digoxin)

Cardiac Glycoside

- Administer after meals; food delays absorption but does not affect total amount absorbed
- Give in fasting state when rapid response is desired
- Do not administer with milk or high-calcium foods; therapeutic effect would be diminished
- High-fiber meals reduce absorption
- Potential for toxicity is increased in magnesium-depleted patients
- Potassium depletion increases ventricular irritability, which digoxin may accentuate
- Increases need for thiamine

DIPHEMANIL METHYLSULFATE (Prantal)

Anticholinergic, Antispasmodic

- Best administered in fasting state; give between meals and at bedtime
- Encourage fluid intake to relieve dry mouth

DIPHENOXYLATE HYDROCHLORIDE WITH ATROPINE SULFATE (Colonil, Lofene, Lomotil)

Antidiarrheal

- Encourage fluid intake to relieve dry mouth, if not contraindicated
- Avoid alcohol; the combination potentiates the depressant effect on the central nervous system

DIPYRIDAMOLE (Persantine)

Coronary Vasodilator

- Best administered at least 1 hour before meals

DOXYCYCLINE (Doxychel, Vibramycin)

Antibiotic

- Ideally administered when the stomach is empty because food decreases absorption slightly
- Can be given with food or milk if gastric irritation occurs
- Encourage fluid intake to reduce risk for esophageal irritation
- Administer with full glass of water to reduce esophageal irritation

ERGOT DERIVATIVES (Hydergine, Methergine, Sansert)

Oxytocic, Antimigraine

- Administer with meals to reduce nausea and vomiting
- Avoid alcohol to reduce headache severity

ERYTHROMYCIN (E-Mycin, Erythrocin, Ilotycin, Robimycin, RP-Mycin)

Antibiotic

- Best administered with full glass of water 2 to 3 hours before meals
- Tablets are coated with an acid-resistant substance to protect the drug from gastric juice; do not administer with acid juices, for example, orange, lemon, or cranberry, carbonated beverages, beer, or wine in amount in excess of 8 ounces

ERYTHROMYCIN STEARATE (Bristamycin, Erypar, Erythrocin Stearate)

Antibiotic

- Best administered 1 hour before or 2 hours after meals; food decreases absorption
- Do not take with acid juices or carbonated beverages; acids decompose tablet prematurely
- Do not crush tablets

ESTRADIOL (Estrace)

Hormone

- Best administered with meals to reduce nausea and vomiting

ESTROGEN, CONJUGATED (Co-Estro, Conest, Ovest, Premarin, Sodestrin)

Hormone

- Best administered with meals to reduce nausea and vomiting

ETHACRYNIC ACID (Edecrin)

Diuretic

- Best administered with meals or milk to reduce gastric irritation
- Avoid alcohol; it worsens orthostatic hypotension
- Increases urinary excretion of magnesium, calcium, and potassium

ETHAMBUTOL HYDROCHLORIDE (Myambutol)

Antitubercular

- Best administered with meals; food decreases absorption slightly but relieves nausea and vomiting

ETHIONAMIDE (Trecator-SC)

Antitubercular

- Best administered after meals to reduce gastric irritation

ETHYL ALCOHOL

Central Nervous System Depressant

- Functions as a vitamin B_6 antagonist or increases vitamin B_6 turnover
- Functions as a folic acid antagonist
- Reduces absorption of thiamine, vitamin B_{12}, and vitamin A
- Depletes body stores of vitamin C
- Increases urinary excretion of zinc, magnesium, and calcium

FENOPROFEN CALCIUM (Nalfon)

Antiinflammatory

- Best administered 30 minutes before or 2 hours after meals; food reduces rate and degree of absorption
- May be given with food or milk to reduce gastrointestinal distress
- Avoid alcohol; it increases gastric irritation

FERROUS GLUCONATE/SULFATE (Entron, Feosol, Fergon, Mol-Iron)

Hematinic

- Best absorbed when given between meals but frequently given with food to reduce gastrointestinal side effects
- Do not administer in conjunction with cereal, eggs, or milk; these foods form insoluble chelates with iron
- Best administered with a source of vitamin C to improve absorption
- Do not crush tablets

FLUOROURACIL (FU, 5-FU, Fluorouracil)

Intravenous Antineoplastic

- Causes alterations in bitter and sour taste sensations
- Causes niacin depletion because it functions as a vitamin B_6 antagonist (vitamin B_6 needed to synthesize niacin from tryptophan)

FURAZOLIDONE (Furoxone)

Antibacterial

- Best given after meals
- Avoid foods that contain tyramine (see monoamine oxidase inhibitors, page 352)
- Encourage fluid intake
- Avoid alcohol; the combination may cause disulfiram-type reactions during treatment and for 4 days after treatment is discontinued (see page 325)

FUROSEMIDE (Lasix)

Diuretic

- Food delays absorption but also prevents gastric irritation
- Reduces carbohydrate tolerance
- Increases urinary excretion of calcium, magnesium, and potassium

GLUTETHIMIDE (Doriden)

Sedative

- Encourage intake of fluids and fiber to prevent constipation
- Avoid alcohol; the combination potentiates the depressant effects on the central nervous system
- Increases turnover of vitamin D and resorption of bone

GLYCOPYRROLATE (Robinul)

Anticholinergic, Antispasmodic

- Best given 30 minutes before meals in the morning, early afternoon, and at bedtime
- Encourage fluid intake to relieve dry mouth and prevent constipation

GRISEOFULVIN (Fulvicin, Grifulvin, Grisactin)

Antibiotic, Antifungal

- Food, especially fat, increases absorption
- Give with meals to increase absorption and to relieve gastric distress
- Causes reduced or altered taste sensations
- Avoid alcohol; the combination produces disulfiram-type reactions (see page 325)

GUANETHIDINE SULFATE (Ismelin)

Antihypertensive

- Avoid alcohol; it potentiates the hypotensive effect

HETACILLIN (Versapen)

Antibiotic

- Best administered 1 hour before or 2 hours after meals; food reduces absorption
- Give with a full glass of water to increase absorption

HEXOCYCLIUM METHYLSULFATE (Tral)

Anticholinergic, Antispasmodic

- Best administered before meals
- Encourage fluid intake to relieve dry mouth

HOMATROPINE METHYLBROMIDE (Ru-Spas # 2, Sed-Tens SE)

Anticholinergic, Antispasmodic

- Best administered before meals and at bedtime
- Encourage fluid intake to relieve dry mouth

HYDRALAZINE HYDROCHLORIDE (Apresoline, Dralzine, Nor-Pres, Rolazine)

Antihypertensive

- Best administered with meals; food increases absorption
- Avoid alcohol; it potentiates the hypotensive effect
- Functions as a vitamin B_6 antagonist and increases turnover of vitamin B_6

HYDROCHLOROTHIAZIDE (Esidrix, HydroDIURIL, Oretic)

Diuretic

- Best administered with meals; food increases absorption and reduces gastrointestinal distress

- Avoid alcohol; it potentiates the hypotensive effect
- Causes decreased carbohydrate tolerance
- Avoid imported (natural) licorice; the combination causes hypokalemia, retention of sodium and water, and alkalosis (aldosterone effect)
- Increases urinary excretion of magnesium, potassium, zinc, and riboflavin

HYDROFLUMETHIAZIDE (Diucardin, Saluron, Salutensin)

Diuretic

- Best administered with meals; food increases absorption

HYDROXYUREA (Hydrea)

Antineoplastic

- Best administered with meals to reduce gastrointestinal side effects

HYOSCYAMINE SULFATE, ATROPINE SULFATE, AND HYOSCINE HYDROBROMIDE WITH PHENOBARBITAL (Donnatal)

Anticholinergic

- Best administered 30 minutes before meals
- Encourage fluid intake to relieve dry mouth

IBUPROFEN (Motrin)

Antiinflammatory

- Best administered 1 hour before or 2 hours after meals; food reduces absorption
- Can be given with food or milk to reduce nausea and vomiting
- Avoid alcohol; the combination increases gastric irritation

INDOMETHACIN (Indocin)

Antiinflammatory, Analgesic, Antipyretic

- Best administered after meals to reduce nausea and vomiting
- Avoid alcohol; the combination increases gastric irritation

INSULIN

Antidiabetic

- Prolonged use reduces salt and sweet sensitivity
- Avoid alcohol; it may reduce gluconeogenesis

ISONIAZID (INH, Isoniazid, Nydrazid)

Antitubercular

- Best given in fasting state; food reduces absorption
- Can be given with food to reduce gastrointestinal distress
- Pyridoxine is usually given with the drug because it depletes body stores of vitamin B_6
- Vitamin B_6 depletion causes niacin deficiency because vitamin B_6 is needed to convert tryptophan to niacin
- Increases need for folic acid
- Increases absorption of iron
- Avoid alcohol; it diminishes the effect of the drug and increases the potential for liver damage

ISOXSUPRINE HYDROCHLORIDE (Isolait, Vasodilan, Vasoprine)

Vasodilator

- Best administered with meals or milk to reduce nausea and vomiting

LEVODOPA (Bendopa, Dopar, Larodopa)

Antiparkinson

- Best administered with small meals to prevent nausea and vomiting, even though food reduces absorption
- Drug effectiveness is decreased by high protein intake
- Avoid foods high in vitamin B_6 (yeast, liver, muscle meats, vegetables, fish, whole grains); vitamin B_6 rapidly reverses the drug's action

- Avoid multivitamin preparations that contain more than 10 to 15 milligrams of vitamin B_6 per tablet
- Avoid fortified cereals that contain 5 milligrams or more of vitamin B_6 per serving
- Increases urinary excretion of sodium and potassium

LINCOMYCIN HYDROCHLORIDE MONOHYDRATE (Lincocin)

Antibiotic

- Best administered 1 hour before or 2 hours after meals; food decreases absorption
- Administer with water, and allow only water 1 to 2 hours before and after drug administration

LITHIUM CARBONATE (Eskalith, Lithane, Lithonate, Lithotabs, Pfi-Lithium)

Antipsychotic

- Best administered with meals; food increases absorption
- Encourage adequate intake of salt and fluids to prevent lithium toxicity
- Drug has strange, unpleasant taste

LOMUSTINE (CeeNU)

Antineoplastic

- Best administered in fasting state to reduce nausea and vomiting
- Encourage fluid intake and small feedings as tolerated

MAGNESIUM OXIDE (Mag-Ox, Oxabid)

Antacid, Cathartic

- Administer with meals; food prevents gastric irritation
- Administer with full glass of water or milk

MECLIZINE HYDROCHLORIDE (Antivert, Bonine, Wehvert)

Antiemetic, Antihistamine

- Avoid alcohol; it potentiates the depressant effects on the central nervous system

MECLOFENAMATE SODIUM (Meclomen)

Antiinflammatory

- Best administered before meals
- May be administered with meals or milk if gastrointestinal distress occurs

MEFENAMIC ACID (Ponstel)

Analgesic, Antipyretic

- Best administered with food or meals to reduce gastric irritation

MELPHALAN (Alkeran)

Antineoplastic

- Best administered 1 hour before or 2 hours after meals
- Can be given with meals to reduce nausea and vomiting

MEPENZOLATE BROMIDE (Cantil)

Anticholinergic

- Best given before meals to prevent interference with absorption

MEPROBAMATE (Bamate, Coprobate, Equanil, Meprospan, Miltown, Robamate)

Antianxiety

- Avoid alcohol; it potentiates the depressant effects on the central nervous system

MERCAPTOPURINE (Purinethol)

Antineoplastic

- Best given with meals
- Encourage fluid intake
- Depletes body stores of vitamin B_6
- Depletes body stores of niacin (vitamin B_6 is needed to synthesis niacin from tryptophan)

METHACYCLINE HYDROCHLORIDE (Rondomycin)

Antibiotic

- Best administered 1 hour before or 2 hours after meals; food reduces absorption
- Do not give with milk or high-calcium foods; calcium would chelate with the drug
- Do not administer pediatric doses with milk formulas or calcium-containing foods

METHANDROSTENOLONE (Dianabol)

Anabolic

- Administer between meals to prevent interference with absorption

METHANTHELINE BROMIDE (Banthine)

Anticholinergic, Antispasmodic

- Best administered 30 minutes to 1 hour before meals and at bedtime to prevent interference with absorption
- Encourage fluid intake to relieve dry mouth

METHAQUALONE (Quāālude, Sopor, Parest)

Sedative, Hypnotic

- Avoid alcohol; it potentiates the depressant effects on the central nervous system

---

METHENAMINE MANDELATE (Mandalay, Mandelamine, Renelate)

Urinary Germicide

- Administer with half-glass of water after meals and at bedtime
- Encourage fluid intake
- Best action achieved in acid urine
- Cranberry juice, ascorbic acid, meat, fish, and fowl produce an acid urine
- Avoid alkaline-ash foods and beverages, namely, fruits, vegetables, milk

---

METHIMAZOLE (Tapazole)

Antithyroid

- Best administered with meals to reduce gastrointestinal side effects
- Decreases taste sensations

METHIONINE (A-D-R, Uranap)

Urinary Deodorant

- Best given 30 minutes before meals to prevent interference with absorption

---

METHOTREXATE

Antineoplastic

- Best administered 1 hour before or 2 hours after meals; food delays absorption
- May be given with food to reduce gastric distress
- Food may be withheld if nausea and vomiting occur
- Avoid alcohol; it increases the risk for hepatotoxicity
- Encourage fluid intake
- Interferes with absorption of vitamin B_{12}

- Functions as a folic acid antagonist; avoid vitamin preparations that contain folic acid
- Causes malabsorption of fat and xylose

METHOXSALEN (Oxsoralen)

Pigment Enhancer

- Best administered with food of meals; food increases absorption and prevents gastrointestinal distress

---

METHSCOPOLAMINE BROMIDE (Pamine)

Anticholinergic

- Best administered when the stomach is empty (30 minutes before meals) to prevent interference with absorption
- Encourage fluid intake to relieve dry mouth

METHYLDOPA (Aldomet)

Antihypertensive

- Avoid alcohol; it potentiates the hypotensive effect
- Encourage fluid intake, if not contraindicated, to relieve dry mouth

---

METHYLPHENIDATE HYDROCHLORIDE (Ritalin)

Central Nervous System Stimulant

- Best administered 30 minutes before meals to prevent interference with absorption
- Avoid beverages containing caffeine, namely, coffee, tea, cola, cocoa

---

METHYLTHIOURACIL (Methiocil)

Antithyroid

- Best administered with food to reduce gastric irritation
- Decreases taste sensations

METOPROLOL TARTRATE (Lopressor)

Antihypertensive

- Best administered with meals; food increases absorption
- Avoid alcohol; it potentiates the depressant effects on the central nervous system

METRONIDAZOLE (Flagyl)

Antiprotozoal

- Best administered with food to reduce gastric irritation
- Avoid alcohol; the combination produces minor disulfiram-type reactions (see page 325)
- Has a metallic taste

MINOCYCLINE HYDROCHLORIDE (Minocin, Vectrin)

Antibiotic

- Administer with full glass of water to prevent esophageal irritation
- Can be given with food or milk if gastric distress occurs; absorption is not appreciably affected by food

MITOTANE (Lysodren)

Antineoplastic

- Best administered with meals

MONOAMINE OXIDASE INHIBITORS (Eutonyl, Marplan, Nardil, Parnate)

Antianxiety

- Best administered 30 minutes before meals to prevent interference with absorption
- Reacts with tyramine in foods to cause severe headaches, hypertension, intracranial hemorrhage and, possibly, death

• Tyramine-rich foods include alcohol, beer, and ale, broad beans, cheeses (Brie, cheddar, Camembert, Stilton) Chianti wine, coffee, chicken livers, chocolate, cola beverages, canned figs, dried fish, licorice, liver, pickled and kippered herring, tea, raisins, sour cream, soy sauce, yogurt, yeast and yeast extracts, and vanilla

NAFCILLIN SODIUM (Unipen)

Antibiotic

• Best administered 1 hour before or 2 hours after meals; food decreases absorption
• Increases urinary excretion of potassium

NALIDIXIC ACID (NegGram)

Urinary Germicide

• Increased blood levels of drug achieved when given in fasting state
• Can be given with food to reduce nausea and vomiting

NAPROXEN (Naprosyn)

Antiinflammatory

• Best administered in fasting state; food reduces absorption
• Can be given with food or milk to reduce gastric distress
• Avoid alcohol; it increases gastric irritation

NEOMYCIN SULFATE (Mycifradin Sulfate, Neobiotic)

Antibiotic

• Reduces absorption of fat and fat-soluble vitamins
• Reduces absorption of nitrogen, lactose, sucrose, calcium, iron, and vitamin B_{12}
• Increases fecal excretion of sodium and potassium

NIACIN (Diacin, Niac, Niacels, Niacinamide, Nicobid)

Hypocholesterolemic

- Administer with cold water to improve ease of swallowing
- Best administered with meals to reduce gastric irritation

NITROFURANTOIN (Cyantin, Furadantin, Furalan, Furatoin, Macrodantin)

Urinary Germicide

- Best administered with meals; food increases absorption and prevents nausea and vomiting

ORAL CONTRACEPTIVES

- Administer with the same meal every day to maintain regular interval and schedule
- Function as folic acid and vitamin B_6 antagonists
- Deplete body stores of riboflavin
- Reduce absorption and increase metabolism of vitamin C
- Increase serum levels of vitamin A

OXACILLIN SODIUM (Bactocill, Prostaphlin)

Antibiotic

- Best administered 1 hour before or 2 hours after meals; food decreases absorption

OXOLINIC ACID (Utibid)

Urinary Germicide

- Best administered with food to reduce gastric distress

OXYPHENBUTAZONE (Oxalid, Tandearil)

Antiinflammatory

- Best administered immediately before or after meals with a glass of milk to reduce gastric irritation
- Avoid alcohol; it increases gastric irritation

OXYPHENONIUM BROMIDE (Antrenyl)

Anticholinergic, Antispasmodic

- Best administered between meals to prevent interference with absorption

OXYTETRACYCLINE (Terramycin)

Antibiotic

- Best administered 1 hour before or 2 hours after meals; food reduces absorption
- Do not administer pediatric doses with milk, milk formulas, or high-calcium foods

PANCREATIN (Elzyme 303, Panteric, Viokase)

Digestant

- Administer with meals for best therapeutic effect; food also prevents nausea and vomiting
- Do not administer with milk or hot foods
- Avoid milk within 1 hour of administration of tablets (enteric coated)

PANCRELIPASE (Cotazym, Ilozyme, Ku-Zyme HP)

Digestant

- Administer with meals for therapeutic effect

PAPAVERINE HYDROCHLORIDE (Cerespan, Pavabid, Vasospan)

Vasodilator

- Administer with meals to prevent nausea and vomiting

PENICILLAMINE (Cuprimine, D-Pen)

Antirheumatic, Heavy-Metal Antagonist

- Best administered when the stomach is empty, 1 hour before or 2 hours after meals
- Causes a general decrease in taste sensations
- Increases need for vitamin B_6
- Increases urinary excretion of zinc, copper, and vitamin B_6

PENICILLIN G, BENZATHINE (Bicillin)

Antibiotic

- Absorption is not appreciably affected by food
- Do not administer with fruit juices, acid foods, beer, wine, or soft drinks

PENICILLIN G POTASSIUM (G-Recillin, Pentids, Pfizerpen)

Antibiotic

- Best administered 1 hour before or 2 hours after meals; food reduces absorption
- Avoid administering with 8 ounces or more of acid juices, for example, orange, cranberry, or pineapple, pale dry ginger ale, and carbonated beverages
- Encourage fluid intake
- Decreases absorption of folic acid, vitamin B_{12}, calcium, and magnesium
- Decreases synthesis of vitamin K; could lead to bleeding
- Inactivates vitamin B_6
- Increases urinary excretion of potassium

PENICILLIN V POTASSIUM (Ledercillin VK, Penapar VK, Pen•Vee K, V-Cillin K)

Antibiotic

- Best administered in fasting state
- May be administered with food; absorption is somewhat decreased

PENTAERYTHRITOL TETRANITRATE (Angitrate, Antora, Corodyl, Peritrate, Vasitol)

Vasodilator

- Best administered in fasting state, 30 minutes before or 1 hour after meals
- Avoid alcohol; it potentiates the hypotensive effect

PENTAZOCINE (Talwin)

Analgesic

- Action is speeded when administered with full glass of water

PEPSIN (Donnazyme, Entozyme, Zypan)

Digestant

- Administer with meals for therapeutic effect and to prevent nausea and vomiting

PHENAZOPYRIDINE HYDROCHLORIDE (Azodine, Azo-Stat, Pyridium, Pyrodiate, Urodine)

Urinary Tract Analgesic

- Best administered 30 minutes to 1 hour before meals

PHENETHICILLIN (Maxipen)

Antibiotic

- Best administered 1 hour before or 2 hours after meals; food decreases absorption

PHENINDIONE (Eridone, Hedulin)

Anticoagulant

- Decreases taste sensation
- Avoid excessive intake of alcohol, which potentiates the anticoagulant effect

PHENMETRAZINE HYDROCHLORIDE (Preludin)

Anorexiant

- Administer 30 minutes before meals for therapeutic effect and to prevent interference with absorption
- Avoid excessive use of caffeine-containing beverages

PHENOBARBITAL (Barbipil, Barbita, Eskabarb, Solu-Barb, Stentol)

Anticonvulsant

- Best administered in fasting state; food delays and decreases absorption
- Can be given with food to reduce gastrointestinal distress
- Avoid alcohol; it potentiates the depressant effects on the central nervous system
- Decreases activity of folic acid and vitamins B_6, B_{12}, D, and K
- Decreases absorption of calcium

PHENOLPHTHALEIN (Alophen, Evac-U-Lax, Ex-Lax, Feen-A-Mint, Phenolax)

Cathartic

- Routine use or abuse affects absorption of vitamin D and calcium

PHENTOLAMINE (Regitine)

Adrenergic Blocker

- Best administered with meals to prevent nausea and vomiting

PHENYLBUTAZONE (Azolid, Butazolidin)

Antiinflammatory

- Best administered before or after meals with full glass of milk to reduce gastric distress
- Avoid alcohol; it increases gastric irritation

PHENYTOIN SODIUM (Dilantin)

Anticonvulsant, Antiarrhythmic

- Best administered with half-glass of water with meals; food increases absorption and reduces nausea and vomiting
- Avoid alcohol; anticonvulsant effect increased with acute alcohol intoxication and decreased with chronic alcoholism
- Decreases taste sensations
- Decreases absorption of vitamin B_{12}, folic acid, and calcium

PIPERAZINE CITRATE (Antepar, Bryrel, Multifuge)

Anthelmintic

- Best administered in nonfasting state to prevent nausea and vomiting

PIPOBROMAN (Vercyte)

Antineoplastic

- Best administered with meals to reduce gastric distress

POTASSIUM COMPOUNDS (K-Lor, K-Lyte, K-10, Kaon, Kay Ciel)

Electrolyte

- Best administered with food or after meals with full glass of water; food delays absorption but reduces gastric irritation
- May be less upsetting to gastrointestinal tract if sipped throughout meal
- Do not administer with milk or milk products
- Potassium chloride affects absorption of vitamin B_{12}

PRAZOSIN HYDROCHLORIDE (Minipress)

Antihypertensive

- Food may delay absorption but reduces gastrointestinal side effects

- Avoid alcohol; it potentiates the hypotensive effect
- Encourage sips of fluid or ice chips to relieve dry mouth

PREDNISONE (Deltasone, Meticorten, Paracort, Prednicen-M, Sterapred)

Adrenocorticosteroid

- Best administered with food to prevent nausea and vomiting
- Decreases absorption of calcium and iron
- Decreases carbohydrate tolerance

PRIMIDONE (Mysoline, Ro-Primidone)

Anticonvulsant

- Decreases absorption of calcium, folic acid, vitamin B_6, and vitamin B_{12}

PROBUCOL (Lorelco)

Antilipemic

- Best administered with food to increase therapeutic effect

PROCARBAZINE HYDROCHLORIDE (Matulane)

Antineoplastic

- Best administered with meals
- Avoid foods that contain tyramine (see monomine oxidase inhibitors, page 352)
- Avoid alcohol; the combination causes disulfiram-type reactions (see page 325)

PROCYCLIDINE HYDROCHLORIDE (Kemadrin)

Antiparkinson, Anticholinergic

- Best administered with meals to reduce gastric distress
- Encourage fluid intake to relieve dry mouth

PROMAZINE HYDROCHLORIDE (Sparine)

Antipsychotic

- Best administered with meals to prevent nausea and vomiting

PROMETHAZINE HYDROCHLORIDE (Phenergan, Quadnite, Remsed, ZiPan)

Antihistamine

- Best administered in nonfasting state to prevent nausea and vomiting

PROPANTHELINE BROMIDE (Pro-Banthine, Robantaline, Ropanth)

Anticholinergic, Antispasmodic

- Best administered 30 minutes before meals and at bedtime; food delays absorption
- Encourage sips of fluid to relieve dry mouth

PROPOXYPHENE HYDROCHLORIDE (Darvon, Dolene, Pargesic-65, Progesic-65)

Analgesic

- Best administered with food; food increases absorption
- Give with a full glass of fluid to speed action
- Avoid alcohol; it potentiates the depressant effects on the central nervous system

PROPRANOLOL HYDROCHLORIDE (Inderal)

Antiarrhythmic, Antihypertensive

- Best administered with food; food increases absorption
- Avoid alcohol; the drug may mask symptoms of alcoholic hypoglycemia

PYRANTEL PAMOATE (Antiminth)

Anthelmintic

- Best administered with food to prevent nausea and vomiting

PYRAZINAMIDE (Tebrazid)

Antitubercular

- Best administered with meals to prevent nausea and vomiting

PYRIMETHAMINE (Daraprim)

Antimalarial

- Best administered with meals to reduce gastric irritation
- Functions as a folic acid antagonist

QUINACRINE HYDROCHLORIDE (Atrabrine)

Antimalarial, Anthelmintic

- As an anthelmintic, best administered when the stomach is empty to increase contact with parasites
- As an antimalarial, best administered after meals with a full glass of water, tea, or fruit juice
- Avoid alcohol; the combination produces minor disulfiram-type reactions (see page 325)

QUINIDINE SULFATE (Cin-Quin, Quinidex, Quinora)

Antiarrhythmic

- Best administered with food to reduce gastric distress
- An alkaline urine decreases excretion of the drug and can lead to quinidine intoxication
- Vegetarian diets, antacids, and more than 1 quart of orange or grapefruit juice daily can produce an alkaline urine; Watch for intake of these foods separately or in combination

RAUWOLFIA and RAUWOLFIA PREPARATIONS
(Raudixin, Rauzide)

Antihypertensive, Antipsychotic

- Best administered with meals, food, or milk to reduce gastric irritation
- Avoid alcohol; it potentiates the depressant effects on the central nervous system
- Encourage fluid intake to relieve dry mouth

RESERPINE (Diupres, Regroton, Serpasil)

Antihypertensive, Antipsychotic

- Drug increases gastric secretions; best given with meals, food, or milk to reduce gastric irritation
- Avoid alcohol; it potentiates the depressant effects on the central nervous system
- Encourage fluid intake to relieve dry mouth

RIBOFLAVIN

Vitamin

- Best administered with meals; food increases absorption

RIFAMPIN (Rifadin, Rimactane)

Antitubercular

- Best administered 1 hour before or 2 hours after meals; food decreases absorption

SALICYLAMIDE (Amid-Sal, Doldram, Salamide, Salrin)

Antipyretic, Analgesic, Antiinflammatory

- Best administered with meals or a full glass of milk to reduce gastric distress
- Avoid alcohol; it increases gastric irritation and bleeding

SPIRONOLACTONE (Aldactone)

Diuretic

- Best administered with food, milk, or meals to prevent nausea and vomiting
- Avoid excessive intake of potassium

STRONG IODINE SOLUTION (Lugol's Solution)

Antithyroid

- Best administered with meals to reduce gastric distress
- Dilute with at least 2 ounces of orange juice or milk to reduce bitterness

SULFASALAZINE (Azulfidine, S.A.S.-500, Sulcolon)

Sulfonamide

- Best administered with full glass of water at mealtimes
- Encourage fluid intake to prevent crystalluria
- Functions as a folic acid antagonist
- Reduces serum levels of iron

SULFINPYRAZONE (Anturane)

Antigout

- Best administered with meals or milk to reduce gastric irritation
- Encourage fluid intake
- Avoid alcohol; it may increase serum levels of urates, and it also increases gastric irritation

SULFONAMIDES (Microsulfon)

Sulfonamide

- Best administered when the stomach is empty; food delays absorption
- Encourage fluid intake to prevent crystalluria

SULFONAMIDES (Gantanol, Gantrisin, Microsulfon, Sonilyn, Sulfstat-Forte, Unisul)

Sulfonamide

- Best administered when the stomach is empty; food delays absorption
- Decreases absorption of folic acid, vitamin B_{12}, calcium, and iron
- Reduces synthesis of vitamin K
- Inactivates vitamin B_6
- Impairs transfer of amino acids during cell synthesis

SULFONAMIDES (Midicel, Sulla)

Sulfonamide

- Best administered after meals

SULINDAC (Clinoril)

Antirheumatic

- Best administered 30 minutes before or 2 hours after meals; food delays absorption
- May be given with meals or milk to reduce gastric irritation

TETRACHLOROETHYLENE

Anthelmintic

- Restrict intake of fats and alcohol before administration; these substances increase absorption and reduce local action

TETRACYCLINES (Achromycin V, Aureomycin, Bristacycline, Cyclopar, Desamycin, Oxlopar, Panmycin, Sumycin, Tetracyn, Tetrex, Uribiotic, Uritet)

Antibiotic

- Best administered when the stomach is empty
- May be given with light meal to reduce gastric distress

- Should not be taken with milk, milk products, or high-calcium foods; calcium impairs absorption
- Withhold antacids, iron, dairy foods, and high-calcium foods for 2 hours after administration of the drug
- Decreases absorption of folic acid, vitamin B_{12}, calcium, magnesium, and iron
- Decreases synthesis of vitamin K
- Inactivates vitamin B_6

THEOPHYLLINE and THEOPHYLLINE COMPOUNDS (Slo-Phyllin, Somophyllin, Theolair)

Adrenergic

- Best administered with a full glass of water 30 to 60 minutes before meals
- May be given with food to reduce nausea and vomiting
- Action is delayed by high-protein meals and speeded by high-carbohydrate meals
- Avoid large amounts of stimulant beverages, namely, coffee, tea, cocoa, and cola

THIOGUANINE

Antineoplastic

- Best administered with meals
- Encourage fluid intake

THYROXINE (Choloxin, Euthroid, Levothroid, Synthroid, Thyrolar)

Hormone

- Decreases absorption of riboflavin by increasing gastrointestinal motility

TOLBUTAMIDE (Orinase)

Antidiabetic

- Best given before breakfast and with meals
- Avoid alcohol; it stimulates production of an enzyme that reduces the life of the drug; the combination also causes disulfiram-type reactions (see page 325)

TOLMETIN SODIUM (Tolectin)

Antiinflammatory

- Best administered 30 minutes before or 2 hours after meals; food delays absorption
- May be given with food or milk to reduce gastric distress
- Avoid alcohol; it increases gastric irritation

TRIAMTERENE (Dyrenium)

Diuretic

- Best administered with meals to prevent nausea
- Avoid high potassium intake
- Functions as a folic acid antagonist
- Reduces serum levels of vitamin B_{12}
- Increases urinary excretion of calcium

TRIHEXYPHENIDYL HYDROCHLORIDE (Artane, Hexaphen, Tremin)

Anticholinergic, Antiparkinson

- Best administered with food or meals
- Give before meals if dry mouth is a problem
- Give after meals if increased salivation or nausea is a problem
- Encourage fluid intake to relieve dry mouth

TROLEANDOMYCIN (Tao)

Antibiotic

- Best administered with full glass of water 1 hour before or 2 hours after meals; food delays absorption

URACIL MUSTARD

Antineoplastic

- Best given with food at bedtime to reduce gastrointestinal side effects

VALPROIC ACID (Depakene)

Anticonvulsant

- Best administered with meals, food, or milk to prevent gastrointestinal side effects
- Avoid alcohol; it potentiates the depressant effects on the central nervous system

WARFARIN (Athrombin-K, Coumadin, Dicumarol, Panwarfin)

Anticoagulant

- Best taken with meals; food increases absorption
- Avoid large amounts of vitamin K in one meal; eliminate turnip greens and spinach from diet; leafy green vegetables increase the prothrombin time
- Avoid high-fat meals; they increase prothrombin activity
- Avoid alcohol; it potentiates the anticoagulant effect with acute intoxication and reduces the effect with chronic use

References

Alcohol-drug interactions. *FDA Drug Bulletin,* June 1979, *9,* 2.

Bauwens, E., & Clemmons, C. Foods that foil drugs. *RN,* September 1978, *41,* 9.

Black, C., Popovich, N., & Black, M. Drug interactions in the GI tract. *American Journal of Nursing,* September 1977, *77,* 9.

Calesnick, B. What patients should know about alcohol and medications. *Consultant,* August 1981, *21,* 8.

Carson, J., Gormican, A. Disease-medication relationships in altered taste sensitivity. *Journal of the American Dietetic Association,* February 1976, *68,* 2.

DiPalma, J. How you can prevent G.I. drug interactions. *RN,* July 1977, *40,* 7.

Feldman, C. Effects of dietary protein and carbohydrate on theophylline metabolism in children. *Pediatrics,* December 1980, *66,* 12.

Giovannitti, C., & Schwinghammer, T. Food & drugs. *Nursing 81,* July 1981, *11,* 7.

Govoni, L., & Hayes, J. *Drugs and nursing implications* (3rd ed.). New York: Appleton-Century-Crofts, 1978.

Green, M., & Harry, J. *Nutrition in contemporary nursing practice.* New York: John Wiley & Sons, 1981.

Howard, R., & Herbold, N. *Nutrition in clinical care.* New York: McGraw-Hill Book Company, 1978.

Kastrup, E., & Boyd, J. (Eds.). *Facts and comparisons.* St. Louis: Facts and Comparisons, 1978.

Krause, M., & Mahan, L. *Food, nutrition and diet therapy* (6th ed.). Philadelphia: W. B. Saunders Company, 1979.

Lambert, M. Drugs and diet interactions. *American Journal of Nursing,* March 1975, *75,* 3.

Lehmann, P. Food and drug interactions. *FDA Consumer,* March 1978, 12, 2.

Leobl, S., Spratto, G., & Heckheimer, E. *The nurse's drug handbook* (2nd ed.). New York: John Wiley & Sons, 1980.

March, D. *Handbook: Interactions of selected drugs with nutritional status in man.* Chicago: American Dietetic Association, 1976.

Professional guide to drugs. Horsham, Pa.: Intermed Communications, 1981.

Robinson, C., & Lawler, M. *Normal and therapeutic nutrition* (15th ed.). New York: Macmillan Publishing Company, 1977.

Rodman, M. Drug interactions you can prevent. *RN,* February 1980, *43,* 2.

Roe, D. Drugs, diet and nutrition. *Contemporary Nutrition,* June 1978, *3,* 6.

Rosenberg, J., & Sangkachand, P. Take with meals ... or not? *RN,* May/June 1981, *44,* 5.

Index

Hospitalized patient: fluid intake, 59–62
  malnutrition, hospital, 58–59
  solid intake, special diets, 62–66
Hydergine, 339
Hydralazine hydrochloride, 343
Hydrating solutions, composition of, 308
Hydrochlorothiazide, 343–344
HydroDIURIL, 343–344
Hydroflumethiazide, 344
Hydroxyglutamic acid, 10
Hydroxyproline, 10
Hydroxyurea, 344
Hygroton, 334
Hyoscyamine sulfate, 344
Hyperalimentation, defined, 320
Hypercholesterolemias, 117–121
Hyperglycemia, stress-induced, with
  burns, 196
Hyperglyceridemias, 120–123
Hyperinsulinism, 162–163
Hyperkinesia, 222–224
Hyperlipidemia, in diabetes, 150
Hyperlipoproteinemias: atherosclerosis,
  123–126
  in diabetes, 162
  hypercholesterolemias, 117–121
  hyperchylomicronemia, 114–116
  hyperglyceridemias, 121–123
Hypertension, 133–135
  and nephrosclerosis, 182–183
Hyperthyroidism, 165–167
Hypertonic intravenous fluids, 308,
  309–310
Hypocalcemia, 247–248
Hypoglycemia, functional, 162–163
Hypoglycemic agents, 150
Hypokalemia, 246–247
Hypomagnesemia, 248–249
Hypothyroidism, 167–169
Hypotonic intravenous fluids, 308

Ibuprofen, 344
Ileostomy, 82–83, 146–147
Illness, diabetes during, 159
Ilotycin, 339
Ilozyme, 354
Immobilization, extended, 233–234
Immunotherapy, cancer, 265
Inderal, 360
Indians, American, 269–270
Indomethacin, 344–345
Infancy, see Pediatric patients
Infant formulas: in cystic fibrosis, 199
  in lactose intolerance, 83–85
Infantile eczema, 210–211
INH, 345
Insulin, 150, 345
  in burns, 196
  food allergies and, 210
  in juvenile diabetes, 153

potassium and, 161
  see also Diabetes mellitus
Insulin shock, in central vein intravenous
  nutrition, 322–323
Interviewing, in nutritional assessment,
  40–44
Intestinal bypass, 147–148
Intralipid 10%, 313
Intravenous hyperalimentation, defined,
  320
Intravenous nutrition, 59
  central vein, 320–323
  peripheral vein, 307
  alcohol, 314–315
  carbohydrates, 309–310
  electrolytes, 316–318
  fats, 312–314
  fluids, 308
  minerals, 316
  protein, 311–312
  vitamins, 315
  total parenteral, 318
Intravenous therapy: burns and, 193–194
  and hyponatremia, 245
  postoperative, 143
Iodine, 21, 28, 292
Iodine solution, administration of, 363
Iron, 21, 28–29
  administration of, 341
  breast feeding and, 284
  in pregnancy, 292
  surgery and, 140
Iron deficiency anemia, 100–106
  diet therapy, 101–104
  nursing implications, 104–106
  pathophysiology, 100–101
  treatment, 101
Irritable bowel syndrome, 88–89
Ismelin, 342
Isocal Complete Liquid Diet, 301
Isolait, 345
Isoleucine, 9
Isoniazid, 345
Isotonic intravenous fluids, 308
Isoxsuprine hydrochloride, 345
Italians, 274

Japanese, 274–275
Jejunoileostomy, 147–148
Jews, 275–276
J-Liberty, 333
Juvenile diabetes mellitus, 152–153,
  155–156

Kaybovite, 335–336
Keflex, 331–332
Kemadrin, 359
Ketoaciduria, branched-chain, 252–253
Ketones, and nervous system, 213
Kidney disorders, see Renal disorders

Proteins: burns and, 192–193, 194
  in diabetes mellitus, 160–161
  dialysis and, 189
  digestion products, 33
  in intravenous nutrition: central vein, 322
    peripheral vein, 311–312
  and kwashiorkor, 243–244
  as nutrients, 5, 8–11
  in pregnancy, 292
  in renal failure, chronic, 186, 188
  stress and, 312
  surgery and, 140
Psychiatric disorders, 224–225
Ptyalin, 32, 33
Puerto Ricans, 278–279
Purine metabolism, and gout, 171–173
Purinethol, 348
Pyelonephritis, chronic, 179
Pyrantel pamoate, 361
Pyrazinimide, 361
Pyridium, 356
Pyrimethamine, 361
Pyrodiate, 356

Quaalude, 348–349
Quadnite, 360
Qualitative diet, in diabetes, 150
Quantitative diet, in diabetes, 150–158
Quinacrine hydrochloride, 361
Quinidine sulfate, 361

Radiation therapy, 260–262
Rauwolfia and preparations, administration of, 362
Recommended daily allowances: fat soluble vitamins, 19, 20, 21
  protein, 11
  vitamin B complex, 14–17
  vitamin C, 18
Regional enteritis, 86–88
Regitine, 357
Regroton, 362
Rela, 331
Religious customs, see Cultural customs
Remsed, 360
Renal disorders: calculi, 179–182
  chronic pyelonephritis, 179
  dialysis, 189–190
  glomerulonephritis: acute, 175–176
    chronic, 176–177
  and hypertension, 133
  nephrogenic diabetes insipidus, 170–171
  nephrosclerosis, 182–183
  nephrotic syndrome, 178–179
  renal failure: acute, 183–185
    chronic, 185–189
  transplantation, 190
Renelate, 349
Replacement intravenous therapy, 307

Reserpine, 362
Respiratory disorders: cystic fibrosis, 198–200
  emphysema, 200–202
  laryngotracheobronchitis, 202–203
  tuberculosis, 203–204
Rheumatoid arthritis, 228–229
Rhodavite, 335–336
Riboflavin, 13, 14, 15
  administration of, 362
  deficiency of, 238–239
Rickets, 241–242
Rifadin, 362
Rifampin, 362
Rimactane, 362
Ringer's solution, composition of, 316
Ritalin, 350
Robamate, 347–348
Robantaline, 360
Robimycin, 339
Robinul, 342
Ro-Chlorozide, 333
Rolax, 330
Rolazine, 343
Rondomycin, 348
Ropanth, 360
Ro-Primidone, 359
Rowe diet, 206–207, 208
RP-Mycin, 339
Ru-Spas #2, 343

Salicylamide, 362
Salicylate radical, and hyperkinesia, 222, 223
Saliva, 32
Salt, 52
Saluron, 344
Salutensin, 344
Sansert, 339
S.A.S.-500, 363
School age children, nutritional considerations, 289
Scurvy, 240–241
Sed-Tens SE, 343
Seizure disorders, 215–217
Selenium, 21, 31
Septra, 335
Serine, 10
Seromycin, 336
Serpasil, 362
Seventh Day Adventists, 279–280
Shock therapy, and caloric needs, 224
Silicon, 21, 31
Sippy diet, 85
Skeletal disorders, see Musculoskeletal disorders
Skin fold measurement, 39
Slo-Phyllin, 365
Social factors, and adult diet, 297–298
Sodestrin, 340